T0271319

STEIN'S RESEARCH
in Occupational Therapy

The seventh edition of this best-selling text continues to provide occupational therapy students and researchers with expert guidance on conducting research, from the formulation of a research hypothesis to collecting, analyzing, and interpreting data.

Now updated in line with the latest ACOTE Standards, the new edition has been thoroughly revised. Of note is a new chapter on the capstone project and the integration of the hierarchical Research Pyramid to enhance the book's usability for researchers, instructors, and students. It also features a new chapter focused on using research literature to inform clinical reasoning, highlighting the benefits of scoping reviews, systemic reviews, meta analyses, and meta synthesis, as well as updated tests and evaluations which can be used as outcome instruments. There are also further contemporary examples of both quantitative and qualitative research, additions to the glossary of terms and statistics, and updated references throughout.

Offering insightful guidance on conducting research from start to finish, this invaluable resource will be essential reading for any occupational therapy student or researcher.

Martin S. Rice, PhD, OTR/L, FAOTA is Professor and Director of the School of Occupational Therapy at the Texas Woman's University. He has been in occupational therapy academia for about 30 years and has served on the editorial boards and as a reviewer for rehabilitation and occupational therapy peer-reviewed journals. He has published over 50 articles and has given over 100 presentations regionally, nationally, and internationally. Some of Dr. Rice's favorite occupations include bicycling and hiking in the great outdoors.

George Tomlin, PhD, OTR/L, FAOTA is Emeritus Professor of Occupational Therapy at the University of Puget Sound. His 38 years of teaching occupational therapy has resulted in about 40 publications and 90 presentations. He has collaborated with Prof. Dr. Bernhard Borgetto at the University of Applied Sciences in Hildesheim, Germany on advancing the Research Pyramid evidence model, and with Dr. Leona Gray at the Glasgow Caledonian University, Scotland on case study epistemology. He is a founding member of the Global Occupational Therapy Think Tank, and has volunteered for over 15 years for the National Board for Certification in Occupational Therapy.

Franklin Stein, PhD, OTR/L, FAOTA is currently Emeritus Professor from the University of South Dakota and former Founding Editor of Occupational Therapy International. He has taught courses as a tenured professor at Boston University, University of Wisconsin-Milwaukee, University of Manitoba, and University of South Dakota. Besides six previous editions of *Clinical Research in Occupational Therapy*, he is the author of six other books and over 70 scholarly articles related to rehabilitation and psychosocial research.

STEIN'S RESEARCH
in Occupational Therapy
7TH EDITION

Martin S. Rice, George Tomlin, and Franklin Stein

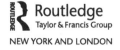
Routledge
Taylor & Francis Group

NEW YORK AND LONDON

Seventh edition published 2025
by Routledge
605 Third Avenue, New York, NY 10158

and by Routledge
4 Park Square, Milton Park, Abingdon, Oxon, OX14 4RN

Routledge is an imprint of the Taylor & Francis Group, an informa business

© 2025 Martin S. Rice, George Tomlin and Franklin Stein

The right of Martin S. Rice, George Tomlin and Franklin Stein to be identified as authors of this work has been asserted in accordance with sections 77 and 78 of the Copyright, Designs and Patents Act 1988.

All rights reserved. No part of this book may be reprinted or reproduced or utilised in any form or by any electronic, mechanical, or other means, now known or hereafter invented, including photocopying and recording, or in any information storage or retrieval system, without permission in writing from the publishers.

Trademark notice: Product or corporate names may be trademarks or registered trademarks and are used only for identification and explanation without intent to infringe.

First edition published by Cengage Learning 2000

Sixth edition published by SLACK Incorporated 2019

ISBN: 9781638221388 (hbk)
ISBN: 9781032885247 (pbk)
ISBN: 9781003523154 (ebk)

DOI: 10.4324/9781003523154

Typeset in Minion
by codeMantra

Contents

ACKNOWLEDGMENTS

I would like to thank my colleagues and students who have supported me in this endeavor. In particular, I am grateful for the help of Brianna Jones, my graduate assistant who worked many hours assisting me in organizing references. This has been an effortful journey with my good friends, colleagues, and co-authors, Franklin Stein and George Tomlin. I stand in awe of their deep knowledge of occupational therapy, research, and general wisdom. I also want to thank Judith Parker Kent for her contribution to the capstone chapter. Lastly, I am grateful for my wife, Carol Getz Rice, PhD, OTR whose insights, wisdom, and love have supported me, not only in this work, but also for the decades of sticking by my side.

Amor Semper Vincentem

—*Martin S Rice*, *PhD, OTR/L, FAOTA*

For the seventh edition, I would like to thank four colleagues who helped update the assessments in Chapter 11: Tatiana Kaminsky, PhD, OTR/L (geriatrics), Chih-Huang Yu, PhD, OTR/L (physical disabilities), Renee Watling, PhD, OTR/L, FAOTA (pediatrics), and Aimee Piller, PhD, OTR/L, FAOTA (pediatrics). I would also like to thank the many students I have learned from over the years, who have taught me that every discipline has its realm of knowledge, and then a parallel realm of knowledge about how to *teach* that original knowledge. Finally, I would like to express my thanks to my spouse Sybille, whose occupational therapy experience is a deep and steady sounding board for my own investigations.

Ethos Anthropos daimon

—*George Tomlin*, *PhD, OTR/L, FAOTA*

In 1973 I was at Boston University as an Associate Professor teaching a course in research methodology to graduate students in Physical and Occupational Therapy, Dietetics and Human Kinetics. I felt at that point that a book on research design for Allied Health students was needed. In 1974 I was granted a sabbatical by Boston University primarily as an opportunity to write a textbook for Allied Health students. For the sabbatical I was appointed as a Visiting Scholar at Cambridge University in England which gave me access and interactions with professors in the Math and Statistics Department. I also spent much time in the university library and the Wellcome Museum of Medicine in London where I referenced sources on the history of medical research. It was an inspiring experience and enabled me to complete the book entitled *Anatomy of Research in Allied Health* in 1976, published by Shenkman/Wiley. For almost 50 years the book has undergone six major revisions. In this seventh edition, Martin Rice, George Tomlin, and Judith Parker have made outstanding contributions maintaining the rigor of the book while making it student friendly. The book has been thoroughly updated applying George Tomlin's Research Pyramid.

I am also grateful for all my former colleagues and students at Boston University, University of Wisconsin-Milwaukee, University of Manitoba and the University of South Dakota for their feedback and support. Of course, Jennie and my family have been staunch supporters of my work and have endured all the moving and travels.

Nil Sine Magno Labore

—*Franklin Stein*, *PhD, OTR/L, FAOTA*

PREFACE TO THE SEVENTH EDITION

In this new edition Dr. George Tomlin and I continue to have the pleasure of working with our good friend and mentor, Dr. Franklin Stein. The idea for this text was conceived by Dr. Stein more than 50 years ago and culminated in the first edition of this book, *Anatomy of Research in Allied Health*, published by Schenkman Publishing Company in Cambridge, Massachusetts, and John Wiley and Sons in 1976. As such this text, in one form or another, has been in print for nearly 50 years. This was the first textbook authored by an occupational therapist on research methodology. Dr. Stein wanted to write a text to demonstrate how the health science professions, including occupational therapy, were part of medical progress throughout the world. Furthermore, he felt that occupational therapy was very much tied to the knowledge base of scientific medicine. In the first edition, Dr. Stein wrote, "The overall purposes of the book are two-fold. One is to assist clinicians and students in the health fields to become effective evaluators and consumers of published research and two is to facilitate research skills by communicating the process of research and the abilities needed to plan and implement a research project" (Stein, 1976, p. viii). These goals are still relevant and appropriate today.

Dr. Tomlin, Professor Emeritus in the School of Occupational Therapy at the University of Puget Sound continues to share his invaluable knowledge, his profound thinking, and his remarkable acumen for scientific method, statistical expertise, and research methodology. In writing the seventh edition of this textbook, Drs. Tomlin and Stein and myself are somewhat like the legs of a three-legged stool. We've depended on each other's support in developing this edition, which reflects the most radical change from previous editions.

While Dr. Tomlin and I met some years ago and have been good friends since we first met, Dr. Stein and I have known each other for two decades. Dr. Stein has been a good friend and mentor for all of these years and I've come to love and appreciate his love for the profession. A wise person once said, "If you want to end up like someone, become friends with that person." Not only has Dr. Stein modeled a level of professionalism that I deeply respect, his level of community involvement is remarkable. Dr. Stein is the epitome of a true gentleman and scholar.

As mentioned above, the seventh edition brings numerous changes, improvements, and enhancements. Some of the more noteworthy changes include:

1. The organizational framework provided by the Research Pyramid (Borgetto et al., 2007; Tomlin & Borgetto, 2011).

2. The addition of a totally new introductory chapter on the relevance of research to occupational therapy.

3. The addition of a chapter introducing the Research Pyramid.

4. The addition of a chapter on the scholarship of the occupational therapy doctoral capstone with the input of Dr. Judith Parker Kent as a co-author on that chapter.

5. Thoroughly updated and re-written chapters on the scientific method, research design, and statistics.

6. Revision and additions to the glossary of terms and statistics.

7. Updated example of the IRB informed consent template from Texas Woman's University.

8. Updated landmarks in the history of occupational therapy.

9. In general, the seventh edition enables the graduate student and clinical researcher to carry out a research study from the formulation of a research hypothesis to collecting data in user-friendly, step-by-step procedures.

10. Out of respect for the legacy of this textbook, which has enriched the profession of occupational therapy for 50 years, Dr. Tomlin and I insisted on re-titling the text as *Stein's Research in Occupational Therapy* in honor of Dr. Franklin Stein.

INTRODUCTION

A Manifesto for a Great Research Text for Occupational Therapy

The first edition of this text was published in 1976. At that time, it was the first textbook on clinical research in the allied health professions. Since then, numerous texts have been published about research from the perspective of clinical practice in occupational therapy, physical therapy, and speech and language pathology and audiology. The current edition, the seventh, is a collaborative effort where the three authors combine their expertise as professors, researchers, and clinicians. In preparing this edition, we raised the question: What characterizes a good textbook in occupational therapy research? In reviewing other textbooks and re-examining the strengths and weaknesses of this text, we proposed the following points:

1. The textbook should be practical, well-written, and easily understood by researchers, practitioners and students. Complex concepts should be explained carefully and presented in a logical step-by-step sequence.

2. Within the context of the text, there should be many examples from the current scientific literature, as well as hypothetical examples explaining theoretical concepts and research principles. The text should come from a pragmatic perspective that presents feasible ideas for best practice.

3. The text should be a resource for further study in related areas. References should be liberally found throughout the text so that the researcher can readily locate resources in designing and implementing a research study.

4. Statistical procedures and tests should be clearly explained in a stepwise procedure. The concept underlying the statistical technique should be emphasized. Although there are a number of available statistical software options, it is important for the student to understand how the statistical results are derived. The student should have a strong background in descriptive statistics before learning inferential statistics.

5. In the textbook, there should be an example of a research proposal that can serve as a model for the researcher. The research proposal should be clearly described and realistically implemented.

6. The textbook should be comprehensive and include a number of different research models that are appropriate for research in occupational therapy.

7. Qualitative, as well as quantitative research models should be described with examples from the literature. Both models are appropriate and relevant. The research design is judged on its own merits as far as validity and application to practice.

8. An important emphasis in research is in raising relevant, significant, and feasible research questions. The researcher should be encouraged to ask questions that generate intellectual interest and curiosity. Research should be a process of discovery and intellectual excitement.

9. The individual who is designing and carrying out a research study should see the relationship between one's research study and one's professional role, whether it be a practitioner, administrator, educator, or researcher. Basic research and applied research are equally important in leading to effective interventions. However, collecting data alone without purpose is not appropriate.

10. The research text should help the student to develop a critical view of research. The student should be able to read the literature with a critical eye and carry over this knowledge to occupational therapy practice, especially in applying clinical reasoning. The researcher should also be able to critique the research methodology and evaluate the validity and limitations of the study.

11. The researcher should have a strong appreciation of the ethical issues involved with human investigation. Researchers should be able to design an informed consent form and be able to safeguard the research participant from unnecessary psychological or physical risks.

12. There should be a historical perspective in the text that connects the reader to other researchers who laid the foundation for research-validated practice. The development of the occupational therapy profession is a continuation of the scientific and medical revolutions that created the health professions. As health care practitioners, we are dependent on the early research in anatomy and physiology, testing and measurement, medical instrumentations, medicine, and environmental health. The knowledge gained in the basic sciences strongly impacts the occupational therapy profession. As scholars, we know that current practice stands on the shoulders of the past and current researchers in basic and professional practice.

The seventh edition contains many changes and modifications from the sixth edition. While the underlying tenets remain, the inclusion of the levels of scientific evidence research pyramid (Borgetto et al., 2007; Tomlin & Borgetto, 2011) is used as an organizing thread throughout the chapters, many of which have been re-written. Another notable change is the recognition that the occupational therapy doctoral capstone is an excellent vehicle for the profession to grow. This seventh edition includes a chapter on how aspects of the scientific method and scholarly principles can be applied to the capstone project. The content of this textbook's chapters are organized comprehensively to include all the components in research from generating a significant research question, carrying out a literature review, designing a research study including the method and procedures, outlining a statistical analysis of data, and writing a scientific manuscript suitable for submission to a peer-reviewed journal. The final chapter concludes the text with a historical synopsis of scientific milestones from whence occupational therapy emerged and matured.

In writing this seventh edition, the authors developed a conceptual model that serves as a rationale for the text.

1. Although the medical model is an essential component of health care systems throughout the world, it is important to note that, in practice, other interventions exist that are effective and deserve research considerations. For example, alternative medicine has become a significant area of practice outside the traditional allopathic medical model. Historically, the medical model includes arriving at a diagnosis that serves as the basis of treatment. The consideration of educational, psychological, and sociological factors in treatment does not negate the medical model. Effective rehabilitation and habilitation depends on a holistic approach that often includes a combination of approaches and models.

2. The goal of research is to discover, through objective and systematic inquiry, the most effective interventions that can be applied to the client with a condition or disability. Research should be driven by theory and rational explanation.

3. The relationship between research and practice is based on the premise that effective occupational therapy depends on multiple factors, including the occupational therapist's skill, the efficacy of an intervention methodology, the suitability of the intervention given the situation and goals of the client, and environmental factors that affect intervention. Research should strive to understand the relationships among these factors in occupational therapy practice.

4. Doing research and critically evaluating the findings help the student to become an effective occupational therapist. Because occupational therapy practice is dependent on clinical reasoning and decision making, the effective occupational therapist applies the scientific method in practice. The research-oriented practitioner is able to evaluate the literature and incorporate current research findings into practice as appropriate.

1

Research and Occupational Therapy
A Powerful Alliance

Occupational therapy is where science, creativity and compassion collide.

Jessica Kensky (2016), survivor of the Boston Marathon Bombing

OPERATIONAL LEARNING OBJECTIVES

By the end of this chapter, the learner will be able to:

1. Define the importance of research in occupational therapy practice
2. Articulate what evidence-based practice is
3. Compare and contrast the characteristics applied to occupational therapy practitioners and researchers
4. Describe two examples of research that can guide occupational therapy practice

1.1 INTRODUCTION

In the not too distant past, the American Occupational Therapy Association's tag line was "Occupational Therapy: Skills for the Job of Living" (AOTA, 2006). This statement is based on some fundamental assumptions, not the least of which is that occupational therapy practitioners impart, teach, or otherwise equip their clients with the skills and abilities to more fully and with greater success engage in the day-to-day activities uniquely identified as important on an individual basis. A second assumption is that the occupational therapy practitioner has the resources and skills to provide this type of service. How is it that occupational therapists become competent, even excellent at what they do? Indeed, it is not a simple process, nor is it a "one-and-done" endeavor. It occurs through multiple means, including, but not limited to occupational therapy education, continuing education, witnessing other occupational therapists delivering excellent therapy, and maintaining an understanding of current professionally relevant empirical occupational therapy research. This last point speaks to the importance of occupational therapy as a discipline and distinguishes it from being a technical service. Research is defined as the systematic and unbiased investigation into a topic guided by a hypothesis or research question, and collecting data, analyzing that data to determine if the hypothesis and/or research questions are supported or answered. A discipline is a body of knowledge that grows, changes, and adapts based upon newly revealed scientific discoveries, while holding fast to the fundamental tenets of the profession; for example, that the therapeutic power of occupation can facilitate significant improvement in the quality of life for occupational therapy recipients. A discipline based upon empirical research dynamically responds as new research findings point to innovative strategies for therapy. We believe that occupational therapy reflects this dynamism as a discipline, and indeed, its body of knowledge has exponentially grown, informed by the empirical research of the last four decades. For the sake of an effective dissemination of new knowledge, there needs to be good communication between occupational therapy researchers and occupational therapy practitioners. It has been argued that evidence-based practice has three main elements including a judicious blend of published research, practitioner experience and patient preference (Sackett et al., 1996). In an ideal world, all practitioners would base their practice, in part, on what the literature supports as effective and be involved in the research process to help identify and document best practice in occupational therapy. We submit to the reader that this is a continuum and a goal of ours is to impart

knowledge and skills to help the student, practitioner, or researcher in occupational therapy to facilitate the growth of occupational therapy as a discipline and in doing so help humankind through the delivery of efficacious occupational therapy (Figure 1–1). Regardless of where one falls on the continuum, having a degree of engagement with the scholarly research-based literature is a common thread.

Whether you are embarking on your studies to become an occupational therapy practitioner, or are an experienced therapist, educator, or researcher, you need to make decisions based on knowledge and evidence. Peer-reviewed, published empirical research is essential for the healthy future of the profession.

Engagement in the research continuum likely begins during occupational therapy school, in that the Accreditation Council for Occupational Therapy Education (ACOTE) publishes various educational standards pertaining to scholarship and research within occupational therapy education. While a student in an accredited occupational therapy program, research typically takes place within the framework of a research project. Some programs require these to be single-student projects while others structure the research to occur within a multi-student experience. At the time of this writing, there are two entry points to the professional occupational therapy degree; namely the masters and the doctoral levels. At the doctoral level (i.e., the OTD), ACOTE published standards requiring a capstone experience. Many occupational therapy doctoral programs allow for several options to satisfy these ACOTE standards. Typical options include program development, advocacy, leadership, clinical practice skills, and research. The research option provides an excellent opportunity for OTD students to engage in a research project. Depending on how the curriculum is designed, the time to complete the project may be brief, and many faculty mentors have suggested that preliminary work be completed or accomplished prior to the semester when the "capstone semester" actually occurs. For example, it is helpful to have the front matter written (i.e., literature review and methods) and to have the approved institutional review board application in hand prior to the capstone semester in order for the student to have time to collect the data, analyze the data, and write the results, discussion, and conclusion. While the time is limited, there are excellent examples of these capstone research projects that have successfully finished on time and some that have even been accepted for publication in peer-reviewed journals, which in turn supports evidence-based practice.

Over the course of your career you will hear a great deal about "evidence-based practice," currently defined as follows:

> …clinical decisions must include consideration of, firstly, the patient's clinical and physical circumstances to establish what is wrong and what treatment options are available. Secondly, the latter need to be tempered by research evidence concerning the efficacy, effectiveness, and efficiency of the options.

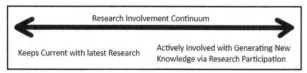

Figure 1–1 Research involvement continuum.

Thirdly, given the likely consequences associated with each option, the clinician must consider the patient's preferences and likely actions (in terms of what interventions she or he is ready and able to accept). Finally, clinical expertise is needed to bring these considerations together and recommend the treatment that the patient is agreeable to accepting.

(Haynes et al., 2002)

It is important as a health care professional to understand that there are two aspects of evidence-based practice that are crucial for the profession: (a) a body of scholarly literature, created through accepted research methods, which supports the effectiveness of what practitioners in the field are doing (evidence-supported practice—for external audiences), and (b) the skills in each practitioner for finding, reading, critiquing, interpreting, and applying the scholarly literature, in order to stay up-to-date in the profession (evidence-informed practice—or how practitioners use scientifically established knowledge). This, in particular speaks to the left end of the "research involvement continuum" seen in Figure 1–1. There will always be multiple factors influencing the decisions therapists make in practice including, but not limited to:

- an understanding of basic science and theories of occupation in humans
- the evaluation data from each client; the goals, priorities, and preferences of the client
- the expertise of colleagues and the practitioner's own experience in the field
- the practical limitations of each work setting
- and even the practitioner's own common sense (both intellectual and emotional).

Additionally, it is essential that clinical reasoning be grounded in the scientific literature.

Such is the complexity of professional reasoning in occupational therapy. As mentioned above, one substantial way of staying up-to date is by reading the discipline's scholarly literature (and that of related disciplines), and by conducting and publishing research about professional practice.

The focus of this textbook, therefore, will be on facilitating skill development for:

(a) analyzing research studies that are applicable for the occupational therapy practitioner, (b) designing and conducting empirical investigations, and (c) and the ability to apply or integrate that knowledge into practice. There is considerable overlap between the three corresponding sets of knowledge, but ultimately they are separate processes, crucial for the long-term development and growth of the profession.

Conducting research has many similarities with professional practice, and several important differences (see Table 1–1). It will be helpful to keep these in mind while working through the chapters of this book.

	RESEARCH	PRACTICE
Similarities	Role is sanctioned by universities and government laws and policies	Role is sanctioned by the National Board for Certification in Occupational Therapy (NBCOT) and state licensing boards
	Essential research design, conduct, analysis and writing skills	Essential evaluation, intervention, and client communication and collaboration skills
	Testing hypotheses	Using trial and error and other investigative techniques in the occupational therapy assessment of a client
	Precise, objective measurement of occupational performance	Precise, objective measurement of occupational performance
	Generating empirical evidence about the hypothesis to test a theory	Generating empirical evidence about client performance and response to intervention
	Critical reasoning skills for analyzing and interpreting the results of studies	Critical reasoning skills for analyzing and interpreting the results of assessments
	Remaining unbiased as an observer and interpreter of data	Remaining unbiased as an observer and interpreter of data
	Solid integrity; putting the rigor of the scientific process above personal gain	Solid integrity; putting the interests of the client above personal gain

TABLE 1–1

RESEARCH AND PRACTICE: SIMILARITIES AND DIFFERENCES

(continued)

	Table 1–1 (Continued)	
Research and Practice: Similarities and Differences		
	Motivation to stay up-to-date	Motivation to stay up-to-date
	Curiosity	Curiosity
Differences	Seeking generalizable knowledge	Seeking to optimize the benefits of intervention for each client
	Carefully planning studies in advance	Each new client may be an unpredictable challenge
	Participants are informed volunteers	Participants are referred, due to an occupational need
	Funding derived from grants or researcher's self-investment	Funding derived from insurance companies, government programs, or client self-pay
	Performing the role of science advocate for the scientific community	Performing the role of client advocate in the client's communities
	Using statistics and techniques of linguistic analysis to extract meaning from data	With one exception (see Chapter 7 on "SCED"), a therapist rarely uses inferential statistics on individual clients
	Success is measured in accepted and cited publications	Success is measured in favorable client outcomes

1.2 Comparison Between Occupational Therapy Practitioners and Occupational Therapy Researchers

In order to practice occupational therapy, occupational therapists are required to graduate from an accredited occupational therapy program, pass the NBCOT exam, and be licensed to practice in a state. Within these boundaries there is quite a lot of flexibility in how our profession is practiced. Similarly, scientific research is considered disciplined inquiry. That is, whether the research is a carefully controlled quantitative experimental study, an observational study, or a deeply involved qualitative study, the method used in the investigation must be a disciplined one, widely accepted by the scholarly community.

As noted in the bottom row of Table 1–1, a scientific study holds little value if it is never published in the scholarly literature. The publication process subjects the paper to scientific scrutiny (i.e., peer review). A refinement of the research manuscript occurs through the peer-review process, and in fact only a fraction of manuscripts submitted actually end up being published. Students, certainly, and newly graduated occupational therapists may be subjected to scrutiny by their supervisor, but an experienced

occupational therapist who has honed their skills will gain the respect and earn the discretion of being a semi-autonomous to independent practitioner. No researcher can become autonomous (free from peer review) and remain a researcher. A necessary part of the research method is placing one's results before the scholarly community for appraisal and critique. A researcher hopes that others will try to replicate these findings (with different participants or in varied contexts) and ultimately build upon them to further knowledge. This is the essence of how a discipline advances. A therapist, on the other hand, does not need to have other therapists validate their therapy by treating the same clients in order to determine that the therapy was selected and performed correctly! The therapist's successful client outcomes will to some degree speak for themselves in persuading referral sources to continue sending clients to them for therapy.

In the end there may be more similarities than differences between being an occupational therapy practitioner and being a researcher. It is the goal of the authors of this text to promote your becoming an excellent evidence-informed therapist, while providing you with the skills to become a researcher who rigorously marshals evidence to support the practices of the field, and perhaps to expand the knowledge base of the profession.

This link between research and practice is crucial for individual occupational therapists and for the profession as a whole. Consider the following examples in which research has directly supported and impacted the practice of occupational therapy. The first example is a study that used a meta-analysis design, which, as explained later in this book, is a type of research that is at the highest level of knowledge. This first example investigated the effectiveness of using functional activity and occupation-based interventions in pediatric populations. The authors concluded that using occupation-based functional activity was more effective than other interventions that did not focus on functional activity and occupation-based interventions (Laverdure & Beisbier, 2021). Specifically, the results of this study provided strong evidence showing improvement in activities of daily living and functional mobility were documented across several studies included in the meta-analysis. The results of this study substantiated the efficacy of occupational therapy's fundamental tenet of the therapeutic power of occupation. Moreover, this study documented the important outcomes seen in the lives of the children who were involved in the studies. Meta-analysis, as explored later in this text, provides the highest level of rigor when investigating a specific construct or independent variable, in this case functional activity and occupation-based interventions. The second example investigated the effectiveness of a forearm rotation orthosis while using the occupational therapy task-oriented approach in a population with hemiparesis due to stroke (Bono et al., 2022). This study measured participant performance on three separate instruments in a pre-test, post-test method including the Wolf Motor Function Test (WMFT), the Motor Activity Log (MAL) and the Canadian Occupational Performance Measure (COPM). The results of this study were that while there were no significant improvements on the WMFT and MAL, there was a significant improvement on the COPM. The authors concluded that using the occupational task-oriented approach in conjunction with a forearm rotation orthosis is effective in improving performance as reported on the COPM in persons who are post-stroke. Because this is a single study, the level of evidence is weaker than the aforementioned meta-analysis, nonetheless, it does provide evidence to help guide clinical reasoning for those occupational therapists who may be treating similar clients. These are just two examples, each providing a different level of evidence, but both are potentially very informative to the decision making of the well-informed occupational therapy practitioner.

This is an exciting time to be in occupational therapy. As the profession continues to develop its knowledge base and occupational therapy practitioners increase their reliance upon this scientific evidence to help guide their practice, the efficacy of what we do and can accomplish will rise to new heights. Most importantly, however, we should judge our efforts to continually polish and refine the efficacy of our practice within the framework of the question that is as old as the profession itself, "But what will it do for the patient?" A discipline that invests in itself to build its knowledge base in order to better serve humankind is a testimony to the noblest of intents, namely to improve humanity one client at a time. We authors are delighted that you are on this journey with us!

1.3 SUMMARY

In this chapter we've discussed the importance and impact that research has upon the discipline of occupational therapy. This chapter also emphasized the role that evidence-based practice has upon the people served by occupational therapy. The similarities and differences between occupational therapy practitioners and researchers were explored. Finally, this chapter gave two contemporary examples from the literature detailing evidence that can inform professional reasoning.

2

The Research Pyramid Model of Research Methods

The Research Pyramid of Borgetto et al. (Borgetto et al., 2007), published in the German language journal Ergoscience, *is the first attempt known to us to… provide a model that treats all evidence important for occupational therapy practice equitably.*

Tomlin and Borgetto (2011)

OPERATIONAL LEARNING OBJECTIVES

By the end of this chapter, the learner will be able to:

1. Describe a three-dimensional model of research methods, the Research Pyramid
2. Articulate the four basic types of methodology in research
3. Describe rigor and level of evidence when categorizing research methods
4. Contrast empirical and non-empirical research
5. Define the systematic review and combination of multiple studies (meta-analysis, meta-synthesis)

DOI: 10.4324/9781003523154-2

2.1 INTRODUCTION

The Research Pyramid model sets up four basic types of exploratory and intervention effectiveness research:

- Descriptive (D)
- Experimental (E)
- Outcomes of therapy/quasi-experimental (O)
- Qualitative (Q)

The base and three sides of the pyramid, respectively, are modeled in Figure 2–1. The Research Pyramid includes a platform at the top where results of multiple studies are combined (meta-analysis, meta-synthesis, mega-synthesis). How this model was derived (Borgetto et al., 2007) will be discussed below.

The Research Pyramid model has the virtue of valuing all types of research at parity, and emphasizes that each type of study has its own strengths and makes its own unique contribution to the body of professional knowledge.

2.2 DESCRIPTIVE RESEARCH

The base of the pyramid, indeed, the foundation of our professional knowledge, consists of observational/measurement studies. In the history of our professional literature, this base began with the case study (or case report, here used interchangeably).

2.2.1 Case Study [Research Pyramid D4]

An honest, comprehensive description of the occupational therapy process as applied by a therapist, and the client's corresponding response, is probably the earliest means by which knowledge in the profession was transmitted. This methodology, still valuable today, has the unique strength of portraying the complexities of the therapeutic interaction, usually over a period of time. It typically conveys extensive quantitative data (from interviews, observations, and measurements by the therapist), as well as the course of reasoning by the therapist. It often contains descriptions of false starts and dead ends made and encountered by the therapist and client in therapy, and how these obstacles were overcome or a successful adaptation was found.

The unique contribution of this methodology is not only that it can provide insights into what is possible in therapy (particularly in new or unusual cases), but also that it is a type of disciplined inquiry (research) that every practitioner can participate in creating. Numerous examples exist in the occupational therapy literature (Peters et al., 2017) on the effects of transcranial direct current stimulation combined with repetitive, task-specific training on an individual who had experienced a stroke ten years prior (Preissner, 2010), on the effects of the Occupational Therapy Task-Oriented Approach on an individual who had had a stroke, even when cognitive limitations were present). In the situation of a newly arising disease or condition (for example, COVID), case studies can be composed and published the fastest, providing guidance for other therapists grappling with similar cases (Mannion & Sullivan, 2021).

2.2.2 Case Series [Research Pyramid D3]

Above the individual case study on the floor of the pyramid is the description of a series of clients with similar diagnoses, challenges, or goals—the case series. The advantage of a case series, compared to a case study, is that it portrays the variety of processes and outcomes that may appear among clients with these challenges. How individual differences called for individualized therapy and resulted in individualized outcomes can be conveyed in a case series study (Rich et al., 2022, on the differing effects of assistive technology on three veterans with COVID-19). General findings across all or most cases in the series strengthen the persuasiveness of the study's conclusions.

2.2.3 Normative Study [also D3]

A normative study is an attempt to capture the typical performance ("central tendency") and range of differences ("variability") in an important skill pertinent to occupational therapy concerns. Usually a single skill, or construct, is carefully (reliably and validly) measured in each person in a sample from a defined population of people. An example skill is finger dexterity in adults (Oxford Grice et al., 2003), or handwriting in children (Fogel et al., 2022). The findings of a normative study can be used by practitioners as a baseline, against which to place the performance of a client and assist in the interpretation of evaluation results.

Specific concerns for this type of research methodology are the careful definition of the population of interest, how the sample was acquired, and the consistency achieved in measuring a trait in many people. Since normative samples often seek to cover a range of ages or other demographic variables, there will be concerns about interpolation (filling in gaps in the data by inference) and extrapolation (projecting patterns outside the range of collected data). Both, when necessary, must be done with care and conclusions kept tentative.

2.2.4 Historical Study [also D3]

A historical research study is conducted with primary records and documents, newspapers, meeting notes,

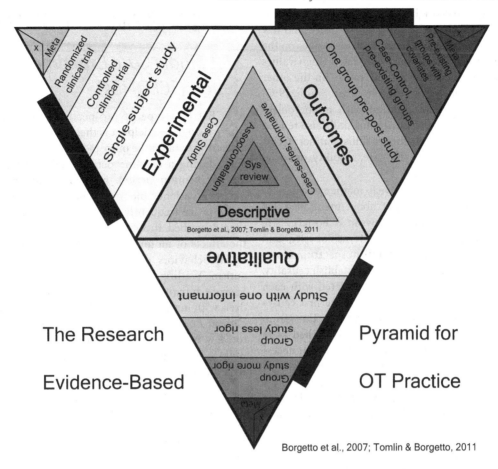

Instructions for the paper pyramid.

For the Research Pyramid paper model: cut out the triangle, keeping the dark edge tabs connected. Cut away the three small triangles marked with "x" at the tips of the outer triangles. Putting the pink "Descriptive" research face at the bottom, fold the yellow "Experimental," blue "Outcomes" and green "Qualitative" triangles upward so that their tips approximate. Fold the three black tabs so as to be at a 90 degree angle inward to their respective faces. Fold the colored tip of each face inward at the small triangle base line. Glue the tabs to each adjacent pyramid face. You may need to use a pencil or chopstick poking inside the pyramid to brace the tab when you apply pressure, in order to get a good bond. Finally fold the three tip triangles together at the top so as to interlock to form a small platform of three colors. Voila! That's the evidence base on which our profession of occupational therapy can most solidly stand.

Figure 2–1 The Research Pyramid for evidence-based OT practice.

emails, and social media artifacts, or through interviews with eyewitnesses or participants, in order to document the details of what has happened and to uncover relationships, influences, and possible causes over time (Pettigrew et al., 2017, on the experience of early occupational therapy by injured soldiers in World War I).

2.2.5 Correlational Study [D2]

In this type of study, more than one variable is collected from each individual in a group. Then these variable data points are analyzed for the extent to which they covary. Another way of putting this is that it is an investigation of whether the values of the variables are **directly** (positively) associated (high values on one variable tend to be accompanied by high values on the other, and low values on one tend to be associated with low values on the other), or **indirectly** (negatively) correlated (high values on one variable associated with low values on the other variable, and vice versa). For example, (Case-Smith, 1995) discovered that preschool children with motor delays who had more developed sensorimotor skills also tended to have more developed fine motor skills, but not necessarily better performance in self-care, mobility, or social engagement.

Correlational studies can reveal mathematical relationships between variables that above-mentioned D4 and D3 methodologies cannot (Lawson & Foster, 2016, on associations among sensory patterns, obesity, and physical activity in children with autism spectrum disorder). Note that they **cannot** be used to establish causality. That is, if two variables are highly correlated with each other, it does not necessarily mean that the first causes the second or that the second causes the first. Thus, from (Case-Smith, 1995), even if fine motor skills had been highly correlated with self-care skills, it would not necessarily follow that therapists could work to enhance fine motor skills and automatically expect to see an improvement in self-care skills. This common pitfall in thinking about correlation studies will be addressed in greater detail in Chapter 5.

2.2.6 Regression Study [D2]

Mathematically, regression is a close relative of correlation. Both attempt to quantify how much the variance in one (or more) variable(s) aligns with, "explains," or predicts the variance in another variable. The most common application of regression is in a study that uses the values of several variables (the independent variables) to predict the values in another variable (the dependent variable). This particular type is thus called multiple regression. It is useful because often in therapy we have obtained measures on some important variables from a client early in the occupational therapy process (typically at the time of the initial evaluation). If we could predict the likely value of a later variable (performance after discharge), that would be useful in formulating an effective intervention and discharge plan (Espín-Tello et al., 2018, on how various aspects of self-esteem in persons with cerebral palsy predict functional capacity).

2.2.7 Systematic Review of Descriptive Studies [D1]

In reality rare, but theoretically possible, is a systematic review of descriptive studies on a given topic. Such a study of studies in the pyramid model would be labeled D1.

2.3 EXPERIMENTAL RESEARCH

2.3.1 Single Case Experimental Design (SCED) [E4]

A SCED is a type of prospective experimental study where a single participant is their own control. It involves collecting data on the outcome measure (dependent variable) during a baseline period, and then again during an intervention period, after manipulating the independent variable (no intervention, then intervention). Designs are frequently more complex than this, as further described in Chapter 7 (Gutman et al., 2012, on the effects of motor-based role-play intervention on the social behaviors of adolescents with high-functioning autism; Watling & Dietz, 2007, on the effects of Ayres' Sensory Integration on undesired behavior in four children with autism spectrum disorder). SCED are used in clinical or community settings where similar cases are too few for group experimental research. Implemented well, SCED may suggest cause-and-effect relationships. An older term for SCED is "single subject design."

2.3.2 Controlled Clinical Trial [E3]

In a controlled clinical trial, two or more pre-existing groups with a similar diagnosis or injury are identified before the data are collected. Each group receives a different intervention. As much as possible, everything else about their care is controlled so as to be the same. Participant outcome performances are measured. Their respective group outcomes are then statistically compared, to determine whether the intervention given to one group was reliably accompanied by a superior outcome.

2.3.3 Randomized Controlled Trial (RCT) [E2]

RCT is the classical prospective, scientific research method. It includes the following characteristics: **random selection** of a sample of participants from a pre-defined population, **random assignment** of participants to at least two different **groups**, **manipulation** of the **independent variable** (intervention versus no intervention or a placebo or "sham" intervention; or one intervention versus a second intervention), **blinding** participants and data gatherers as to the purpose of the study and the membership of participants in which group, and measuring the outcome on one or more **dependent variables**. An RCT attempts to **control** for all extraneous influences on the outcome variables, including researcher and participant biases, and environmental (temperature, stimuli) and chronological (time of day, day of week) artifacts. When control is implemented effectively, claims can be made about a cause-and-effect **relationships** between the independent and dependent variables. In other words, a claim could be made that a certain intervention caused a better outcome in the group of people receiving that intervention, thus that this is a superior intervention to use with clients similar to the group studied (Jackson et al., 1998, where *Lifestyle Redesign* improved social participation in community-dwelling elderly; Madhoun et al., 2020, where mirror therapy improved upper limb motor function in people with subacute cerebrovascular accident; Yu et al. 2021, where an occupational therapy task-oriented approach improved performance and satisfaction with movement in people post-stroke).

A variant of an RCT is the sequential clinical trial. In this study the random assignment to intervention type is made as participants enter the study at different times. It allows for the collection of a greater sample than would be available to the researcher at any one given point in time. The study continues only up to the moment when it is statistically established that one intervention type is superior to the other.

2.3.4 Meta-Analysis of Experimental Studies [E1]

When a sufficient number of experimental studies can be identified, where the studies used similar interventions and similar outcome measures, and when each study has provided adequate information about their outcomes (typically, effect sizes), then a mathematical combination of these studies can be performed (Brown et al., 2018, on the effects of weight loss intervention on people with mental illness). The result is a generalized or average effect size, considering all the studies, including all the respective participants, as a totality. If this average effect size is statistically established as large enough, then one intervention can be claimed to be superior to another, or to be better than doing nothing. See Chapter 10 for more detail.

2.4 OUTCOME (QUASI-EXPERIMENTAL) RESEARCH

2.4.1 Single Group Pre-Post [O4]

In this retrospective or prospective study, one group of participants is studied before and after an intervention is applied (Mathiowetz, 2019, on the effects of meditative movements on people with chronic health conditions). Measurements (pre/post intervention) are made and statistically compared to indicate change over time. The absence of a control group weakens any possible inference as to cause and effect.

2.4.2 Comparison of Two (or More) Pre-Existing Groups (Retrospective or Prospective) [O3]

In this study type, two or more pre-existing groups are compared as to their therapy outcomes, for example Hersch et al. (2012), who found that participation in a cultural heritage group was accompanied by improved quality of life, but no better than in individuals in a typical activity group. Groups in an O3 study may have been pre-defined by a demographic feature (males versus females, younger versus older children) or by a diagnostic feature (medical diagnosis, severity of injury, location of condition or injury). When conducted retrospectively, the study consists of accessing records that were created prior to the planning of the study. When prospective, the study design is planned and then the data are collected. The study may include a control group (the "case-controls"). A difference in outcome performance is then analyzed statistically. If the group difference is found to be statistically significant, then an inference can be made about the pre-existing difference causing the difference in outcome. Alternatively, the difference between the two groups could be which intervention the groups were provided. If a significant difference in outcome is statistically demonstrated, one could claim that the different interventions would reliably cause the different outcomes in the populations from which the samples were drawn. The strength of this claim, however, is weaker than that from an RCT, due to the non-random assignment of people to groups. With the use of non-randomly-assigned groups, it is possible that the groups differed on some important aspect that affected the outcome, and not that the intervention difference itself caused the difference in outcome.

2.4.3 Comparison of Two or More Groups with Statistical Adjustment of Covariates [O2]

A study type that can make a stronger cause-and-effect claim than the O3 studies described above is the two-or-more group comparison, where groups are first balanced or equalized using other information collected besides the independent and dependent variables (called the covariates). For example, Chang et al. (2021), compared two self-selected groups on improvements to cognition, after equating the groups on their pre-existing strength of memory (reciting digits from memory). After this equalization, they found that the group receiving occupational therapy-selected cognitive tasks showed a better immediate recall of information, compared to the group that received nutritional education. Using this approach (often with the statistic analysis of covariance, or ANCOVA) potentially makes for a fairer comparison of the two pre-existing groups. This approach may be implemented prospectively (Chang et al., 2021) or retrospectively.

2.4.4 Meta-Analysis of Outcome Studies [O1]

As with the meta-analysis of experimental studies (see E1, above), a meta-analysis of similar outcome studies may be performed. With sufficient information about effect sizes reported, a similar statistical combination of those effect sizes can be calculated. As with E1 studies, albeit weaker due to the lack of random assignment, a combined claim may be made as to the superiority of one intervention over another. Often, meta-analyses are conducted on a combination of experimental and quasi-experimental studies, in which case they would be labeled E1/O1.

2.5 QUALITATIVE RESEARCH

The types of qualitative research common in therapy studies include the following:

Phenomenology—a study that attempts to describe the *lived experience* of its participants (sometimes called informants) in their own terms, to gain access to the meaning participants ascribe to their experiences.

Ethnography—originally, a study of the behavior, values, and worldview of people of a unique culture. More recently, ethnographic techniques have been applied to a variety of small groups of people, for example: a group with a common diagnosis (spinal cord injury), a group that underwent a certain intervention (e.g., mirror therapy), or a group with a similar institutional experience (residents of an assisted living center). It is, at its core, an **interpretation of the meaning** of the people's behavior, motivation, and beliefs.

Critical theory—a type of qualitative research that seeks to "deconstruct" a social construct (e.g., "disability") and reveal hidden social relations, including power relationships, especially for underrepresented members of society.

The Research Pyramid model puts different qualitative research studies into a rigor hierarchy that cuts across the above-named types of qualitative research. That is, none of the above-named types is held to be better, more rigorous, or more reliable than the others simply based on the type. Instead, the scope of the study (in number of informants or in number of techniques of qualitative rigor applied) is used, as noted below.

2.5.1 Investigation of One Participant [Q4]

A qualitative study of whichever type is conducted, based on the testimony and behavior of one participant. Such a study may nonetheless provide extraordinarily valuable insights for therapists (McCuaig & Frank, 1991, on perceptions of ability and the self in an individual with cerebral palsy).

2.5.2 Investigation of Multiple Participants with Fewer Elements of Rigor [Q3]

When a qualitative study is conducted with multiple informants, but fewer elements of rigor were applied (such as peer checking, triangulation, member checking; see Chapter 9 for more detail) then it is labeled Q3 (Bailliard, 2015, on sensory experiences and mental health among immigrants in the US from Latin America).

2.5.3 Investigation of Multiple Participants with More Elements of Rigor [Q2]

A qualitative study with more informants and elements of rigor is designated Q2 (Leibold et al., 2014, on activities and adaptation in late life depression). The findings of such a study are held to be more dependable.

2.5.4 Meta-Synthesis of Qualitative Studies [Q1]

Over the past 30 years, new techniques have been developed to combine the findings from multiple qualitative studies (Finlayson & Dixon, 2008; Sandelowski & Barroso, 2006). This type of study is called a meta-synthesis (Kokorelias et al., 2020), and is covered in more detail in Chapter 10.

2.6 MIXED METHOD STUDY

When a study uses more than one methodology, usually called a mixed methods design because it combines a quantitative with a qualitative approach, that study is given a combination label, such as "Q3/O2." For example Waldman-Levi et al. (2022) used questionnaire instruments, interviews, and assessments standardized to use video footage to study the playfulness of fathers and their children, and the fathers' perceptions of playfulness.

If a review study combines meta-analysis and meta-synthesis, the Research Pyramid model calls that a "mega-synthesis," and would label it "E1/Q1" or "E1/O1/Q1." To date, no known example of a mega-synthesis has been published in the occupational therapy literature, to the authors' knowledge.

2.7 ORIGIN AND STRUCTURE OF THE RESEARCH PYRAMID

Borgetto and his students, the originators of the Research Pyramid model, deconstructed the traditional single hierarchy evidence model (e.g., AOTA, www.aota.org/career/continuing-education/approved-providers/levels-and-strength-of-evidence). They identified two axes of variation among methodologies: quantitative/qualitative and internal validity/external validity, together forming four quadrants of space. Because rigorous qualitative studies tend to strengthen both internal and external validity, those two qualitative quadrants were collapsed into one. They retained the notion of a hierarchy of rigor **within** each quadrant, that is, stronger methods should be placed at a higher level, creating a meaningful third dimension. The implications were that this more accurate model of evidence in practice forms a three-dimensional object: a base with three sides forming a pyramid shape (see Figure 2–1).

The Research Pyramid model has in common with the single hierarchy model used by AOTA and many other professional health organizations the retention of the vertical dimension as reflecting greater rigor in studies. It differs from the traditional evidence hierarchy in that it places at parity all types of research methodologies. From its structure as a pyramid, it can be inferred that without any one of the main categories of research, the structural integrity of the construction (i.e., the evidence for the profession) is undermined.

The Research Pyramid model represents the history of research method evolution across many disciplines. The formation and communication of knowledge begins (at the base) with descriptive studies ("D"). Over time, as potential weaknesses were observed in descriptive studies (e.g., unknown representativeness of a sample of one), new methodological techniques were developed to mitigate these weaknesses. For example, researchers conducting outcome (quasi-experimental) studies would carefully define how membership was established in one group, or in the two groups to be compared. Great care is taken to perform systematic measurements in a reliable and valid way. Since pre-existing differences may still exist between the two comparison groups, the techniques of randomization were created, or in other words the experimental side of the pyramid was formulated. Finally, due to the limitations of quantitative research as a whole, qualitative research was developed. Here, for example, great effort is made not to presume what the ideas or constructs of importance will be. Rather they are gleaned from study participants as the study progresses. Overall, the E, O, and Q methodologies evolved from descriptive research to create greater rigor, thus greater reliability of findings.

Each new technique of research that strengthens the **internal validity** of the study (accuracy of findings irrespective of how commonplace or applicable the conditions of the study were), however, such as excluding individuals not fitting a homogeneous sample, tends to weaken the study's **external validity** (applicability to a typical professional setting or diagnostic population). Unfortunately, many efforts to strengthen the internal validity of an experimental study render its external validity (generalizability) more problematic. Rigorous therapy schedules, no secondary diagnoses in participants, expensive equipment, highly trained and calibrated therapists providing the intervention in exactly the same way, are all features rarely found in a typical practice setting. In addition, individual variations in people's occupational trajectories, goals, and priorities are powerful influencers of outcomes in therapy. Thus, the expectation that the average therapist will achieve the same intervention effects as in the study (the "effect size"), is not fully justified.

On the other hand, outcome studies conducted in typical, realistic professional settings tend to have greater external validity (their conditions of study are more representative of those in an average practice setting). Lacking certain elements of methodological rigor (such as random assignment to an intervention group, or blinding of participants and outcome measurers), however, means that the internal validity of non-experimental or quasi-experimental studies is thereby weaker. A pre-existing difference between groups or an unknown factor could have been responsible for the observed outcomes, not the difference in intervention itself.

Therefore, the Research Pyramid model holds that all research methodologies are important for considering evidence in practice. Each face (side or floor) of the pyramid contributes unique strengths to the knowledge base of the profession (experimental, outcome, qualitative, descriptive), as noted below:

1   Without experimental studies on an intervention, there is a lack of persuasive evidence that the intervention itself caused the better therapy outcomes (the cause-and-effect claim is weakened).

2   Without outcome studies, there may be no trustworthy applicability of study findings to real life practice, and therapists may find experimental research findings unhelpful.

3   Without qualitative studies therapists and researchers may lack insights into the lived experience of the therapy client; in fact, they may be paying attention to issues that are not as important to clients undergoing therapy.

4   Without descriptive studies, which could be more readily conducted by many therapists, the profession loses the opportunity to enlist large numbers of therapists to lead studies getting findings into the professional knowledge base; there may also be a loss of quick turnaround between the appearance of a new disease or conditions of health and publication of early knowledge, and the inhibition of sharing

new, creative approaches to therapy. There may also be a loss of insights into the complexity of human occupation and professional practice decisions about interventions, such as can be portrayed in comprehensive case studies.

A profession dealing with the complex nature of human occupation can ill afford to neglect any source of knowledge or insight.

The Research Pyramid is particularly well-suited to organizing published evidence for the purpose of *evidence-informed practice*, that is, practicing therapists improving their practice with published findings. It aligns research evidence types to the types of professional reasoning important for therapists in making practice decisions (Tomlin & Borgetto, 2011; described by Fleming, 1991). Procedural reasoning—the selection of appropriate evaluation instruments and intervention approaches—can be well supported by experimental research findings. Conditional reasoning, or deciding about feasible outcomes for a particular client, is well-informed by outcome/quasi-experimental research that is more likely to have been conducted in realistic settings under typical conditions. Interactive reasoning, or making decisions about how best to interact therapeutically with the client, is well-informed by qualitative research, which illuminates the lived experience of clients (in daily life or in therapy settings). Finally, insights from descriptive research can support all three types of decision making.

It should be noted that the Research Pyramid was designed to sort out research methodologies for **empirical** studies (generating new data) about therapy **interventions**, or the content and process of therapeutic interventions. Other types of studies that are not covered in the Research Pyramid model but that are valuable for the profession include (a) studies of tests and measurement instruments ("methodological" studies), (b) literature/scoping reviews, portraying the "state of the literature" on a given subject, (c) effectiveness studies of an entire program, department, agency, or organization ("evaluation" studies), and (d) economic, management, or policy studies. These studies are not categorized by the Research Pyramid model, nor are published "expert opinions" or "practice guidelines," because these are not empirical studies.

Some types of research, furthermore, such as survey research, participatory action research (PAR), heuristic research, or operations research, are not named for the methodology type they use. Thus, they are also not separately categorized in the Research Pyramid model. A PAR study may be implemented using any or all of the methodological types of research noted above. Likewise, most types of methodology can be implemented in a **prospective** way (study planned before data are collected) or in a **retrospective** way (data were already documented; they are "mined" for the purpose of the study). Thus, there is no distinct Research Pyramid label for these approaches to research studies. Instead, they would be labeled with

the appropriate label for the main methodology they used (correlational, D2; ethnographic, Q2).

The Research Pyramid can be applied in any profession where the human element is paramount, among them education, psychology, social work, nursing, speech pathology, physical therapy, and the practice of medicine, in addition to its application in occupational therapy. Indeed, it has begun to be used in many of these disciplines (Coburn et al., 2022—behavioral neuroscience; Lindström, 2023—medicine; Österholm et al., 2022—health services; Warner et al., 2021—palliative care).

Due to its developmental structure, we have chosen to use the Research Pyramid to organize the subsequent chapters of this textbook on research methodologies. In each of the following chapters on methodologies, we will present (a) the strengths and weaknesses of each method type in the following order: descriptive, experimental, outcome, qualitative; (b) the corresponding statistical or qualitative analytic procedures that are appropriately used with that methodology; and (c) conclude with a chapter on "studies of studies," or meta-analysis and meta-synthesis, and systematic evidence reviews.

A comparison and translation table between AOTA's level of evidence hierarchy and that of the Research Pyramid can be found in Figure 2–2.

Translation Table for Evidence Levels of AOTA, Research Pyramid

Pyramid Level	AOTA Level
Q4	no equivalent
Q3	no equivalent
Q2	no equivalent
Q1	no equivalent
E4	4
E3	2B
E2	1B
E1	1A
O4	3B
O3	2B
O2	2B
O1	2A
D4	5
D3	4
D2	no equivalent
D1	no equivalent
no equivalent	5- expert opinion, narrative reviews, consensus statements

AOTA Level	Pyramid Level
IA	E1
1B	E2
2A	O1
2B	O2, O3
3A	O1
3B	O4
4	E4, D3, D2
5	D4; no equivalent for expert opinion

Figure 2–2 Translation Table for Evidence Levels of AOTA, Research Pyramid

3

Descriptive Research

Statistical interpretation depends not only on statistical ideas, but also on "ordinary" thinking. Clear thinking is not only indispensable in interpreting statistics, but is often sufficient even in the absence of specific statistical knowledge.

Wallis et al. (2014)

OPERATIONAL LEARNING OBJECTIVES

By the end of this chapter, the learner will be able to:
1. Describe the basic types of descriptive research
2. Describe the place of descriptive research in the Research Pyramid model
3. List the strengths and limitations of descriptive research methodologies
4. Define key terms associated with descriptive statistics
5. Understand concepts of measurement and of data
6. Understand the difference between discrete and continuous data
7. Describe the relationship between sampling and the Central Limit Theorem
8. Differentiate common assumptions for parametric inferential statistics
9. Differentiate between parametric and non-parametric statistical tests

In this chapter and in following Chapters 5 through 10, the same sequence of content will be used. First, material on that chapter's research method will be presented, then the statistical or other analytic tools commonly used with that method, and finally one or more examples of published articles that used this method will be offered.

3.1 Descriptive Research Methodologies and the Research Pyramid

This chapter focuses on descriptive studies (the floor of the Research Pyramid) and the descriptive statistics that are used in these studies. The sequence used will be case study (pyramid level D4), then case series/developmental study/normative study/longitudinal study (level D3). Correlational/regression studies (level D2) are placed in their own chapter (Chapter 5), as they are a transitional type of study between descriptive and quasi-experimental (outcome) studies. Note that when longitudinal studies contain statistical group comparisons over time, they should be categorized as an outcome study (one group, pre-post: O4), which is covered in Chapter 8.

3.2 Case Study (Pyramid Level D4)

A case study is a concentrated inquiry about one person, case, event, institution, or team. It is fundamentally descriptive, in that there is no manipulation of the environment of the case or control exerted over the conditions in the case. It is an attempt to comprehensively detect and then describe the important features of the case. In this chapter case study and the more medically focused name case report will be taken as synonyms.

For the sake of evidence-based practice in occupational therapy, a case study would be the accurate and comprehensive description of the occupational therapy process between one client and one practitioner. Ideally the description would include material conveying the professional reasoning of the therapist as well as the therapeutic use of self. This descriptive approach represents the earliest and most direct means of conveying empirical data (and thus professional knowledge) from one therapist to another. In this type of study researchers (often the therapists themselves) can examine the role of factors and the interactions among factors in the response of the client to the provided intervention. Such a detailed examination of the complexity of factors affecting an actual human being is difficult to investigate in a group experimental study. This strength of a case study represents the unique contribution of case studies to

the professional knowledge base. Case studies have another advantage for conveying information about new diseases such as COVID-19 (Wilcox et al., 2021), or about new intervention approaches using occupational therapy in drug addiction (Ribeiro et al., 2019), or even about new inventions for therapy such as the telescopic robotic arm for use with an individual with a spinal cord injury (Sledziewski et al., 2012). A case study may even illustrate the application of a specific theory in therapy (Bouteloup & Beltran, 2007).

Case studies display certain disadvantages as a research methodology. There is an unknown amount of bias in the practitioner delivering the intervention, particularly when the therapist is also the author of the case study. As the therapist, the person may be predisposed to seeing a favorable outcome in the client. Apart from the intrinsic authenticity in the description of the occupational therapy process, there are usually no means of ascertaining how biased the therapist may have been. Careful reporting of pre- and post-standardized, quantitative measurements, for example with joint range of motion measurements, may be the best way to mitigate bias. In the matter of external validity, or how generalizable the findings of the case study are to other similar clients, there can be no statistical inference made. It is rare that the client in a case study is randomly selected from a pool of equally suitable clients. Even if the client had been selected in this way, there can be little mathematical confidence of representativeness with a sample of one. Nonetheless, readers can make their own appraisals of the value the insights of a case study may hold for the professional practice of other therapists. Especially in cases of difficult diseases, intractable conditions, or severe injuries, the mere demonstration that positive outcomes from therapy were achieved **once** indicates that it is **possible**.

As the interest in case studies increases across many disciplines (education, psychology, nursing), criteria of rigor in the composition of a case study have become more important. Well-recognized are the CARE guidelines (Gagnier et al., 2013). These guidelines were designed with a medical intervention in mind, but they fit very well to the occupational therapy process (www.care-statement.org/checklist).

The purposes served by a published case study may be (a) to describe success in the intervention for a client in a rare or challenging case, (b) to illustrate how empirical evidence from other studies can be applied to a new case, (c) to describe the application of a new theory to the occupational therapy process decisions for a client, (d) to introduce a new invention or intervention approach and how a client responded to it, (e) how occupational therapy can be combined with interventions from another discipline to good effect, and (f) to explore relationships that can generate further correlational, experimental, or qualitative research.

Most investigators, in reporting a case study, use a chronological outline starting from the client's first interaction with a therapist and continuing through discharge from services. A topical approach is another way to organize data. For example, in a case study of a client with osteoarthritis, the investigator may want to report data under subject headings, such as possible etiological factors (genetic vulnerabilities, joint injuries, allergies, emotional stresses, endocrine disorders) or interventions (occupational therapy, physical therapy, pharmacological, and psychological). An interpretive discussion including implications for wider professional practice follows the reporting of results. Box 3–1 gives an example of a case study and how to extract its contents and place them in an evidence table.

BOX 3-1. EXAMPLE OF QUALITATIVE CASE STUDY

1. Bibliographical Notation

Chan, A. S., Tsang, H. W., & Li, S. M. (2009). Case report of integrated supported employment for a person with severe mental illness. *American Journal of Occupational Therapy, 63*, 238–244.

2. Abstract

OBJECTIVE: We illustrate the implementation of an integrated supported employment (ISE) program that augments the individual placement and support model with social skills training in helping people with severe mental illness (SMI) achieve and maintain employment.

METHOD: A case illustration demonstrates how ISE helped a 41-year-old woman with SMI to get and keep a job with support from an employment specialist. An independent, blinded assessor conducted data collection of employment information, including self-efficacy and quality of life, at pretreatment and at 3-month, 7-month, 11-month, and 15-month follow-up assessments.

RESULTS: The participant eventually stayed in a job for 8 months and reported improved self-efficacy and quality of life.

CONCLUSION: The case report suggests that ISE could improve the employment outcomes of people with SMI. Moreover, changes in the participant's self-efficacy and quality of life were shown to be driven by the successful employment experience.

3. Justification and Need for Study

The author documents the need for individuals with severe mental illness to obtain and maintain competitive employment since only 15% to 30 % are employed. A protocol for the integrated supported employment program was tested and evaluated with one individual diagnosed with depression.

4. Literature Review

Twenty-nine references were cited in the study. Primary sources came from *Community Mental Health Journal, American Journal of Occupational Therapy, Psychiatric Rehabilitation Journal, American Journal of Psychiatry, Schizophrenia Bulletin, British Journal of Medical Psychology, Psychiatric Services, Psychiatric Quarterly, Archives of General Psychiatry, Social Indicators Research, Psychiatry: Interpersonal and Biological Processes, Social Psychiatry and Psychiatric Epidemiology, Journal of Nervous and Mental Disease, Journal of Behavior Therapy and Experimental Psychiatry, International Journal of Psychosocial Rehabilitation, Psychologia,* and the *American Journal of Rehabilitation.*

5. Research Hypothesis or Guiding Questions

The authors assessed how integrated supported employment can improve the employment outcome of an adult individual with chronic depression.

6. Methods

The integrated supported employment program was operationally defined applying vocational assessment, individual employment plan, social skills training, vocational placement and follow-along support. The program was in place for 7 months.

7. Results

The individual stayed in her job for 8 months. She expressed that she was satisfied in her job and was able to maintain a good relationship with her supervisor and co-workers.

(continued)

BOX 3-1. EXAMPLE OF QUALITATIVE CASE STUDY (CONTINUED)

8. Conclusions

The authors felt that the program supported the application of integrated supported employment program and was developing an e-learning package for clinicians.

9. Limitations of the Study

Since this was a qualitative study without a control group more research is needed to validate the conclusions. The protocol developed in the study needs to be replicated to assess its applicability in a wide range of vocational rehabilitation programs.

10. Major References Cited in the Study

Bond, G. R. (2004). Supported employment: Evidence for an evidence-based practice. *Psychiatric Rehabilitation Journal, 27*, 345–359.

Drake, R. E., McHugo, G. J., Bebout, R. R., Becker, D. R., Becker, D. R. et al. (1999). A randomized clinical trial of supported employment for inner-city patients with severe mental illness. *Archives of General Psychiatry, 56*, 627–633.

McGurk, S. R, Mueser, K. T., & Pascaris, A. (2005). Cognitive training and supported employment of persons with severe mental illness: One year results from a randomized controlled trial. *Schizophrenia Bulletin, 31*, 898–909.

3.3 CASE SERIES (PYRAMID LEVEL D3)

If multiple clients are available to the researcher and they are similar to each other, a case series study should be possible. In purpose and contribution to occupational therapy, they are similar to a case study, with one important addition. As soon as a second similar case is available, then the researcher may seek insights by examining similarities and differences between the two (or more) cases. Why did the intervention work well for some people but not as well for others? CARE Guidelines can be employed with each person in a case series, in order to similarly strengthen the rigor of the study. In this kind of study it is important to report if any possible participants were excluded from the series, and why. Without transparency in this step it would be difficult for the reader to make an accurate appraisal of the study's generalizability.

3.4 DEVELOPMENTAL RESEARCH (PYRAMID LEVEL D3)

Nearly 100 years have passed since Gesell asserted that "observation, with conditions so clearly defined that they can be duplicated and so delimited that only a single variable remains for study is scientifically a goal to work toward" (Gesell, 1928). This description remains the benchmark for research on child development. Developmental observation research is concerned with the rigorous investigations into the process, stages, and hierarchical steps in human development. How does speech develop? What are the sequential stages in the areas of language, ambulation, psychosocial development, cognition? These and other questions are examples of research problems that lend themselves to developmental observation methods. The investigator seeks to identify the processes involved in development, the approximate ages when landmarks are reached, and the biopsychosocial factors that shape development.

A key assumption in developmental research is that human behavior unfolds at critical stages. In Table 3–1, some examples of approximate ages are given for achieving a developmental landmark. The typical child is expected to pass a test item related to chronological age. The child's rate of development is relative to the norm response for specific chronological age groups. For example the Denver Developmental Screening Test (Frankenburg et al., 1992) makes the assumption that human development progresses in a linear direction influenced by genetically based parameters. In this model, the child is ready at specific ages to learn to walk, play games cooperatively with other children, speak, write, and perform many other developmental tasks. Environmental experiences provide the opportunities for development to occur. Muluk et al. (2016) studied the language development of children aged 5 to 27 months using the DDST-II.

3.4.1 Stating the Guiding Question

The first task of the researcher is to state a research question that focuses and guides the generation of data. Piaget

TABLE 3–1

DENVER DEVELOPMENTAL SCREENING TEST—II

DEVELOPMENTAL SKILLS	HIERARCHICAL SEQUENTIAL ACTIVITIES FROM BIRTH TO 6 YEARS
Gross motor:	Lifts head at 2 months to walks backward (heel to toe) at 6 years
Fine motor:	Visually tracks objects to midline at 2 months to draws a man with six distinct parts at 6 years
Language:	Responds to bell at 2 months to defines six words at 6 years
Personal-social:	Regards face at 2 months to dresses without supervision at 5 years

Note: From normative data, age levels were established as to when children develop individual skills. Normal limits (upper and lower) were validated for each hierarchical activity.
Source: Adapted from The Denver Developmental Screening Test–II (DDST–II) by Frankenburg et al. (1990). © 1990 Denver Developmental Materials. The DDST is also available as an online tool at www.denverii.com/

TABLE 3–2

SUGGESTED AREAS FOR RESEARCH QUESTIONS

AREAS OF DEVELOPMENT	EXAMPLES OF RESEARCH QUESTIONS
Social:	What are the sequential stages that lead to cooperative play in children?
Emotional:	What are the origins of anxiety?
Cognitive:	What types of logic are used by 3-year-old children?
Language:	What is the most favorable age for learning a second language?
Academic:	What cognitive processes are related to reading?
Moral:	What factors facilitate moral learning in 8-year-old children?
Motor:	What are the sequential stages of development in eye-hand coordination?
Feeding:	What is the relationship between obesity in infancy and obesity in adolescence?

(2010), in the first sentence of his book *The Language and Thought of the Child*, wrote: "The question which we shall attempt to answer in this book may be stated as follows: What are the needs which a child tends to satisfy when he talks?" (p. 1). Gesell et al. (1934), in their research on infant behavior, also began with a guiding question: "When does this orthogenetic patterning of the human individual begin?" (p. 9).

The potential areas for research using developmental observation are considerable. An outline of the broad scope of development and specific research questions, listed in Table 3–2, demonstrates the wide spectrum of developmental research.

The questions listed in Table 3–2 represent only a fraction of the potential research appropriate for developmental observation. The aspect of development selected by a researcher and the research questions generated provide the engine for the study. The justification and need for the study are based on practical and clinical issues.

3.4.2 Need for Study in Developmental Observation

For the occupational therapist, developmental research provides a bedrock for evaluating clients and interpreting the results. Does this individual demonstrate development within typical limits? To answer this question, norms pertaining to development are needed. Developmental studies therefore provide benchmarks for interpreting developmental levels and devising sequential intervention programs. In children with developmental disabilities, such as cerebral palsy, intellectual disability, autism, or severe social deprivation, data from developmental observations can be used by therapists to monitor progress in response to the intervention. The rationale behind this approach is that development progresses sequentially and in a hierarchical fashion in the typical child, but can be delayed, incomplete, or impaired in the child with a developmental disability. The developmental therapist reconstructs the sequential stages in one or more aspects of development and facilitates the child's progress through each stage. Steps along a linear developmental progression are programmed for the individual child starting at the current level of performance.

The results of developmental observation research have a direct effect on evaluating and treating children with developmental disabilities. After delineating the need for the study, the researcher designs an observational method for collecting data.

3.4.3 Observational Methods for Collecting Data

The technique of observation of infant behavior is not a subject that lends itself to free and easy generalization. Nor does the question, *what is the best technique?*, permit a simple answer. Observation methods must vary considerably with the age of the infant, and of course with the objectives in view (Gesell, 1928).

The observational method that the developmental researcher selects should provide objective descriptive data that are representative of the child's repertoire of behavior. This is accomplished by providing the child with a stimulus that will elicit the desired behavior, schematically represented in Figure 3–1.

The researcher selects the stimulus after operationally defining the area of development in terms of the behavioral response. Tests for assessing a child's level of development such as the *Bayley Scales of Infant Development–3* (Bayley, 2006), the Mullen Scales of Early Learning (Mullen, 1995), and the *Miller Assessment for Preschoolers* (Schoen & Miller, 1985) are examples of this method. In the BSID–3, cognitive abilities are operationally defined by the following tasks:

6 months—plays with single object—banging it

9 months—relational acts emerge (e.g., placing spoon in cup; placing lid on pot)

2 years—symbolic play (e.g., pretend to drink from a cup)

3 years—symbolic play more complex (e.g., pretend to call someone on make-believe phone

DEVELOPMENTAL FACTORS	OPERATIONAL DEFINITION
Object Permanence	An object is wrapped in a sheet of paper while the child is watching. The child is asked to find the object.
Manual Dexterity	Child puts pegs into a peg board in a timed or untimed condition. The time taken to complete the task is age specific.

Questions arise in this context. How does the researcher know that all aspects of a developmental factor are being considered and that the operational definition of a developmental factor is valid? These questions are pertinent in developmental research, and they call for a rationale from the investigator.

In reporting developmental data, the researcher should describe factors in the child that may have affected the results. These factors include age, gender, intelligence, education, socioeconomic status, family structure, and experiences. The identification and control of these factors by inclusion in the research reduces ambiguity in interpreting the results.

As well as operationally defining the developmental factors and identifying variables within the child, the

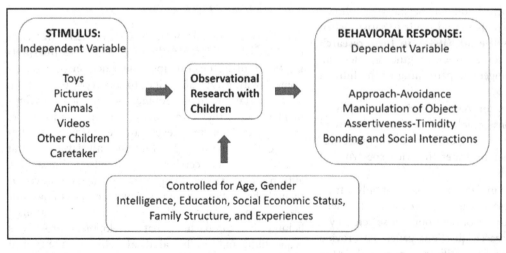

Figure 3–1 Schematic representation of observational research. Notice that participants are provided with stimuli so as to elicit a response. The data docketed are the behaviors elicited by the stimuli.

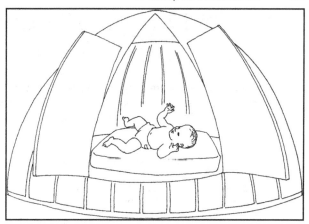

Figure 3–3 Illustration of a photographic dome used by Gesell (1928) in observational research.

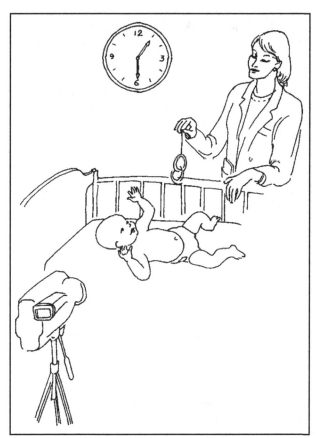

Figure 3–2 Position of the camera and baby when taking observational data.

researcher must construct an objective environment for collecting valid data. Examples of study environments in developmental research are shown in Figures 3–2 and 3–3. Arrangements for observation are part of a standard procedure. Adaptations in this method include the use of a photographic dome as developed by Gesell (1928) or the use of study rooms with one–way mirrors, where the observer is not seen by the subject. Box 3–2 gives an example of a study using developmental research.

BOX 3-2. EXAMPLE OF DEVELOPMENTAL OBSERVATION

1. Bibliographic Notation

Kawaguchi, H., Murakami, B., Kawai, M. (2010) Behavioral characteristics of children with high functioning pervasive developmental disorders during a game. *Journal of Epidemiology, 20*(Suppl. 2), S490–S497.

2. Abstract

BACKGROUND: To evaluate children's sociability through their behavior, we compared the motion features of children with high functioning pervasive developmental disorders (HFPDD) and typical development (TD) during a game. We selected 'Jenga' as the game because this is an interactive game played by two people.

METHODS: We observed the behavior of 7 children with HFPDD and 10 children with TD. An optical motion capture system was used to follow the movement of 3-dimensional position markers attached to caps worn by the players.

RESULTS: The range of head motion of the children with HFPDD was narrower than that of the control group, especially in the X-axis direction (perpendicular to the line connecting the two players). In each game, we calculated the range of motion in the X-axis of each child and divided that Figure by the matched adult player's range. The average ratios of children with HFPDD and TD were 0.64 and 0.89 (number of games are 61 and 18), and the difference of these two ratios is significant (P < 0.001).

CONCLUSIONS: This ratio has sensitivity to identify HFPDD children and could be useful in their child care.

3. Justification and Need for Study

"We attempted to derive a behavioral indicator connected to sociability based on comparing the behavioral characteristics of two groups of children, children who are socially challenged (with high functioning pervasive developmental disorders (HFPDD)) and those who are not (children with typical development (TD))" (p. 491).

(continued)

Box 3-2. Example of Developmental Observation (continued)

4. Literature Review

The authors cited 45 references from the literature. Journals cited included *Journal of Epidemiology, Trends in Cognitive Science, Brain Imaging Behavior, Child Development, Science, Journal of Child Psychiatry and Psychology, Developmental Psychology, Perceptual and Motor Skills, Japanese Journal of Child Adolescent Psychiatry* and *Early Development and Parent.* The majority of articles were published in the last ten years.

5. Research Hypothesis or Guiding Question

The authors sought evidence to demonstrate that children with HFPDD as compared to a normal typical group of children responded differently in their social behavior as observed in playing a Japanese game.

6. Methods

Six video cameras, two microphones, and an optical motion capture system set up inside an observation room recorded the social interaction of the participants.

7. Results

The results of the observations indicated that HFPDD children have problems conveying their interests through movement and seemed to have difficulty in non-verbal communication.

8. Conclusions

"Making the assumption that children with developmental disorders are creating communicative signals, if we make efforts to pick up those signals, and educate widely with this objective, we may be able to create a society where children with developmental disorders can live comfortably" (p. S497).

9. Limitations of the Study

Further research is needed to replicate the study with another group of children with HFPDD to determine if the methodology is reliable and valid in observing children at play.

10. Major References Cited in the Study

Frith, C. D., & Frith, U. (2006). The neuronal basis of mentalizing. *Neuron, 50,* 531–534.

Ozonoff, S., & Miller, J. N. (1995) Teaching theory of mind: A new approach to social skills training for individuals with autism. *Journal of Autism and Developmental Disorders, 25,* 415–433.

Rogers, S. J., Hepburn, S. L., Stackhouse, T., & Wehner, E. (2003). Imitation performance in toddlers with autism and those with other developmental disorders. *Journal of Child Psychiatry and Psychology, 44,* 763–781.

Sallows, G. O., & Graupner, T. D. (2005) Intensive behavioral treatment for children with autism: Four-year outcome and predictors. *American Journal of Mental Retardation, 110,* 417–438.

Yamamoto, J., Kakutani, A., & Terada, M. (2001) Establishing joint visual attention and pointing in autistic children with no functional language. *Perceptual Motor Skills, 92,* 755–770.

3.5 Longitudinal Research (Prospective Designs, Pyramid Level D3)

Are there developmental factors that over a period of time cause changes in a person's anatomical and physiological processes, predisposing that person to illness? Do occupationally enriched environments result in improved independence in instrumental activities of daily living in high school graduates? Does a sedentary lifestyle in the adolescent years influence the type of occupations in which people engage across the lifespan? Does early intervention influence high school graduation rates? What is the prognosis for high-risk children who come from socially disadvantaged environments? What is the relationship between occupational hazards and the later onset of disease? These problems are all affected by time factors.

Longitudinal research is a method used in observing the effects of independent variables on dependent variables over an extended period of time. The investigator uses longitudinal research to predict an outcome based on the presence of presumed causative factors. For example, a team of researchers may study groups of individuals over a period of 20 years from young adult to middle age and observe whether certain groups are more vulnerable to heart disease than other groups. In occupational therapy, a researcher may examine the long-term effects of sensory integration therapy on academic achievement in children with learning disabilities. Box 3–3 provides an example of longitudinal research investigating the influence of age upon rehabilitation success in persons with traumatic brain injury.

BOX 3-3. EXAMPLE OF LONGITUDINAL STUDY

1. Bibliographic Notation

Sendroy-Terrill, M., Whiteneck, G. G., & Brooks, C. A. (2010). Aging with traumatic brain injury: Cross-sectional follow-up of people receiving inpatient rehabilitation over more than 3 decades. *Archives of Physical Medicine and Rehabilitation, 91*, 489–497.

2. Abstract

OBJECTIVE: To investigate aging with traumatic brain injury (TBI) by determining if long-term outcomes after TBI are predicted by years postinjury and age at injury after controlling for the severity of the injury and sex.

DESIGN: Cross-sectional follow-up telephone survey.

SETTING: Community residents who had received initial treatment in a comprehensive inpatient rehabilitation hospital.

PARTICIPANTS: Survivors of TBI (N = 243) stratified by years postinjury (in seven 5-year cohorts ranging from 1 to over 30 years postinjury) and by age at injury (in 2 cohorts of people injured before or after age 30).

INTERVENTIONS: None.

MAIN OUTCOME MEASURES: Measures of postconcussive symptoms, major secondary conditions including fatigue (*Modified Fatigue Impact Scale*), physical and cognitive activity limitations (*FIM, Alertness Behavior Subscale of the Sickness Impact Profile, Medical Outcomes Study 12–Item Health Status Survey Short Form*), societal participation restrictions (*Craig Handicap Assessment and Reporting Technique*), environmental barriers (*Craig Hospital Inventory of Environmental Factors*), and perceived quality of life (*Satisfaction with Life Scale*).

RESULTS: Most problems identified by the outcome measures were reported by one fourth to one half of the study participants. Increasing decades postinjury predicted declines in physical and cognitive functioning, declines in societal participation, and increases in contractures. Increasing age at injury predicted declines in functional independence, increases in fatigue, declines in societal participation, and declines in perceived environmental barriers.

CONCLUSIONS: This investigation has increased our understanding of the aging process after TBI by demonstrating that both components of aging (years postinjury and age at injury) are predictive of several outcomes after TBI.

Key Words: brain injuries, brain injury, chronic, follow-up studies, outcomes assessment (health care), rehabilitation

3. Justification and Need for Study

The purpose of this descriptive exploratory study was to determine whether age at injury is associated with progressive functional decline. This hypothesis has important intervention implications, particularly because the advent of neuroprotective therapies for dementia will make it important to identify people at risk for cognitive decline in late life.

4. Literature Review

The authors did an extensive review of the literature with 54 references cited. Examples of the journals cited included: *Archives of Physical Medicine and Rehabilitation, Brain Injury, Annals of Neurology, Journal of Head Rehabilitation Trauma, Archives in Neurology, Neurorehabilitation, Journal of Neurology, Journal of Trauma,* and *Journal of the American Medical Association.*

5. Research Hypothesis or Guiding Question

The primary hypothesis stated that older patients show greater decline in neurological function over the first 5 years after TBI than younger patients.

(continued)

BOX 3-3. EXAMPLE OF LONGITUDINAL STUDY (CONTINUED)

6. Methods

The study was identified as a longitudinal cohort study. It included participants who met the following criteria: (a) age of 16 years or older at the time of traumatic brain injury, (b) arrival at a hospital emergency department within 8 hours after injury, (c) receipt of acute and rehabilitation treatment at a traumatic brain injury model system (TBIMS) affiliated hospitals, (d) complete Disability Rating Scale (DRS) 25 scores taken at 1- and 5-year follow-up evaluations, and (e) provision of informed consent directly or by proxy. At the time of this investigation 1127 patients were eligible to receive a 5-year post-TBI DRS evaluation specified in the TBIMS protocol, and 624 (55%) patients had complete DRS data 5 years post-TBI. Four hundred twenty-eight patients had complete DRS outcome data at both year 1 and year 5 (38%) and constituted the cohort analyzed here.

7. Results

All three age groups improved between admission and rehabilitation through year 5, and the magnitude, or slope, of improvement among the three age groups was similar through the first year postinjury. Paired-sample t-test results show significant improvement in functioning as measured by the four outcome measures (i.e., DRS, *FIM*, cognitive domain of the *FIM*, *Extended Glasgow Outcome* Scale; GOS-E) over time among the youngest group. In addition, the intermediate group showed significant improvement on the DRS, and the oldest did not show significant improvement on any of the outcome measures. Change scores for the outcome measures were examined as a marker of the magnitude of improvement between year 1 and year 5. The two younger groups showed greater change in DRS than the oldest group, and there were no differences in magnitude of change among the other outcome measures.

8. Conclusions

The study supported the primary hypothesis that older survivors of TBI show greater functional decline than younger survivors. Results from this study show that younger survivors of TBI showed significant improvement in disability ratings between the first and fifth years postinjury, whereas older counterparts did not show significant improvement in outcome measures over the same time period. Furthermore, the results suggest older survivors have a higher risk of functional decline than younger survivors, because patients 26 years or younger showed a lower rate of decline over a 4-year span than older patients.

9. Limitations of the Study

One limitation of the study was the potential for systematic bias created by subjects lost to follow-up. Employment could be overestimated because of the loss of subjects with prior histories of substance abuse. Another limitation of the present investigation is that it is difficult to determine whether the decline in disability rating over time experienced by the oldest group is attributed to disabling effects of brain injury or simply decline associated with normative aging. Future studies may need to incorporate an orthopedic control group separated into age groups.

10. Major References Cited in the Study

Consensus Conference. (1999). Rehabilitation of persons with traumatic brain injury (NIH Consensus Development Panel on Rehabilitation of Persons with Traumatic Brain Injury). *Journal of the American Medical Association, 282,* 974–983.

Flanagan, S. R., Hibbard, M. R., & Gordon, W. A. (2005). The impact of age on traumatic brain injury. *Physical Medicine and Rehabilitation Clinics of North America, 16,* 163–177.

Thurman, D. J., Alverson, C., Dunn, K. A., Guerrero, J., & Sniezek, J. E. (1999). Traumatic brain injury in the United States: A public health perspective. *Journal of Head Trauma Rehabilitation, 14,* 602–615.

Whitnall, L., McMillan, T. M., Murray, G. D., & Teasdale, G. M. (2006). Disability in young people and adults after head injury: 5–7 year follow up of a prospective cohort study. *Journal of Neurology, Neurosurgery, and Psychiatry, 77,* 640–645.

3.6 NORMATIVE RESEARCH (PYRAMID LEVEL D3)

Definition: Normative research is a systematic attempt to build tables of data displaying the typical performance of individuals on specified tasks, or the quantities of a trait evident in people of various demographic factors. For example, a table of norms for dominant hand grip strength would show the central tendency (the mean, usually) and variability of the trait (standard deviation typically, and sometimes also the standard error of the mean) in boys and girls of various ages (Mathiowetz et al., 1986). It was found important to list the sexes separately because there is a systematic difference in grip strength between the sexes. Ages needed to be listed sequentially because grip strength increases with age. With such a table, any future therapist measuring a child's grip strength, knowing the child's age and sex, could look up to see how that child compares with the norms for the child's age and sex. Given the mean for those demographics and the standard deviation, many forms for this comparison could be expressed: percentiles, z-scores, or even the useful "within normal limits," which might be defined as the mean plus or minus 1.5 standard deviations. (See the remainder of this chapter for more detail on finding these descriptive statistics.)

Normative studies, where a measurement is made on a group of individuals, require many participants in order to provide for a table of stable normative estimates. At a minimum there should be six participants contributing to each cell of the table (e.g., from the example above, at least 6 boys between the ages of 4 and 4.5 years of age). The faster the trait is developing in typically growing individuals, the smaller the age categories need to be in order to fairly capture the moving normative value. Needless to say, for a normative table with many cells, the study may require hundreds of individuals to capture the norms accurately.

3.7 DESCRIPTIVE STATISTICS (FOR USE WITH PYRAMID LEVELS D4 AND D3)

Descriptive statistics can be considered to be foundational to statistics in that they are used to characterize, quantitatively, a participant group. They characterize the central tendency of the group (mean, median, mode) and the variability of data within the group (standard deviation, variance, range, interquartile). More specifically, descriptive statistics can help portray various participant group characteristics by quantifying aspects of those characteristics or by providing the frequency (e.g., number of times of occurrence) of participant behaviors. Examples of participant characteristics are the average age or height of a participant group, or perhaps the average length of stay in a health care setting a participant group may have experienced. The frequency of participant behaviors may include the average number of times a group of school children share a toy with another child during recess. Descriptive statistics are reported in nearly every published quantitative study and are also very common in qualitative studies. Indeed, there are many studies that are "descriptive" in nature and exclusively report descriptive statistics. An example

is Chang et al. (2023) investigating the preparatory activities of daily living for rest and sleep in a sample of individuals residing in long-term care facilities. In this study, 29 residents were observed and their activities associated with rest, sleep preparation, and sleep participation were listed and categories were developed. Examples from the list provided within each category included "listened to radio," "got dressed for bed," and "went to bed," respectively. Additionally, it was reported that the average time sleeping was 10.22 hours per night and participants rested an average of 4.77 hours per day. Chang et al. (2023) concluded that occupational therapists are especially suited to facilitate occupational performance in activities associated with rest and sleep preparation.

Note that when only descriptive statistics are used in a study, and there appear differences between sub-groups in the study (e.g., in the mean values between clients with left versus right CVA), no statistical claim can be made about whether this difference is statistically significant. Such claims can only be made on the basis of inferential statistics, which are covered later in Chapters 4, 5, and 6.

3.8 STUDY DESIGN INCLUDING APPLICABILITY/FEATURES AND INHERENT LIMITATIONS

As the name implies, "descriptive statistics" describe. While intuitive comparisons may be possible with descriptive statistics, they are not designed to statistically analyze the differences between groups or conditions. For instance, an average score of one group may be higher or lower than that of a second group, but the differences are limited to observation only. As we will see in later chapters, though, when mathematically combining specific descriptive statistics together, for example, the respective means, variances, and sizes of multiple groups, it is possible to make statistical comparisons, inferentially. That is, it is possible to statistically compare one group with another by testing a probability hypothesis: how likely was it, given the data, that these differences appeared by chance? As such, the reader can see that descriptive statistics have utility in and of themselves to "describe," but can also be used in combination with more advanced statistical calculations to test research hypotheses.

There are many foundational concepts presented in this part of the chapter. Many of these concepts are commonly referred to in quantitative research articles published in peer-reviewed journals. Thus, the key terms and concepts used in this section and denoted as such and in the chapters that follow should be reviewed in the glossary.

3.9 Concept of Measurement and Numbers: Data

Before we explore specific types of descriptive statistics, an introduction to data and what types of data exist is helpful. First of note is that the word "data," technically, is plural, whereas the much less common word, "datum," is singular. One can find instances, though, where data is used as a singular.

Data in statistics are derived from empirical observations. These observations are the result of a standardized measurement procedure, such as simple counting, interviews, observations, standardized test results, or machine monitoring of physiological functions. *Measurement* is the assignment of numbers to the characteristics of objects, persons, or events according to rules. Measurement transforms certain attributes of the world into numbers, which can then be summarized, organized, and analyzed by statistical procedures.

The properties or characteristics of objects, persons, or events are called *variables* (e.g., height, weight, sitting balance). A variable can assume two or more different values, reflecting the fact that objects, persons, or events vary in the extent they show certain characteristics. This concept of *individual differences* is central to most scientific disciplines. One of the purposes of statistics is to reflect and summarize such individual differences in the values of variables.

3.10 Measurement Scales

Measurement scales are a system for the numerical representation of the values of a variable. Four basic types of measurement scales are distinguished in statistics:

3.10.1 Nominal Scale Data

Nominal scale measurement is the most discrete and simplest level of data. With nominal scale data, observations are arranged into various classes or categories. Observations falling into the same class or category are considered qualitatively equivalent, whereas observations in different classes are considered qualitatively different. Eye color, for example, as classified into blue, brown, hazel, or gray, is an example of nominal scale data. Ideally each item to be classified falls into one and only one category.

Numbers are usually assigned to each class or category, but these numbers merely reflect different labels for the classes or categories. The numbers do not reflect arithmetical magnitude or order; they only distinguish one class or category from another.

With nominal scale measurement, categories and classes are determined, and a count is made of the number of observations in each category. Because nominal data constitute the most elementary level of measurement, the only arithmetic operation that can be performed on the numerical data is counting the number of observations in a category and then documenting proportions or percentages among categories. Examples of nominal scale data in health research include diagnostic categories, subspecialization areas, geographic locations, leisure interests, and health care settings (e.g., hospital, nursing home, or rehabilitation clinic).

3.10.2 Ordinal Scale Data

Ordinal scale data is the next level of measurement where objects or individuals are not only distinguished from one another and are able to be sorted into categories, but also are arranged in order or rank. The numerical values of a variable are arranged in a meaningful order to indicate a hierarchy of the values of the variable or to show relative position. Examples of ordinal scale data are birth order among siblings, the order of finish in a race, or the relative academic standing of university students in a class. The numbers assigned in the above examples not only distinguish between individuals, but also indicate the order or rank of the individuals relative to one another.

The major limitation of ordinal scales is the inability to make inferences about the degree of difference between values on the scale. Numbers assigned in ordinal scale measurement have the properties of both distinctness and order, but the difference between the numbers may not be equal. For example, the difference in time between 1st and 3rd place in a race may not be equivalent to the difference between 25th and 27th place in the race. There may be wide or narrow differences between each pair of ranks. With ordinal scale data, it is only possible to state that one individual or object ranks above or below another. Examples in health care include the amount of assistance needed (dependent, maximal assist, moderate assist, minimal assist, touch cues, verbal cues, independent), muscle strength categories (good, fair, poor), the severity of illness or injury (severe, moderate, mild), and the degree of pain (1 through 10 as perceived, where the differences between ratings are not necessarily equal).

3.10.3 Interval Scale Data

Interval scale measurement extends ordinal scales by adding the characteristic that differences between scale values are equal. Thus, the difference between each pair of variable scores (1 to 2, 3 to 4…) is equal in amount to that trait. With interval measurement, numbers serve two purposes: (a) to convey the order of the observations, and (b) to indicate the distance or degree of differences between observations. Numbers are assigned so that equal differences in the numbers correspond to equal differences in the property or attribute measured. However, the zero point of the interval scale can be placed arbitrarily and does not indicate total absence of the property measured.

Examples of interval scale data are calendar years and the temperature scales of Celsius and Fahrenheit. In a temperature scale, the difference between 10 and 15°C is the same quantitative difference as between 20 and 25°C, but 20°C is not twice as warm as 10°C because 0°C is not a true zero point, representing the absence of all heat.

Interval scales are important in scientific research. Many human characteristics and attributes, such as intelligence scores, range of motion, dexterity, coordination, and standard scores, are scales with approximately equal intervals. In addition, more sophisticated inferential statistical procedures may be performed with interval scale data as compared with nominal and ordinal scale data.

3.10.4 Ratio Scale Data

Ratio scale data is the highest level of measurement and includes the maximum amount of information. The ratio scale is named as such because the ratio of numbers on the scale is meaningful. Because there is a genuine zero point, equal ratios between scale values have equal meaning (i.e., the ratio 40:20 is equivalent to 100:50 or 120:60, that is, twice as much of the attribute). The zero point on a ratio scale indicates total absence of the property measured. With ratio scale data, all arithmetic operations (addition, subtraction, multiplication, and division) are possible and meaningful. The measurements for such variables as height, weight, heart rate, and respiratory rate are all ratio scaled. Figure 3–4 illustrates the differences between the four basic types of measurement scales, and Table 3–3 illustrates their characteristics and properties.

In the foregoing example (Table 3–4) of measurable variables, numbers can be assigned to indicate the degree of improvement, strength, perceptual ability, and quality of life. Rating scales can also be devised using a continuum of measurement, equal intervals, or item ranking. Likert-type scales using descriptor adjectives is another alternative. In this scale, it is not assumed that there are equal intervals between numbers (e.g., 1 to 2 is not assumed to be the same distance as 2 to 3) or that there is an absolute zero. Nonetheless, measurement at this level is an improvement over a practitioner non-empirically stating, on the basis of their opinion of an intervention, that the client has either improved or not improved.

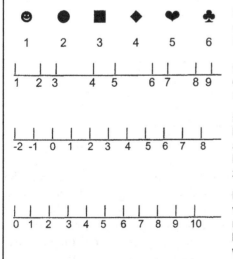

Nominal scale: Numbers act as labels only, indicating differences in kind (e.g., identification numbers).

Ordinal scale: Numbers represent rank ordering. Differences between rank are not equidistant (e.g., grade levels).

Interval scale: Equal differences between values represent equal amounts, but ratios have no meaning because of the arbitrary location of the zero point (e.g., temperature).

Ratio scale: Equal differences between values represent equal amounts. Equal ratios of values are also equivalent because of a genuine zero point (e.g., weight scale).

Figure 3–4 Differences between the four measurement scales are illustrated.

TABLE 3–3

CLASSIFICATION OF SCALES OF MEASUREMENT

MEASUREMENT SCALE	TYPE OF VARIABLE	RESEARCHER APPLICATION	PURPOSES	EXAMPLES
Nominal	Discrete	Sorting of items	Establishing mutually exclusive groups	Occupations, diagnostic groups
Ordinal	Discrete	Rank ordering of items	Determination of greater or lesser	Patient improvement, clinical performance of students
Interval	Continuous	Equal ordering of items	Establishing equal intervals on a continuum	Intelligence, perceptual-motor abilities, work capacities
Ratio	Continuous	Equal ordering of items with an absolute zero point	Establishing continuous measurement with zero point	Range of motion, muscle strength, weight, height, auditory and visual acuity

TABLE 3–4

MEASURABLE VARIABLES

VARIABLE TO BE TESTED	EXAMPLES OF MEASURING INSTRUMENTS
Hand strength:	Dynamometer
Range of motion:	Goniometer
Attitudes toward individuals with disabilities:	Attitudes Toward Disabled Persons Scale
Clinical performance of students:	Fieldwork Performance Evaluation for the Occupational Therapy Student
Psychological improvement:	Tennessee Test of Self Concept (TTSC)
Social values and life goals:	Life Satisfaction Index (LSI)
Stress management:	Stress Management Questionnaire (SMQ)
Sensory integration:	Sensory Integration and Praxis Tests (SIPT)
Cognitive functioning:	Allen's Cognitive Level (ACL)
Self-care:	Functional Independence Measure (FIM)
Developmental levels:	Miller Function & Participation Scales (M-FUN)
Eye-hand coordination:	Developmental Test of Visual-Motor Integration (VMI)
Perceptual ability:	Test of Visual Perceptual Scales (non-motor) (TVPS)
Instrumental activities of daily living:	Executive Function Performance Test
Hand function:	Jebsen-Taylor Hand-Function Test (JTHFT)

3.11 TABLE OF PERCENTAGE

Statistical analysis begins with organizing data into summary tables and diagrams. In descriptive studies such as survey research, tabular summaries of data provide the results. For example, Table 3–5 summarizes data from three different mental health diagnostic groups who were earning at least minimum wage.

The table reports the percentage of people employed and earning at least minimum wage who either had a single or who had multiple hospital admissions. The data are also stratified by age group. Three striking trends can be observed in this table. First, there is an inverse relationship between age and employment. Second, males have a higher employment rate than females, and third, higher employment rates are associated with single admissions compared to multiple admissions. Nonetheless, the descriptive statistics that displayed these relationships do not allow for a statistical claim that the differences are probably real.

TABLE 3-5

PERCENTAGE EARNING MINIMUM WAGE OR ABOVE IN THE THREE DIAGNOSTIC GROUPS AND IN THE GENERAL POPULATION IN DECEMBER 2010

AGE GROUP		SCHIZOPHRENIA		OTHER NONAFFECTIVE PSYCHOSIS		BIPOLAR AFFECTIVE DISORDER		GENERAL POPULATION
		SINGLE ADMISSION (% EMPLOYED)	MULTIPLE ADMISSIONS (% EMPLOYED)	SINGLE ADMISSION (% EMPLOYED)	MULTIPLE ADMISSIONS (% EMPLOYED)	SINGLE ADMISSION (% EMPLOYED)	MULTIPLE ADMISSIONS (% EMPLOYED)	
Total category, N		4449	15510	5277	6097	1561	2779	3835979
20–29	Males	17.9%	8.0%	30.5%	17.9%	34.0%	25.6%	47.6%
	Females	13.8%	5.2%	23.7%	10.9%	35.0%	18.8%	37.9%
30–39	Males	19.1%	8.3%	37.1%	30.5%	52.1%	40.2%	64.0%
	Females	12.0%	5.3%	29.8%	12.3%	43.8%	29.5%	47.1%
40–49	Males	13.3%	6.7%	30.8%	21.3%	36.6%	33.5%	63.7%
	Females	5.8%	5.0%	20.7%	9.5%	33.6%	23.6%	48.5%
50–65	Males	7.5%	3.3%	21.4%	15.8%	27.6%	17.3%	48.4%
	Females	5.9%	2.5%	13.6%	5.0%	15.2%	14.0%	36.2%

Source: Davidson et al. (2015).

TABLE 3–6			
PERCENTAGE OF RESPONDENTS REQUIRED TO PERFORM MANUAL TRANSFERS AND PERCENTAGE OF THOSE WHO SUSTAINED AN INJURY WHILE TRANSFERRING A PATIENT IN THEIR FACILITY			
FACILITY	NUMBER OF RESPONDENTS (*N*)	RESPONDENTS REQUIRED TO PERFORM MANUAL TRANSFERS (%)	RESPONDENTS WHO SUSTAINED INJURY DUE TO MANUALLY TRANSFERRING OF PATIENT WITHIN THE PAST YEAR (%)
Acute care	19	100.0	10.0
Home health	14	100.0	0.0
LTC/SNF	87	92.0	4.6
Hospital inpatient rehab.	34	91.2	11.8
Private practice	8	87.5	0.0
Community center	8	87.5	25.0
Outpatient rehab.	29	82.8	3.3
School system	48	60.4	4.2
Psych-based	5	60.0	0.0
Work hardening/industrial rehab.	7	57.1	0.0
Academia	10	30.0	0.0
Source: Rice et al. (2011)			

Yet another method of displaying data is to compare results between periods of time, distances, or settings. For example, Table 3–6 lists numerous settings where occupational therapists work and the frequency of distribution in percentage across categories of settings. When examining the data, the reader can note that some relatively low injury rates are evenly distributed across the various settings (e.g., home health, out-patient rehabilitation, psych-based, and work hardening), whereas other injury rates are greater within other types of settings (e.g., acute care, LTC/SNF, hospital inpatient rehab, and community centers). While descriptive studies do not offer causation-based conclusions, frequency distribution differences like these may suggest differing factors associated with risk exposure are involved specific to the setting or types of settings.

The above examples demonstrate the importance of descriptive statistics in summarizing results from a research study. A number of methods can be used to describe data. Some of the most frequently used methods for organizing descriptive data are discussed in the following section.

3.12 FREQUENCY DISTRIBUTION TABLE

A *frequency distribution table* is organized into columns of data that include the number or frequency of cases (and the equivalent percentages) that fall into a designated category. In the research study represented below, a frequency distribution table portrays the age and gender of the population sampled in the study.

The first column of a frequency distribution table includes the class intervals (in this example, age group by years). It could also represent data such as range of motion in degrees, scores on perceptual tests, or diastolic blood pressure. The class intervals are separated into equal 10-year intervals in the above example (e.g., 15–24 and 25–34). The second column of a frequency distribution includes the number of cases tallied for each class intervals (e.g., 36 males between the ages of 5 and 14). The third column includes the percentage of cases within a class interval, of the total number of individuals in the study. For example, there are 52 females in the class interval of 25 to 34, which represents 52 from a total of 228 females in the study, or 22.8%, which may be rounded to 23%. We can also determine the *cumulative frequency* of each class interval and the *cumulative relative frequency* with the data provided in the study. Table 3–7 shows data organized into a frequency distribution table to include relative frequency and cumulative relative frequency for males only.

In summary:

- *Class interval* is the category of score values in a distribution. The number of class intervals is determined by the number of participants in the study and the range of values or scores.

TABLE 3–7

FREQUENCY DISTRIBUTION FOR MALES

CLASS INTERVAL	FREQUENCY (F)	RELATIVE F (%)	CUMULATIVE F	CUMULATIVE RF (%)
5 – 14	36	6	36	6
15 – 24	147	24	183	30
25 – 34	200	33	383	63
35 – 44	105	17	488	80
45 – 54	60	10	548	90
55 – 64	41	7	589	97
>65	21	3	610	100
Unknown	4	.006	614	100
Total	**614**	**100%**	**614**	**100%**

- *Frequency of cases* includes the total number of cases within an assigned class interval.
- *Relative frequency* or *percentage* is the percentage of cases falling within the class interval and is calculated by dividing the number of cases within the class interval by the total number of cases in the distribution.
- *Cumulative frequency* represents the total number of scores within a class interval that is added cumulatively from the lowest up to that interval. The grand total of the cumulative frequency equals the total number of scores or cases in the distribution.

- *Cumulative relative frequency* or *cumulative percentage* is the percentage of cases added from the lowest class interval through the highest selected class interval. When the top interval is selected, the cumulative percentage should equal 100%.

3.12.1 Constructing a Frequency Distribution Table

The table below displays hypothetical ungrouped raw scores on resting heart rate for 50 healthy young adults.

Step 1. *Record raw scores from ungrouped data.*

PERSON	SCORE	PERSON	SCORE	PERSON	SCORE	PERSON	SCORE
01	54	14	67	27	54	40	79
02	72	15	74	28	73	41	85
03	80	16	76	29	72	42	52
04	53	17	79	30	78	43	56
05	75	18	77	31	78	44	67
06	53	19	48	32	56	45	55
07	78	20	76	33	80	46	79
08	47	21	47	34	84	47	81
09	72	22	50	35	72	48	72
10	54	23	65	36	68	49	67
11	66	24	83	37	57	50	71
12	68	25	55	38	57		
13	68	26	76	39	63		

Step 2. *Identify the highest and lowest values in the distribution.* Persons 08 and 21 have heart rate scores of 47 (lowest score, or the minimum). Subject 41 has a heart rate score of 85 (highest score, or the maximum).

Step 3. *Calculate the range (highest score to lowest score).* In our example, the range is 85 – 47 = 38.

Step 4. *Determine the number of class intervals.* The determination of the number of class intervals depends on the number of scores in the frequency distribution and the range of scores. Too many or too few class intervals may not give adequate information to describe the distribution. Determining the number of class intervals is a trial-and-error process. For example, compare the three frequency distributions using the same scores but with class intervals of too many, too few, and approximately correct. Most researchers constructing frequency distributions establish 6 to 15 class intervals as a general rule.

Step 5. *Determine the size of a class interval.* The size of the class interval is determined through estimation by dividing the range of scores by the number of class intervals. Using the same example, the range of 38 is divided by 13 (the number of class intervals) to yield a class interval size of 3. It is recommended that an odd number be selected for the class interval so that the midpoint of the class interval is a whole number. For example, the midpoint of the

class interval of 83–85 is 84. Later, in calculating group means from a frequency distribution table, the reader will find that it is easier to work with whole numbers than with fractions.

On the other hand, if we determine that the size of a class interval in the previous example is 5, how many class intervals would be established? In this case the range of scores (38) is divided by the size of the class intervals (5) to arrive at 8 class intervals.

CL	MIDPOINT
81–85	83
76–80	78
71–75	73
66–70	68
61–65	63
56–60	58
51–55	53
46–50	48

Step 6. *Tally the number of scores within each class interval.* Check to determine if the number of tallies total up to the number of scores in the frequency distribution.

CLASS INTERVAL	REAL LIMITS*	MIDPOINT	TALLY	f	Cf
83–85	82.5–85.5	84	|||	3	50
80–82	79.5–82.5	81	|||	3	47
77–79	76.5–79.5	78	||||||	7	44
74–76	73.5–76.5	75	|||||	5	37
71–73	70.5–73.5	72	||||||	7	32
68–70	67.5–70.5	69	||	2	25
65–67	64.5–67.5	66	||||||	6	23
62–64	61.5–64.5	63			1	17
59–61	58.5–61.5	6	0	0	16
56–58	55.5–58.5	57	||||	4	16
53–55	52.5–55.5	54	||||||	7	12
50–52	49.5–52.5	51	||	2	5
47–49	46.5–49.5	48	|||	3	3
Total				**50**	**50**

*Defining the upper and lower real limits of the class intervals is described below.

The upper real limit of a class interval is the highest value contained in the interval. Conversely, the lower real limit of a class interval is the lowest value contained in the interval. In dealing with numbers having at least two decimals, round the number up to include it in the nearest class interval. For example, 82.50 or above would be tallied in the class interval 83–85. On the other hand, 82.44 would be tallied into the class interval 80–82 as shown in the example.

Step 7. *Determine the relative frequency or percentage.* Calculate the relative frequency of the scores in each class interval by dividing the number of cases or scores in the class interval by the number of cases in the entire frequency distribution. This is illustrated in Table 3–8.

Relative Frequency = frequency of cases in the class interval / total cases in the frequency distribution

Step 8. *Determine cumulative frequency.* Calculate the cumulative frequency by adding the total frequency in each class interval consecutively from the **lowest class interval to the highest**. In the previous example, the number of cases in the class interval 83–85 is 3. This number is added to the number of cases in the class interval 80–82, which is also 3, giving a cumulative frequency of 6. The completed frequency distribution table is shown in Table 3–9.

Summary of construction of frequency distribution table:

1. Organize raw scores from ungrouped data by arranging values from the lowest to the highest scores.
2. Identify the lowest and highest scores in the distribution.
3. Calculate the range, which is the difference or distance from the lowest to the highest scores in the distribution.
4. Determine the number of class intervals, using the rule of selecting within a range of 6 to 15 categories of intervals.
5. Determine the size of each class interval. First estimate the size of class intervals by dividing the range by the number of class intervals. Try to select an odd number so that the midpoint of the class interval will be a whole number.
6. Count or tally the number of scores within each class interval.

TABLE 3–8				
FREQUENCY DISTRIBUTION OF HEART RATE SCORES FOR HYPOTHETICAL POPULATION				
CI	MIDPOINT	FREQUENCY	CUMULATIVE FREQUENCY	RELATIVE FREQUENCY (%)
83–85	84	3	50	6
80–82	81	3	47	6
77–79	78	7	47	14
74–76	75	5	37	10
71–73	72	7	32	14
68–70	69	2	25	4
65–67	66	6	23	12
62–64	63	1	17	2
59–61	60	0	16	0
56–58	57	4	16	8
53–55	54	7	12	14
50–52	51	2	5	4
47–49	48	3	3	6

TABLE 3–9					
FREQUENCY DISTRIBUTION OF HEART RATE SCORES FOR HYPOTHETICAL POPULATION					
CI	MIDPOINT	FREQUENCY	CUMULATIVE FREQUENCY	RELATIVE FREQUENCY (%)	CUMULATIVE RELATIVE FREQUENCY%
83–85	84	3	50	6	6
80–82	81	3	47	6	12
77–79	78	7	47	14	26
74–76	75	5	37	10	36
71–73	72	7	32	14	50
68–70	69	2	25	4	54
65–67	66	6	23	12	66
62–64	63	1	17	2	68
59–61	60	0	16	0	68
56–58	57	4	16	8	76
53–55	54	7	12	14	90
50–52	51	2	5	4	94
47–49	48	3	3	6	100

7. Calculate the relative frequency or percentage of scores in each class interval.

8. Calculate the cumulative frequency by adding in succession the frequencies in each class interval. Check that the number of cases counted in succession is equal to the total number of cases or scores in the distribution.

9. Determine the cumulative relative frequency, which is the percentage of cumulative frequency sitting in each class interval. It is **customary to start from the lowest class interval when calculating cumulative values**.

3.13 GRAPHS AND OTHER PICTORIAL REPRESENTATIONS

In addition to presenting data in tables, many researchers use pictorial presentations to display results and describe data. These presentations can be in the form of frequency polygons, histographs, bar graphs, pie graphs, and stem and leaf plots.

3.13.1 Frequency Polygon

A frequency polygon is a line graph displaying the frequency of data by categories. The categories compared are on the horizontal axis (abscissa), and the frequencies of occurrences are on the vertical axis (ordinate).

The frequency polygon in Figure 3–5 shows the percentile of respective body mass index (BMI) for US males and females from 2009 through 2018. The BMIs are listed on the x-axis, the **abscissa**, and the year groupings are on the y-axis, the **ordinate**. Observations from this Figure illustrate that BMIs included in the 50th percentile or smaller remained relatively stable through the years, however, the BMIs within percentiles greater than 50 tended to increase, particularly from 2011 through 2014, indicating that this population may be becoming more obese.

3.13.2 Histograms and Bar Graphs

Histograms and bar graphs are often used by investigators to display frequency of data within categories, similar to frequency polygons. In histograms, the bars are attached to each other, whereas in bar graphs, each bar is detached from the others, as in Figure 3–6. The distinction sometimes is based on aesthetic reasons. Figure 3–6 illustrates the number of reported injuries by occupational therapy practitioners to various body parts due to manually transferring patients.

Constructing a Frequency Polygon, Histogram, or Bar Graph

A frequency polygon, histogram, or bar graph graphically depicts the data provided in a frequency distribution table. The data provided in the *Frequency Distribution of Heart Rate Scores* in Table 3–9 will be used in the following examples.

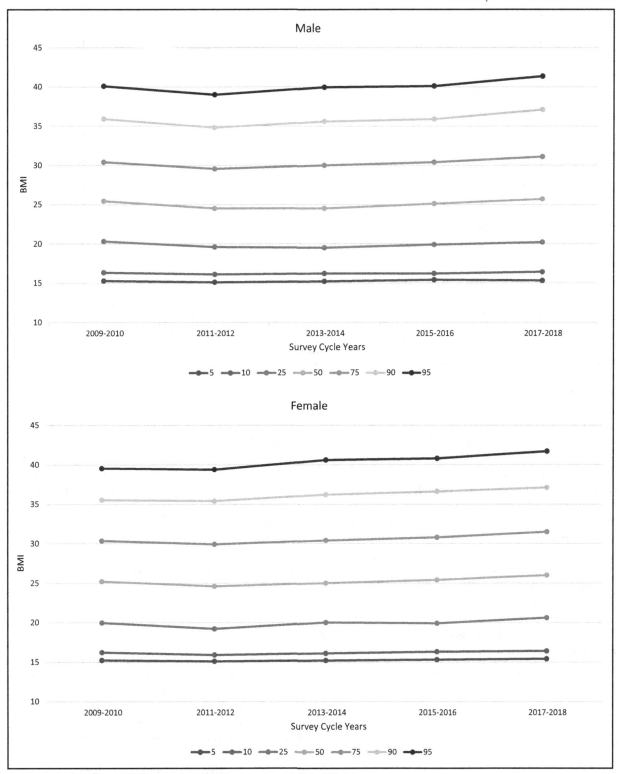

Figure 3–5 Selected weighted percentiles of BMI by survey cycle: NHANES 2009 to 2018.

Source: Ogden et al. (2020) CL, Fryar CD, Martin CB, Freedman DS, Carroll MD, Gu Q, Hales CM. Trends in obesity prevalence by race and Hispanic origin—1999–2000 to 2017–2018. JAMA 324(12):1208–10. 2020. doi:10.1001/jama.2020.14590.

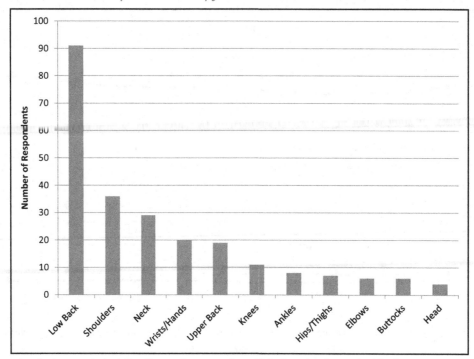

Figure 3–6 Example of a bar graph depicting the maximum number of injuries related to various body parts associated with manually transferring patients.
Source: Rice et al. (2011).

Step 1. *Identify the x-axis (abscissa) and the y-axis (ordinate).* This is illustrated in Figure 3–7.

Step 2. *Label the abscissa descriptively.* In the example in Table 3–9, the heart rate values range from the lowest score of 47 to the highest of 85. The midpoints of each class interval are located on the abscissa (Figure 3–8). The class intervals are extended on both ends to include zero frequency intervals. The lowest class interval with zero frequency is 44–46 with a midpoint of 45. The highest class interval with zero frequency is 86–88 with a midpoint of 87. There are now 15 class intervals including the zero frequency intervals.

Step 3. *Organize the ordinate into frequency of occurrence.* In the previous example, frequencies of occurrence range from 0 to 7. As a rule, the number of class intervals for

frequency should be between 8 and 15. In this case, there will be 8 class intervals including 0.

The frequency polygon is depicted in Figure 3–8 with the data from Table 3–9. The histogram is depicted in Figure 3–9 with the same data used in constructing the frequency polygon.

Many software programs exist that create many graph styles. For instance, spreadsheet programs often have a graphing module as well as a statistical module that can conveniently facilitate the creation of graphs.

3.13.3 Cumulative Frequency Distribution Polygon

A cumulative frequency distribution polygon is a line graph that shows the total number of observations or cases up to the upper real limit of a given class interval. For example, in Section 3.11.2, Step 8, determining cumulative frequency, the data for the heart rates of 50 subjects are displayed. In Figure 3–10, the cumulative frequency distribution polygon is constructed from the previous table of hypothetical heart rate values (Table 3–9).

Cumulative frequency curves are useful in specifying the individual's relative position or standing in a total distribution of scores. For example, someone with a heart rate of 80 in the above distribution is in the 94th percentile or upper 6% of the distribution. Cumulative frequency curves often are useful in plotting group data, such as grip strength, range of motion, blood pressure, and

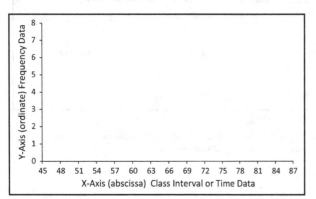

Figure 3–7 Parts of a frequency polygon, histogram, or bar graph. The frequency data are plotted along the vertical axis or ordinate (y-axis), While the class intervals or time data are plotted along the horizontal axis or abscissa (x-axis).

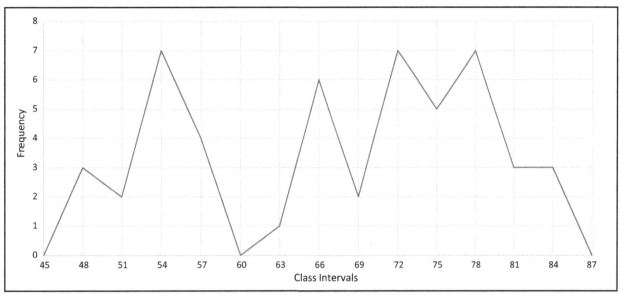

Figure 3–8 Frequency distribution polygon illustrating the frequencies of heart rate scores for a hypothetical population. The data used to plot this polygon are from Table 3–9.

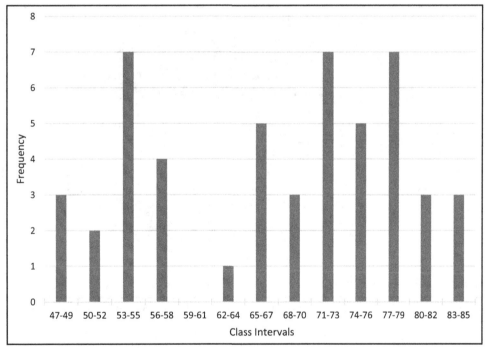

Figure 3–9 Bar graph of heart scores in a hypothetical population. The data from Table 3–9 and depicted in Figure 3–8 in a frequency polygon are depicted in a bar graph here.

achievement test scores. Individual test data plotted on a cumulative frequency curve can be used to evaluate an individual's function and diagnosis.

In designing a cumulative frequency curve, the ordinate axis is used to display cumulative frequencies, cumulative percentages, or cumulative proportions. The abscissa shows the score values as midpoints or individual scores.

The shape of the cumulative frequency curve reflects the form or shape of the original frequency distribution.

As a general rule, the cumulative frequency curve will have the greatest slope or most rapid rate of rise at the point where there is the greatest accumulation of the scores in the original frequency distribution. The cumulative frequency curve levels off and shows the lowest slope for the class intervals when there are fewer scores. Cumulative curves do not describe variations in the data as well as histograms and should not be used to draw conclusions about the form or shape of the data. The original frequency distribution is best used for this purpose.

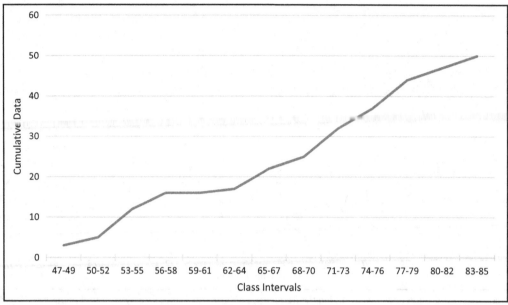

Figure 3–10 Cumulative frequency distribution polygon using data from Table 3–9.

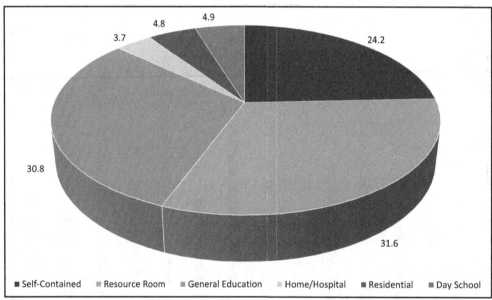

- Self-Contained   ■ Resource Room   ■ General Education   ■ Home/Hospital   ■ Residential   ■ Day School

Figure 3–11 An example of a statistical pie graph that illustrates the hypothetical percentages of specialty practice areas of women physicians.

3.13.4 Statistical Pie

A statistical pie is a pictorial representation of the relative percentage of discrete values, or nominal categories, for a variable, such as health professions, distributions of disease, occupational role functions, types of work injuries, or treatment techniques applied. It is particularly useful to quickly assess the relative percentage of each category. In Figure 3–11, the percentage of students with special needs in each type of educational placement is graphically displayed in a statistical pie.

Constructing a Statistical Pie

Step 1. *Make sure the statistical pie is relevant for describing data.* The statistical pie is appropriate when there are between 3 and 10 discrete categories. If there are more than 10 categories, the data will be better presented in a frequency distribution table. The data collected should be categorical and inclusive. For example, data collected regarding the cause of death should include all major causes for a designated population and should add up to 100%. Unknown causes should be included in the statistical pie.

Step 2. *First organize data into a frequency distribution table deriving relative percentages for each category.* In the hypothetical example below, specialty areas for female physicians are described. A sample of 250 female physicians was surveyed.

MEDICAL SPECIALTY	FREQUENCY	RELATIVE PERCENT
Pediatrics	84	33.6
Psychiatry and Neurology	34	13.7
Internal Medicine	25	10.0
Anesthesiology	23	9.1
Pathology	22	8.6
General Surgery	4	1.6
Other	58	23.4
Totals	**250**	**100**

Step 3. *Transform relative percent into the degrees of a circle, which is the proportion of 360 degrees.* The relative percent is multiplied by 360 degrees.

Step 4. *Use software with graphing capabilities to construct the pie chart.* Divide the statistical pie with a protractor into seven segments running clockwise starting with the largest category at 12 o'clock, which in this example is pediatrics (33.6% or 121°), other (23.4% or 84°), and psychiatry and neurology (13.7% or 49°). Continue with the other specialty areas in completing the 360° circle.

Step 5. *Label each segment category with the relative percent rather than the degrees of arc.* The completed statistical pie is shown in Figure 3–12.

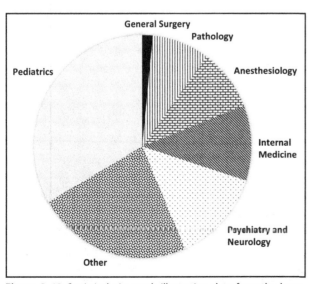

Figure 3–12 Statistical pie graph illustrating data from the hypothetical data of women physicians.

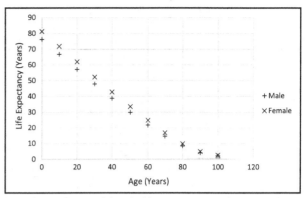

Figure 3–13 Male and female life expectancy in the United States for all races in 2019.

3.13.5 Scatter Diagrams

A scatter diagram is a graphic representation of the relationship between two variables. In this example, the scatter plot depicts the relationship between age (presumed independent variable) and life expectancy (presumed dependent variable) in males and females between the age of zero and 100 years (Figure 3–13). The size of the class interval for age (x-axis) is 20 years, and the size of the class interval for life expectancy (y-axis) is 10 years. The highest life expectancy is approximately 80 for females and is a few years less for males. This is associated with the youngest age on the y-axis (zero). Visual examination of scatter diagrams often reveals a trend. In Figure 3–13, the trend is that as age increases, the life expectancy (meaning the number of years one is expected to continue to live at a given age) decreases. The points located on the scatter diagrams are coordinates in which the two variables intersect. For example, in this graph, the expected life expectancy at age 100 is approximately 2 years.

Constructing a Scatter Diagram

In a hypothetical example a researcher collects the following data, examining the relationship between grip strength as measured by a Jamar dynamometer and functional activities of daily living (ADL) scores as measured by the Klein-Bell Test for clients with muscular dystrophy.

Step 1. *Record raw data for hypothetical example of grip strength and ADL scores in patients with muscular dystrophy.*

PARTICIPANTT	GRIP STRENGTH (ABSCISSA)	ADL SCORE (ORDINATE)
01	15	20
02	40	95
03	30	50
04	30	80
05	10	20

06	25	15
07	10	15
08	20	42
09	20	15
10	15	75
11	10	70
12	30	60
13	20	45
14	10	30
15	40	85

Step 2. *Determine the range along the abscissa (grip strength) and ordinate (ADL scores).* The range for grip strength is 30 (highest value, 40, minus lowest value, 10). The range for ADL scores is 80 (highest value, 95, minus lowest value, 15).

Step 3. *Determine the number of the class intervals for each variable.* Using the convention of 6 to 15 class intervals, we would establish 8 class intervals for grip strength with the size of the interval being 5. The actual score values are 5, 10, 15, 20, 25, 30, 35, 40 (along the abscissa). For ADL scores, the class interval is 20 with a range from 15 to 95. The actual score values plotted along the ordinate are 0, 20, 40, 60, 80, and 100.

Step 4. *Design the scatter diagram (illustrated in Figure 3–14) with the score value on the abscissa (grip strength) and ordinate (ADL scores).* For example, Participant 01 had a grip strength score of 15 and an ADL score of 20. The investigator plots the coordinates for all 15 participants.

In the above example, a *positive relationship* is noted because higher scores on one variable tend to be associated with higher scores on the other variable. A negative or inverse relationship is obtained when higher scores on one variable tend to occur with lower scores on the other variable. The degree of relationship between the two variables, or the *correlation coefficient*, will be discussed in Chapter 5.

3.14 Measures of Central Tendency

The first step in organizing data is usually to design a frequency distribution table or graph. The table or graph provides information concerning the form of the data. The properties of a set of data can be further described by calculating a summary statistic, such as a measure of central tendency. Measures of central tendency describe "typical" or "average" values in a distribution of data. An index of central tendency provides one value that best captures the distribution as a whole. There are generally three ways to do this:

1. *Mode:* The most frequent score in a distribution.
2. *Median:* The point halfway between the top and bottom halves of a distribution (50th percentile).
3. *Mean:* The arithmetic average of all the scores ($\bar{X}$ or M).

3.14.1 Mode

The mode is the easiest measure of central tendency to find and the simplest to interpret. It may be used to describe any distribution, whether the data is nominal, ordinal, interval, or ratio.

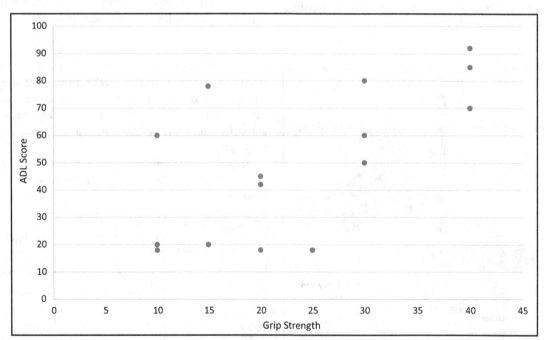

Figure 3–14 Example of a scattergram. Hypothetical example showing the relationship between grip strength and ADL scores in clients with muscular dystrophy.

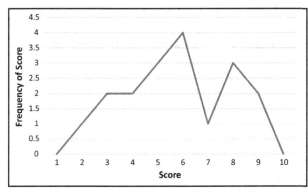

Figure 3–15 Illustration of a mode. The highest point is the mode.

Definition. The mode is the most frequent score (raw or ungrouped data) or the midpoint of the interval containing the most scores (grouped data). In a frequency distribution graph, the mode is the highest peak in the graph. Figure 3–15 illustrates the mode using the following data on a distribution of scores in which there is only one mode:

SCORE (X)	FREQUENCY OF SCORE (f)	
3	1	
4	2	
5	2	
6	4	Mode = 6
7	2	
8	3	
9	2	

There is no mode in a distribution of scores if all the scores occur with the same frequency (Figure 3–16). For example:

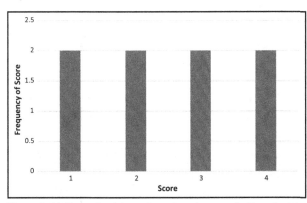

Figure 3–16 Example of data where there is no mode. Note that the frequency of each score is the same.

SCORE (X)	FREQUENCY OF SCORE (F)
1	2
2	2

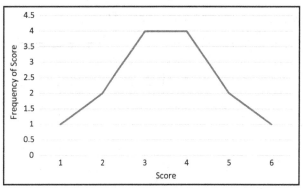

Figure 3–17 Example illustrating the mode when the data has two adjacent numbers with the same frequencies. In this case, the mode is equal to the average of the two adjacent numbers (e.g., (3 + 4) / 2 = 3.5).

3	2
4	2

When two adjacent scores have the same frequency and this frequency is higher than any other scores in the distribution, the mode is the average of the two adjacent scores (Figure 3–17). For example:

SCORE (X)	FREQUENCY OF SCORE (f)	
1	1	
2	2	
3	4	
		Mode = 3.5
4	4	
5	2	
6	1	

For grouped data, it is necessary to first calculate the midpoint of each class interval before computing the mode. The mode is then the midpoint of the interval containing the most scores (Figure 3–18).

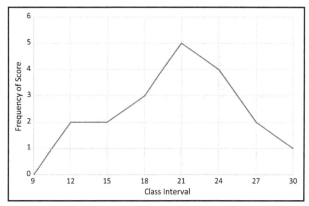

Figure 3–18 Example of a mode when grouped data are used.

CLASS INTERVAL	MIDPOINT	FREQUENCY OF SCORES (f)	
10–12	11	2	
13–15	14	2	
16–18	17	3	
19–21	20	5	Mode = 20
22–24	23	4	
25–27	26	2	
28–30	29	1	

The mode is the simplest measure of central tendency but it has two primary limitations:

1. Frequency distributions may have more than one mode, such as a bimodal or even tri-modal distribution. In this case, there may be ambiguity about which mode to report, especially if the two (or more) peaks in the distribution are nearly equal. Often one mode is reported as the *primary* or major mode (slightly higher peak), and the other peak reported as the *secondary* or minor mode (Figure 3–19).

2. When data are grouped, the mode is sensitive to the size and number of class intervals. By changing the class intervals for a distribution, the mode will change—sometimes drastically.

3.14.2 Median

A second and more sophisticated measure of central tendency is the median. The median is appropriate as a measure of central tendency for ordinal, interval, or ratio data but not for nominal (categorical) data from which the mode is the only measure of central tendency that can be calculated.

Definition. The median is the 50th percentile in an ordered group of scores, that is, the point in an array of scores that has 50% of the cases below it and 50% of the cases above it. The median divides the ranked scores into halves, with one half of the scores below the median and one half of the scores above the median.

The calculation of the median is a simple procedure for raw or ungrouped data:

Step 1. *When the number of cases, N, is odd, the median is the score of case (N + 1) / 2 after scores are ranked (either in ascending or descending order).* For example, consider the following array of nine scores:

6, 2, 17, 5, 11, 8, 3, 13, 10

To calculate the median, the nine scores are ranked in order as follows:

RANK OF SCORE	SCORE	FREQUENCY	
1	2	1	
2	3	1	4 scores below median
3	5	1	
4	6	1	
5	**8**	**1**	**Median = 8**
6	10	1	
7	11	1	
8	13	1	4 scores above median
9	17	1	

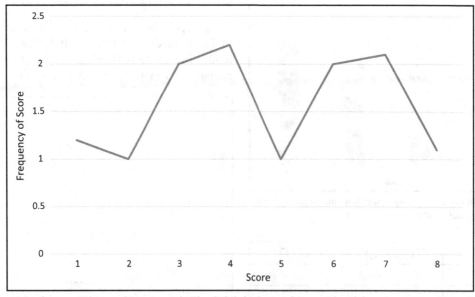

Figure 3–19 Example of scores with an ambiguous mode. The slightly higher peak is considered the primary or major mode, while the next highest peak is considered the secondary or minor mode.

Median = (score for rank N + 1) / 2
        = (score for rank 9 + 1) / 2
        = score for rank 5.

Therefore, the median is equal to the score for rank #5, which is equal to the score of 8.

Step 2. *When N is even, the median is the score midway between the scores after all scores are ranked.* For example, consider the following scores ($N = 8$):

2, 1, 10, 7, 0, 15, 8, 5

The first step in calculating the median is again to rank order the scores.

RANK OF SCORE	SCORE	FREQUENCY	
1	0	1	
2	l	1	3 scores below median
3	2	1	
4	5	1	
			Median = 6 (midpoint of 5 and 7)
5	7	1	
6	8	1	
7	10	1	3 scores above median
8	15	1	

For *grouped data*, the median is the point in a distribution at or below which exactly 50% of the cases fall. The median is calculated by constructing a cumulative frequency distribution. The median is then calculated from the cumulative frequency distribution with the following formula:

$$\text{Median} = LL + \left(w_i \left[\frac{(\frac{N}{2}) - cf}{f_i} \right] \right)$$

Where:
LL = lower real limit of the median interval
w_i = width of class interval
N = number of cases
cf = cumulative frequency up to the median interval
f_i = frequency within the median interval

The first stage in calculating the median is to construct a cumulative frequency distribution beginning with the lowest class interval and proceeding in ascending order to the highest class interval. The next step is to locate the interval that contains the 50th percentile or the median by examining the cumulative frequency column. For example:

CLASS INTERVAL	REAL LIMITS	f	Cf	CUMULATIVE PERCENTILE	
12–14	11.5–14.5	2	2	10	
15–17	14.5–17.5	4	6	20	
18–20	17.5–20.5	3	9	45	
21–23	**20.5–23.5**	**5**	**14**	**70**	**The median is in the class interval in which the 50th percentile rests.**
24–26	23.5–26.5	3	17	85	
27–29	26.5–29.5	2	19	95	
30–32	30.5–32.5	1	20	100	

Inspection of the above cumulative frequency distribution shows that the median or 50th percentile must fall in the class interval of 21–23 because the previous interval of 18–20 has accumulated only 9 of the 20 total cases, that is, 45%, or the 45th percentile.

LL = lower real limit of median interval = 20.5
w_i = width of class interval = 3
N = total number of cases in the frequency distribution = 20

cf = cumulative frequency *up to* median interval = 9 (starting from the lowest to the highest score)
f_i = frequency within median interval = 5

Therefore:

$$\text{Median} = LL + \left(w_i \left[\frac{\left[\left(\frac{N}{2} \right) - cf \right]}{f_i} \right] \right)$$

$$= 20.5 + \left((3)\frac{\left[\left(\frac{20}{2}\right)-9\right]}{5} \right)$$

$$= 20.5 + \left[3\,(1/5)\right]$$
$$= 20.5 + 3\,(.20)$$
$$= 20.5 + .6$$
$$= 21.1$$

The above formula can be used to calculate the median for any grouped frequency distribution, as well as for ungrouped distributions (with or without tied scores).

Calculation of the Raw Score from the Percentile Rank. A modification of the formula allows a generalized method for calculating raw scores corresponding to a given percentile rank (PR).

$$LL + \left[(w_i) \left(\frac{\left\{ \left[\frac{(PR)(N)}{100} \right] - cf \right\}}{f_i} \right) \right]$$

Where:

LL = lower real limit of the interval containing the given raw score, that is, (PR) (N) / 100
w_i = width of the class interval
PR = percentile rank
N = number of cases in the distribution
cf = cumulative frequency up to the given class interval containing the raw score
f_i = number of cases within the class interval containing the raw score.

In the next example, what is the raw score corresponding to the 90th percentile rank?

Raw score *(rs)* at 90th percentile rank =

$$26.5 + \left[(3) \left(\frac{\left\{ \left[\frac{(90)(N)}{100} \right] - cf \right\}}{f_i} \right) \right]$$

Where:

LL = 26.5 cf = 17
w_i = 3 f_i = 2
N = 20   PR = 90

$$rs = 5 + \left[(3) \left(\frac{\left\{ \left[\frac{(90)(20)}{100} \right] - 17 \right\}}{2} \right) \right]$$

$rs = 26.5 + [(3) *\{[(1800 / 100) - 17] / 2\}]$
$rs = 26.5 + \{(3) * [(18 - 17) / 2]\}$
$rs = 26.5 + 3\,(1 / 2)$
$rs = 26.5 + 1.5$

Therefore, a PR of 90 corresponds to a raw score of 28.

Calculation of the PR From the Raw Score. A researcher may also want to calculate the PR from the raw score. For example, given a raw score of 19 in a group distribution (see above data), what is the PR?

$$PR = \frac{\left[(f_i)(rs - LL) \right] + \left[(w_i)(cf) \right]}{(N)(w_i)}$$

Where:

f_i = 3 rs = 19
LL = 17.5 w_i = 3
cf = 6 N = 20

$$PR = \frac{\left[(3)(19 - 17.5) \right] + \left[(3)(6) \right]}{\left[(20)(3) \right]}$$

$$= \{[(3)\,(1.5) - 17.5] + (18)]\}/ 60$$
$$= (4.5 + 18) / 60$$
$$= 22.5 / 60$$
$$= 37.5 \text{ PR}$$

Therefore, a raw score of 19 equals a percentile rank of 37.5.

3.14.3 Mean

The mean is the most widely used and familiar index of central tendency. The mean is the arithmetic average of all the scores in a distribution and is calculated by summing all scores and dividing by the total number of scores.

The general formula for the mean $(\overline{X})$ is

$$\overline{X} = X_1 + X_2 + X_3 \ldots X_n / N$$
$$\overline{X} = \Sigma X / N$$

Where:

X_1 = first raw score
X_2 = second raw score
X_3 = third raw score
X_n = *nth* raw score
Σ = summation or sum of
N = number of subjects in the distribution

The mean may be conceptualized as a "center of gravity" or "balance point" in which the scores or "weights" on one side exactly balance the scores or weights on the other side. Each weight represents a score from a distribution of scores. The arithmetic mean of all the scores or weights is the center of gravity or balance point.

The deviation of scores in one direction exactly equals the deviation of scores in the other direction.

Calculating the Mean with Raw or Ungrouped Data. The mean is readily calculated for a distribution of raw scores in which each score occurs only once. The mean is simply the sum of the raw scores divided by the number of scores. For example, consider the following distribution of eight scores:

3, 6, 7, 8, 11, 15, 16, 22

$\Sigma X = 88$
$N = S$
$\bar{X} = \Sigma X / N$
$\quad = (3 + 6 + 7 + 8 + 11 + 15 + 16 + 22) / 8$
$\quad = 88 / 8$
$\quad = 11.0$

The mean or average value is calculated as 11.0.

For ungrouped data with a small sample of scores, the above procedure may be used to calculate the mean. Alternatively, for grouped data, a frequency distribution should be set up. Then the mean is calculated from the frequency distribution table by multiplying each score by the frequency of occurrence and summing the total across all scores before dividing by the total number of scores.

In the following example, several scores occur more than once:

2, 3, 3, 4, 5, 5, 6, 6, 6, 7, 8, 8, 9, 9, 9

Step 1. *The first stage in computing the mean is to form a frequency distribution table.*

X	f	fX
2	1	2
3	2	6
4	1	4
5	2	10
6	3	18
7	1	7
8	2	16
9	3	27
		$\Sigma (fX) = 90$

The number in the third column is obtained by multiplying each raw score by the frequency of occurrence. The symbol *fX* represents the product of the scores multiplied by the frequency of scores. This column is then summed and divided by the total number of scores, in this example, 15 scores.

$\bar{X} = \Sigma fX / N$

So:
$\Sigma fX = 90$
$\quad N = 15$
$\quad\quad = 90 / 15$
$\quad\quad = 6.0$

Calculating the Mean for Grouped Data. When working with grouped data, first find the midpoint of each score interval before calculating the mean.

The general formula to determine the mean for grouped data is

$\bar{X} = \Sigma fX / N$

As an example, consider the following scores grouped into six class intervals:

CLASS INTERVAL	MIDPOINT (X)	f	fX
3–5	4	2	8
6–8	7	1	7
9–11	10	4	40
12–14	13	6	78
15–17	16	3	48
18–20	19	4	76
		$\Sigma f = 20$	$\Sigma fX = 257$

Therefore,
$\bar{X} = 257 / 20$
$\bar{X} = 12.85$

In the above example, the midpoint of each class interval (X) was multiplied by the frequency in each interval. This product was summed over all the class intervals to give a value equal to 257. This value (ΣfX) is then divided by the total number of scores or the sum of the frequencies (i.e., $\Sigma f = 20$) to yield the final calculated mean of 12.85.

The mean calculated from a grouped frequency distribution will differ slightly from the mean calculated from raw scores. When scores are grouped, information is lost and a certain amount of inaccuracy introduced. As a general rule, the coarser the grouping of scores, the more the grouped mean will differ from the raw score mean. Nonetheless, for most situations in which 10 to 20 class intervals are typically used, the agreement is close enough between the two calculated means.

Comparing the Mode, Median, and Mean

1. As a measure of central tendency, the mean takes into account all the scores of the distribution and is affected by each single value. One extreme score or "outlier" can influence the mean to a large degree,

especially with small samples. For example, in the following distribution of ten scores, both the mean and median have a value of 6.0; when an extreme score of 50 is added as the eleventh score, the mean dramatically increases to 10.0, while the median changes only to 7.0:

Scores: 2, 3, 4, 4, 5, 7, 8, 8, 9, 10
Mean = 6.0   Median = 6.0

The mean is changed when an extreme score of 50 is added:

Scores: 2, 3, 4, 4, 5, 7, 8, 8, 9, 10, 50
Mean = 10.0 Median = 7.0

Therefore, when extreme scores or outliers are present in a frequency distribution of scores, the median may be a more appropriate measure of central tendency than the mean.

2. In distributions that are symmetrical in shape, the mean equals the median, and both are equal to the mode if the distribution is unimodal. This is illustrated in Figure 3–20.

3. In distributions that are symmetrical but not unimodal, it is important to report the mode, mean, and median to provide a clearer picture of the shape and central tendency of the distribution. In Figure 3–21, which depicts a bimodal distribution, there are two modes (at 28 and 40) that should be noted: the mean equals the median and both equal 34.

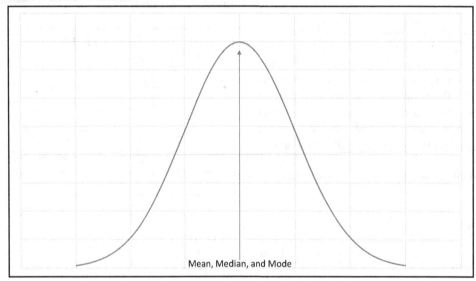

Figure 3–20 The normal unimodal curve depicting the mean, median, and mode. All three fall at the same place on a bell-shaped curve.

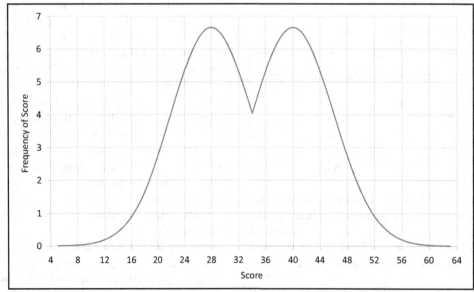

Figure 3–21 Comparison of mean, median, and mode in a bimodal distribution. The two modes have the value of 28 and 38. The median and the mean have the same value, 34.

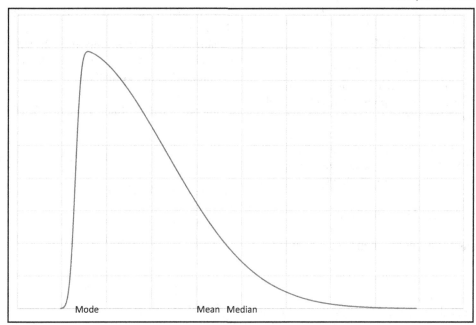

Figure 3–22 A positively skewed distribution. Notice that the Figure is pulled to the left, indicating that the scores with the largest frequencies are at the lower end of the distribution.

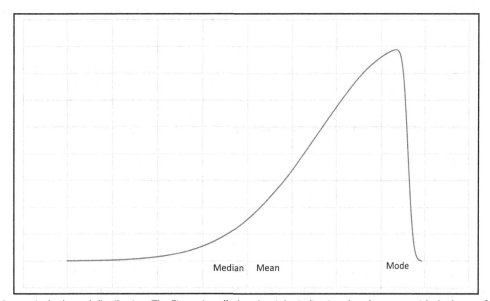

Figure 3–23 A negatively skewed distribution. The Figure is pulled to the right, indicating that the scores with the largest frequencies are at the upper end of the distribution.

4. In distributions that are skewed to the left or right, the mode, median, and mean will have different values. Note that the mean is pulled either to the right or to the left by the outliers or extreme scores on one end of the skewed distribution. The median is the preferred measure of central tendency for skewed distributions, especially as the degree of skewness increases. Figures 3–22 and 3–23 illustrate the locations of the three measures of central tendency for right- and left-skewed distributions.

Common descriptive statistics often cited in regard to public health documents include those under the umbrella term "Vital Statistics."

3.15 VITAL STATISTICS

The quality of a health care system in a country is usually described by vital statistics such as the infant mortality rate, rates of illnesses and diseases, life expectancy, and mortality rates from specific diseases. In justifying the need for a research study in a clinical area, the researcher first reports the incidence and prevalence rates of a disability or illness to establish the importance of the study. The following are some of the most common vital statistics.

3.15.1 Crude Mortality (Death) or Morbidity (Disease) Rates

The crude mortality or morbidity rate is calculated by dividing the frequency of deaths or illnesses by the total number of individuals in the population. This number is then multiplied by 1,000, 10,000, or 100,000 so it can be used as a comparative Figure. For example, if a certain population has a mortality rate of 9.3 per 1,000 population per year, how does this compare with another population where there are 180,000 deaths in a population of 24,000,000?

Calculation of Crude Mortality Rate

Crude death rate = (180,000 / 24,000,000) (1,000)
$$= .0075 \times 1,000$$
$$= 7.5 \text{ per } 1,000 \text{ population}$$

In this hypothetical case, the investigator would conclude that there is a lesser mortality rate in the sample of 180,000 deaths per 24,000,000 population than in the 9.3 per 1,000 population.

3.15.2 Prevalence and Incidence Rates of Disability or Disease

The terms *prevalence rate* and *incidence rate* are often confused with each other. Prevalence rate refers to the number or proportion of a population who have a given condition. Incidence rate is the number of new cases of a condition within a given time period.

In 2012 the estimated population in the United States was about 313,000,000. In that same year there were an estimated 1,218,400 people in the United States living with HIV infection (www.cdc.gov/hiv/pdf/statistics_2012_HIV_Surveillance_Report_vol_24.pdf). In the same year, the estimated incidence for new cases of HIV infection was about 48,000 (Division of HIV/AIDS Prevention, 2014).

Calculation of Prevalence and Incidence Rates

Incidence rate = (48,000 / 313,000,000) (100,000)
$$= .000153 (100,000)$$
$$= 15.3 \text{ per } 100,000 \text{ population}$$
Prevalence rate = (1,218,400 / 313,000,000) (100,000)
$$= .0038 (100,000)$$
$$= 380 \text{ per } 100,000 \text{ population}$$

3.15.3 Adjusted Rate

Researchers are also interested in obtaining statistics for specific populations. In these examples, the calculation of rates is adjusted. For example, an investigator is interested in comparing infant mortality rates adjusted for gender. In a hypothetical population there are 40,000

births of males and 35,000 births of females. In this population, 150 males and 180 females die at birth. What are the adjusted infant mortality rates for females compared with the total crude rates per 1,000 population?

Calculation of Crude Rate

Crude rate = [(150 + 180) / (40,000 + 35,000)] [1,000]
$$= (330 / 75,000) (1,000)$$
$$= (.0044) (1,000)$$
$$= 4.4 \text{ per } 1,000 \text{ (for both males and females)}$$

Adjusted Rate for Females

Adjusted rate = (180 / 35,000) (1,000)
$$= (.0051) (1000)$$
$$= 5.14 \text{ per } 1,000$$

For this hypothetical example, it appears that the infant mortality rate is higher in females compared with the total population.

3.16 MEASURES OF VARIABILITY

Measures of variability are descriptive statistics that indicate how scores in a distribution differ from each other and from the mean. For example, in a distribution with the scores 7, 7, 7, 7, the measure of variability is 0 because the scores do not differ from each other and from the mean of 7. The measure of variability increases from zero as the scores vary from each other and from the mean. The *measures of variability* are the range, variance, and standard deviation.

3.16.1 Range

The *range* is the value derived from subtracting the smallest score in the distribution from the largest score. In the distribution 21, 23, 24, 26, 28, 30, the range is 9. The range is a crude measure of variability because only the highest and the lowest scores of a distribution are used in the calculation.

3.16.2 Variance

The *variance* is a measure of the variability of scores in a distribution that takes into account all the scores in that distribution. The computational formula for the variance is:

$$s^2 = \frac{\left[N\Sigma X^2 - (\Sigma X)^2 \right]}{N}(N-1)$$

Where:

N = total number of subjects or scores in the distribution

$\sum X^2$ = raw scores are squared and then the values are totaled

$(\sum X)^2$ = the value which equals the square of the summation of the scores.

Example of Calculating the Variance

PARTICIPANT	SCORE (X)	X^2
01	2	4
02	4	16
03	7	49
04	9	81
05	10	100
06	12	144
07	14	196
$N = 7$	$\sum X = 58$	$\sum X^2 = 590$

Computational Formula for the Variance

$s^2 = [N \sum X^2 - (\sum X)^2] / [N (N - 1)]$
$s^2 = [(7)(590) - (58)^2] / [7 (7 - 1)]$
$s^2 = [4130 - 3364] / 42$
$s^2 = 766 / 42$
$s^2 = 18.238$

3.16.3 Standard Deviation

The *standard deviation is* the square root of the variance. In the example above, the variance equals 18.23. Therefore, the standard deviation equals 4.27. The standard deviation is a useful value in that it carries the same units as the mean (the units of the original measurements: kilograms, centimeters, seconds, degrees). It is also used in inferential statistics, such as the *t*-test.

3.17 STEM AND LEAF DISPLAYS

A stem and leaf display is a method of displaying data that was developed by Tukey (1977) and is an alternative to the frequency distribution. It derives its name from its display: any given number is divided into two parts, a stem and a leaf. The first part, the stem, represents a large class into which the number falls, while the second number, the leaf, designates the actual placement in the larger class. For example, the number 15 can be divided into 1 (the stem) and 5 (the leaf), while the number 216 can be divided into 2 or 21 (the stem) and 16 or 6 (the leaf). When the stem and leaves are displayed in a column, the researcher can easily visualize the organization of the

data. The researcher is able to identify the specific scores obtained, as well as the frequency of the class of scores.

An example of unpublished data helps to explain the concept. Pre- and post-test data were collected to determine the change in understanding of collaboration techniques. The pre- and post-test scores are in Table 3–10.

In constructing a stem and leaf plot, the first step is to rank order the data. Table 3–11 tabulates the rank ordered data from Table 3–10.

Once the data are rank ordered the next step is to list the "stems," which in our case is the first digit of the scores, for example 1, 2, 3, 4, 5, and 6. Then for the leaves, place the second digit to their respective stems according to their size. Once completed, the stem and leaf plot can be seen in Table 3–12.

Once the data are organized into a stem and leaf display, a graph is drawn, allowing the researcher to visualize the structure of the data. The whisker is a line that connects the hinges to the extremes. An example of this is seen in Figure 3–24. An examination of the two box plots in this Figure reveals that there is little difference between the two scores. Although the upper extreme and

TABLE 3–10
HYPOTHETICAL PRE- AND POST-TEST DATA

PARTICIPANT	PRE-TEST SCORE	POST-TEST SCORE
1	39	39
2	46	48
3	15	18
4	12	18
5	64	69
6	24	22
7	54	57
8	55	59
9	33	35
10	37	39
11	35	38
12	41	43
13	63	66
14	42	44
15	43	46
16	27	24
17	35	38
18	52	55
19	25	24
20	41	43

TABLE 3–11			
RANK ORDERED PRE- AND POST-TEST DATA			
PRE-TEST		POST-TEST	
SCORE	RANK	SCORE	RANK
12	1	18	1
15	2	18	2
24	3	22	3
25	4	24	4
27	5	24	5
33	6	35	6
35	7	38	7
35	8	38	8
37	9	39	9
39	10	39	10
41	11	43	11
41	12	43	12
42	13	44	13
43	14	46	14
46	15	48	15
52	16	55	16
54	17	57	17
55	18	59	18
63	19	66	19
64	20	69	20

TABLE 3–12			
STEM AND LEAF PLOT USING DATA FROM TABLE 3—10			
PRE-TEST		POST-TEST	
STEM	LEAF	STEM	LEAF
1	89	1	13
2	457	2	244
3	3579	3	58899
4	11236	4	33468
5	245	5	579
6	12	6	69

the upper hinge are higher on the post-test, the medians, lower extreme, and lower hinge are similar. There is more variability on the post-test.

3.18 Z-SCORES AND THE NORMAL CURVE

The z-scores are summary values that indicate the distance between a raw score and the mean, using standard deviation units. For example, a z-score of 0 (zero) is equal to the mean. The z-scores are important to describe the relative standing of a raw score. For example, a raw score of 40 is equal to a z-score of +1 in a normal distribution with a mean equal to 30 and one standard deviation equal to 10. Figure 3–25 illustrates the z-score for a raw score of 40.

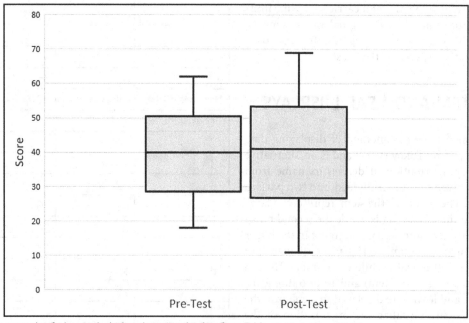

Figure 3–24 An example of a box and whisker plot using the data from Tables 3–10, 3–11, and 3–12.

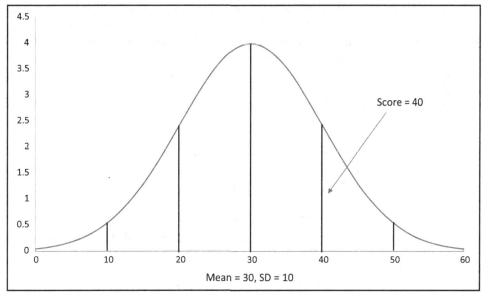

Figure 3–25 Normal curve depicting raw score of 40, mean of 30, SD of 10. Notice that a raw score of 40 lies one standard deviation above the mean (e.g., *z*-score of + 1) and at a percentile of 84.

In this example, a raw score of 40 is equal to a percentile rank of 84, which means that an individual with a *z*-score of +1 did better than, or is above, 84% of the individuals in that distribution.

The formula for calculating *z*-scores is:

z = (raw score – mean) / standard deviation, or
  $z = (\text{rs} - \bar{X}) / \text{SD}$

In the above example:

$z = [40 - 30] / 10$
$z = 10 / 10$
$z = +1$

The *z*-scores can be positive or negative depending on whether the raw score is above or below the mean. These scores are widely used in psychometric testing and are helpful in interpreting raw scores.

3.19 Central Limit Theorem: Normality and the Normal (Gaussian) Curve

Many human characteristics, for example height, given a large enough population, will show a frequency distribution that is what is known as a "normal curve." A normal curve is also known as a "bell-shaped" curve, because, indeed, that is what it appears to be (Figure 3–25). Another term for this is the Gaussian distribution. Researchers take samples from this population, and from the characteristics of the sample (mean and

standard deviation, usually) make inferences about those values in the greater population itself. These values are called the parameters of the population. No researcher can be confident that the one sample drawn for that one study accurately reflects the greater population. That is, such samples are subject to sampling error.

Imagine researchers taking repeated samples from the population. The means of some of them will be above the population mean, and of others will be below the population mean. A few sample means might be right on the population mean. If these sample mean values were plotted in a frequency distribution graph, they, too, would create a normal curve. In other words, most sample means will be close to the population mean. The farther from the population mean the sample mean turned out to be, the fewer times the researcher would have drawn a sample of that extreme of a mean.

The Central Limit Theorem states that, even when the population distribution is not normal (is skewed from a perfect bell-shaped curve), the sampling distribution described above will be a normal curve. The Central Limit Theorem is a powerful theorem in statistics, because it allows us, through the use of statistical probability formulas, to make calculations telling us how confident we can be that one single sample is representative of the population. This logic can also be applied when we are applying statistics to the question of whether one intervention is truly better than another. The Central Limit Theorem assures us that we can accurately calculate the probability that the difference between the two sample group means reflects a real difference in the means of the corresponding populations. This process of statistical inference about differences will be covered in detail in Chapters 4, 5, and 6.

For the occupational therapist, one of the most difficult decisions is to decide whether a client's physiological, physical, or psychological function is within normal limits. What is normal blood pressure, heart rate, muscle strength, height, visual-perceptual function, or intelligence? Is normality a function of personality or behavior or is it a statistical value?

When an individual goes to a physician for a physical examination, the physiological and neurological functions are tested to determine whether they are within normal limits. Predetermined values are used by the physician to compare with the patient's results. Individual differences within a range of normality are accepted by the physician in determining that a function is normal. The same judgments are made by the occupational therapist in testing range of motion in a specific joint, or in evaluating muscle strength, or many other characteristics of human function.

On the other hand, the statistician's definition of normality and abnormality will depend on the frequency of occurrences within designated class intervals. Abnormality is interpreted by the statistician as a deviation from the mean value, such as 1 or 2 standard deviation units from the mean of a normally distributed variable. In research, scores or values that are abnormal are considered to be outliers or scores that vary widely from expected values. Many times those outliers or abnormal scores are considered at odds with the rest of the values in a distribution. Consider the scatter diagram in Figure 3–26. Four of the five scores are consistent with a positive relationship with the X and Y variables. However, one coordinate (50, 5) seems to be an outlier and does not fit into the pattern. The outlier or abnormal score should be discussed separately by the researcher.

The normal curve (Figure 3–27) is the statistician's guide for examining the relationship between normal values and outliers. In the normal curve it is expected that 68% of the cases will lie within −1 to +1 standard deviation units of the mean and 96% of the cases will lie within −2 to +2 standard deviations of the mean. If we know that a characteristic is normally distributed, then by calculating

the mean and standard deviation of a population, we will be able to determine how many of the cases will be within −2 to +2 standard deviation units from the mean. For example, if we know that the resting heart rate is normally distributed and that the mean value for adults is 72 beats per minute with a standard deviation of 5, then we can determine the percentile ranks from the raw scores. For example, what is the PR of an individual with a resting heart rate score of 78?

The normal curve in Figure 3–27 shows the relationship between the raw score of 78 and the normal values for resting heart rate. We estimate that, based on the diagram, the PR for a raw score of 78 will be slightly above the 88th PR.

Calculation of PR. First calculate z-scores from raw scores:

$$z = (rs − \bar{X})\,SD_z$$
$$= (78 − 72) / 5$$
$$= 6 / 5 = 1.2$$
$$z = +1.2$$

Look up the percentile rank from the statistical table (C–2 in the appendices) for the z-score of +1.2. Note that in Table C–2, a z-score of +1.2 is equal to the percentile rank of .8849.

Earlier in this chapter, a discussion about the utility of descriptive statistics was made in reference to comparative statistics. What is meant by "comparative statistics" is loosely encapsulated by the quantitative statistics represented on the Experimental and Outcomes sides of the Research Pyramid. Many of these statistics can be grouped together in what is known as inferential statistics. Inferential statistics infer, which is markedly different from descriptive statistics, which describe. Inferential statistics can generally be sub-categorized into parametric or non-parametric statistics. For many parametric statistics, there is one or more non-parametric statistics

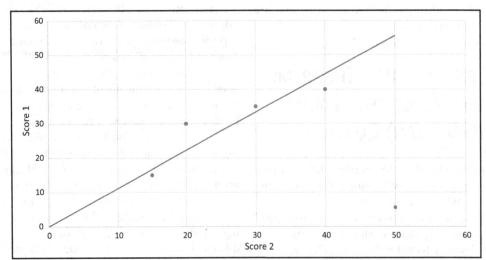

Figure 3–26 Scattergram showing an outlier at the coordinates of 50, 5. The outlier is the score that appears to be markedly different from the other scores.

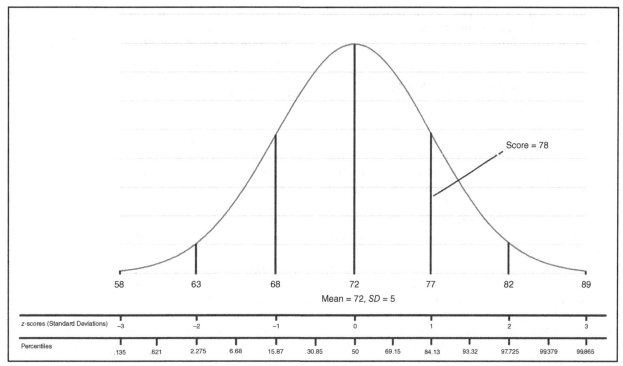

58   63   68   72   77   82   89

Mean = 72, *SD* = 5

| z-scores (Standard Deviations) | –3 | | –2 | | –1 | | 0 | | 1 | | 2 | | 3 |

| Percentiles | .135 | .621 | 2.275 | 6.68 | 15.87 | 30.85 | 50 | 69.15 | 84.13 | 93.32 | 97.725 | 99.379 | 99.865 |

Figure 3–27 Normal curve depicting the relationship between the heart beat rate of 78 when the mean is 72 and the standard deviation is 5. What is the *z*-score of this heart beat? Is it above or below normal?

that can be used to test the same hypotheses as the parametric statistics are. The differences between parametric and non-parametric statistics are based on the differing underlying assumptions upon which they are respectively based. Parametric statistics are more tightly conditioned than non-parametric statistics. While there are nuances unique to each type of parametric statistic, generally speaking, the assumptions include the following:

1. The sample is a random selection or is representative of the target population.
2. Each data point occurrence is independent from other data point occurrences.
3. The variances (or the standard deviations) in the compared groups are approximately the same.
4. The sizes of the two groups are approximately equal.

The first assumption states that participants recruited for the study are reflective of the general population from which they were recruited. Often this can be accomplished by randomly selecting participants from the pool of potential participants, thereby avoiding bias. The second and third assumptions are somewhat related in that the recruited participants should not be related in any way, that is, correlated with other members of the participant pool. If they were, then there would likely be unequal variances amongst the experimental groups. An example would be if participants were randomly recruited from area hospitals from across the state, however, a third of the participants all came from the same hospital and were assigned to the same group,

and moreover, they all were treated by the same occupational therapist compared to the other group where the participants came from all different locations from across the state. It is possible that the participants treated by the same occupational therapist would behave in a similar fashion, whereas the participants who each had their own unique therapist would have more variability in their respective behavior and therefore be more representative of the larger population within that state. The fourth assumption of near equal-sized groups has to do with the accuracy of the probability calculation of the statistic (how the formula arrives at the exact *p* value for a statistical test).

Given the above discussion of the Central Limit Theorem and sampling distributions always being normal, it is noteworthy to see the connection to inferential statistics. When researchers can ensure that all of the underlying assumptions are satisfied, then best practice is to use the parametric statistic that is most appropriate for the study design. This practice is commonly followed because parametric statistics are the most powerful statistic to use in most cases. Additionally, most parametric statistics require that the data are continuous variables, though there are some exceptions to this general rule. The *t*-test is robust to certain violations of its assumptions. Explaining why is beyond the scope of this text, though. If any of the underlying assumptions are markedly violated, then best practice is to use a non-parametric statistic that is most suited for the research design. For most parametric statistics, there are comparable non-parametric statistics. In the following chapters, examples of both parametric and non-parametric statistics appropriate to the chapter topic will be discussed in turn.

3.20 Chapter Summary

This section of the chapter introduced the concept of descriptive statistics, first by defining common statistical concepts and defining various types of data. Descriptive statistics, as the phrase indicates, describe. They portray characteristics of the variables of concern in research studies. At the most basic level, they provide a means to make simple observational comparisons. Despite them being the most basic type of statistic, they have great utility in providing key information for most research studies and can be either the main type of analysis or can be an adjunct alongside inferential statistics used to analyze hypotheses and research questions. A variety of examples for displaying descriptive statistics were discussed including frequency distributions, statistical pies, and scatter diagrams. Finally, concepts associated with the measures of central tendency were discussed including the Central Limit Theorem and descriptive statistics associated with vital statistics.

This chapter detailed methods to calculate many examples of descriptive statistics including but not limited to mean, mode, median, variance, and standard deviation. Additionally, many examples of how to graphically display descriptive data were detailed. The authors feel that it is important to understand the fundamentals associated with calculating and producing these descriptive statistics and their graphical representation, hence the detailed content presented in this chapter. It is also commonplace to generate these same statistics and Figures using software. Using software can be much more time-efficient and is the optimal method chosen by the majority of scholars. Using statistical software, though, without understanding the underlying fundamentals can lead to errors and misinterpretations in a study. It is pedagogically sound for students to truly understand the inherent meaning of these descriptive statistics and their graphical representation. As such, it is recommended to first review the material in this chapter and then explore the use of software to more efficiently generate the desired calculated descriptive statistics and any generated Figures for data portrayal.

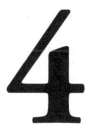

Inferential Statistics
Testing the Null Hypothesis

Inferential statistics—how are they different from descriptive statistics? Definition: "…a rigorous form of inductive inference… about population parameters… based on sample statistics."

Ferguson and Takane (1989, p. 145)

OPERATIONAL LEARNING OBJECTIVES

By the end of this chapter, the learner will be able to:

1. Define inferential statistics
2. Understand the difference between descriptive and inferential statistics
3. Articulate the concept of sampling regarding research participants
4. Apply confidence intervals in statistical analysis planning
5. Differentiate between Type I and Type II errors
6. Calculate effect size
7. Consider power analyses in determining sample size

DOI: 10.4324/9781003523154-4

Virtually all research studies use samples from theoretical larger groups (usually of people). The power of inferential statistics is that they can tell us something, solely from the samples in the study, about the populations from which these samples were drawn. Using the data in the samples (the sample statistics), conclusions can be drawn about the populations the samples were selected from (the population parameters). Based on certain mathematical assumptions, the inferential statistics allow for a quantification of the confidence the researcher can have in the study findings, as explained below.

4.1 SAMPLING/SAMPLING DISTRIBUTIONS/STANDARD ERROR OF THE MEAN

One of the most under-appreciated aspects of research studies in occupational therapy and health studies in general is that of sampling. Perhaps that is because therapists work mostly with small, special populations, and researchers are satisfied with any sample of volunteers they can recruit for a study. Nonetheless, how the sample was formed ("drawn from its population") has a profound effect on the interpretation of the findings of a study. It greatly affects how one study's findings can be generalized to other settings and other groups.

One oft-overlooked step in the process of sampling is a consideration of the ideal population. Which theoretical group of individuals is the researcher interested in? This ideal population could be as large in scope as all the people on earth who have a diagnosis of cerebral palsy (CP). It could be much narrower, if the researcher is only interested in those individuals with CP who attended one hospital clinic in the past year. If there is no intention to generalize the findings beyond the study itself, then defining the ideal population more narrowly is fine.

Whatever the definition of the ideal population, though, there are the practicalities of systematically finding members of that population. How is the researcher to obtain access to (theoretically) every member of the ideal population? For example, with the mobility in society, every ideal population is constantly gaining and losing members. Some members of the ideal population may in fact not be reachable by any feasible means. Thus, researchers will work with, and draw their samples from, the *accessible* population. This population might consist of a list of all the names and addresses of families whose children attend public schools in a single district, accurate as of the first of September in the year of the study. Whatever the findings are of a study drawing its sample from that accessible population, they can only directly be generalized back to this accessible population. They should not be applied to children who are home-schooled, for example, unless they are included in the address list of district pupils.

For the ability to directly generalize the findings from a sample back to the entire accessible population, the sample should be drawn through a probability or random procedure, explained below, thus giving high confidence that the sample is representative of the population. A non-probability or perhaps biased procedure for sampling would be taking a sample from the most convenient pool of individuals, for example, from a single school. Another type of non-probability sampling is quota sampling, where quotas are set by demographic characteristics, such as, participants will be sought until there are ten individuals in each age category (0–5 years, 6–10 years, 11–15 years) and each race/ethnicity grouping (African-American, Asian-American, Hispanic-American, Caucasian-American) for a total of $10 \times 3 \times 4$ or 120 individuals. Another non-probability sampling method is snowballing or cascading sampling. In this approach, individuals are recruited from the referrals of the first few volunteers, until saturation is reached (no more new individuals are being referred), or until the desired number of volunteers has been secured. For any of the non-probability methods of sampling it is very problematic to generalize directly to a larger population. The researcher cannot be confident that everyone in that larger population had an equal chance of being selected for the study.

In contrast, probability sampling provides that equal opportunity for participation in the study, which allows for a more direct generalization of the findings (strengthening external validity). Probability sampling comes in several types, as noted below.

1. Simple random sample—participants are invited to the study through a random number table or a software random number generator, ensuring every member of the accessible population (everyone on the list of potential participants) had an equal chance of being selected for the study.

2. Systematic random sample—here the sample is recruited from, for example, every tenth person on the list being invited to participate. The invitation list is generated more easily, but the resulting sample is probably not as representative of the accessible population as a simple random sample would be.

3. Stratified random sampling—when it is important for the research purpose to form sub-samples of equal size from demographic layers (or strata) of a population, this sampling method may be used. Within each stratum invitees are selected by a simple random sampling method. The final sample is a better representative of each stratum, though it may be less representative of the overall accessible population made up by all the strata.

4. Cluster sampling—if simple random sampling would be prohibitively expensive (ending up with the recruitment of individuals from all over a large country), clustering may be used. The accessible population is divided into clusters (e.g., regional schools). First a certain number of clusters are

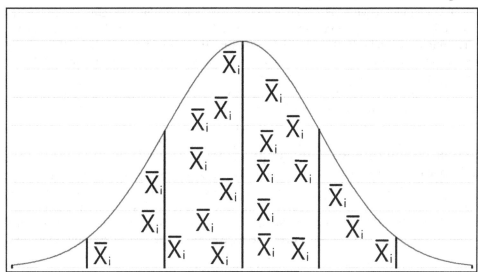

Figure 4–1 Normal curve distribution full of sample populations.

randomly sampled from the entire list of clusters. Then from within these geographically tighter clusters, simple random samples of individuals are drawn. According to the structure of the clusters, and how much variability there is among the clusters, the likely representativeness of the final sample can be estimated (Sudman, 1976).

5. Disproportional sampling—Occasionally a researcher will use this type of sampling, when it is more important to determine differences between sub-groups of the accessible population than to determine the parameters of the accessible population as a whole. The disproportion comes about because a larger percentage of one sub-group must be sampled since that sub-group is smaller than another. The aim is to have sub-group samples of equal size, for more accurate statistical comparison. The representativeness of the findings for the accessible population as a whole is thereby weakened, to the degree that the sub-groups do truly vary among themselves on the dependent variable.

Taking one sample from a population can never give certainty about the characteristics of that population. The sample just drawn may have in it a combination of individuals that is not representative of the population. They may be faster or slower. They may be stronger or weaker. In general, the sample mean may be above or below that of the population. It might be exactly on the population mean. It cannot be known, from one sample, which of these sampling errors it may have.

Imagine taking repeated samples, though, and plotting their means on a number line. The shape of that plot gives us a sampling distribution (see Figure 4–1). Some samples will have means above the population mean. Some will have means below that mean. There will be more samples, however, whose mean is closer to the population mean, than

samples whose mean is very far away from the population mean (although there will be a few of these with large errors). As we take more samples, the mean of the sample means will get closer and closer to the population mean. After all, if it had been possible to sample everybody once, the whole population would have been measured, so then of course the sample mean is the same as the population mean! It rarely happens that everyone in the theoretical population is sampled for a study. Therefore, we must rely on the shape of the sampling distribution to show something about the population mean. As noted in Chapter 3, the Central Limit Theorem indicates that the shape of the sampling distribution is a normal curve, and its mean is the population mean, *even if the distribution of values in the population is non-normal.* Another way of putting this claim is this: if there were enough statistics from samples, the population parameter could be specified to a more exact degree.

The standard deviation of the normal curve formed by the sampling distribution, called the **standard error of the mean**, is an estimate of the variability shown among sample means. Sample means drawn from a population will vary more if:

1. the population has greater **variability** (which is reflected by larger standard deviations in the samples) OR

2. the size of the sample we draw is **small** (the estimates of the population mean will be less accurate with a small sample).

Thus, the formula for the standard error of the mean (SEM):

SEM = *SD* / square root of *n*

where *SD* is the standard deviation among the scores in the sample, and *n* is the number of scores (people) in the sample.

Therefore, with a given sample it cannot be known what the population parameter is (usually, for the population mean), however, even just one sample can indicate the amount of confidence the researcher could have in the accuracy of the sample. The less varied the scores in the sample, the less probable it is that the population scores vary greatly. This fact alone indicates that our sample is likely to be more accurate. Likewise, if the sample is large, the less likely it is that the sample ended up with individuals who were all above the population average (yielding an overestimate of the population parameter), or who were all below the population average (yielding an underestimate of the population mean). The simple formula of the SEM quantifies how accurate the sample is likely to be.

4.2 CONFIDENCE INTERVALS

A clear understanding of the origin of the SEM allows a better understanding of confidence intervals (CI), which are often used in research studies to report the findings. Of course, if there was only one sample ever drawn from a population and studied, and if there were no Central Limit Theorem or concept of SEM, all the researcher could do is make a point estimate of the population mean: taking that one sample mean as the best estimate of the population mean ("taking X-bar to estimate Mu," in statistical language). It would be helpful to know, though, how far off this point estimate is likely to be, given the characteristics of the sample. In other words, a range around the sample mean is constructed, called an interval estimate, so that the researcher could be 95% or 99% confident that this **confidence interval** has captured the population mean. To calculate this interval estimate (the CI), two decisions must first be made by the researcher:

1. *Do I have a large or small sample?*

More than 30 is generally considered **large** (use the z distribution in the CI formula); 30 or less is generally considered **small** (then use the t distribution in the CI formula)

With a sample of more than 30 the probability is notably greater that the sample accurately reflects the population.

2. *How confident do I need to be that my estimate contains the population mean?*

Quite confident is OK (use a **95%** confidence interval)

I need to be all but certain (use a **99%** confidence interval)

The formula for confidence intervals (CI) is:

CI = (Sample Mean) $\pm$ (z or t value) $\times$ (Standard Error of the Mean)

The Sample Mean is found by averaging the scores in the sample. The Standard Error of the Mean is calculated by dividing the *SD* of the sample by the square root of *n*, the number of individuals in the sample, as noted above.

For large samples (> 30) use z, and find the appropriate z value in Table C–2, as follows:

For a **95% CI**, look in Table C–2 for the cell with **.97500** in it. That amount, the 97.5th percentile (47.5% between 0 and z plus 50% below 0), slices off 2.5% of the normal curve in the upper tail. Slicing another 2.5% off the lower tail would leave 95% of cases. The corresponding value of z to .9750 is 1.9 (from the row) plus 0.06 (from the column) or **1.96**, the number we want for the formula. Put another way, one needs to move 1.96 standard deviations above and below the mean in a normal curve to capture 95% of the cases in the distribution represented by the curve. What this means in practice is that in only 5% of the times you would draw a sample over 30 in size from its population would the researcher end up with a sample whose mean is outside the CI. Conversely, 95% of the time the researcher draws a sample of this large size from the population, the population mean will fall within the CI generated around the sample mean (using the SEM of the sample and that z value from the table).

For a **99% CI**, look in Table C–2 for the entry **.99506**. The 99.5th percentile slices 0.5% from the upper tail, and adding 0.5% from the lower tail gives a total of 1%, which leaves 99% of the cases. The corresponding value of z is **2.58**, the number we want for the formula this time. In other words, if the researcher wants to have 99% confidence that the CI has captured the population mean, 2.58 SD must be marked off above and below the mean, and multiplied by the SEM derived from that sample.

For small samples, the researcher uses a t-value instead of z. The appropriate t value is found in Table C–3. Assume an alpha = .05 in a two-tailed test. Remember that *df* (degrees of freedom) = sample size –1, in this situation. If the sample size is 20, your sample mean is 35.2, the Standard Error of the Mean is 4.5, and a 95% CI is desired, then the formula: 35.2 $\pm$ (2.093) $\times$ (4.5) is used, where 2.093 is the Table C–3 entry for *df* = 19, alpha =.05, two-tailed. That makes 35.2 $\pm$ 9.42 as the CI. Put another way, the chance is 95% that the population mean is between 25.8 (35.2–9.42) and 44.6 (35.2 + 9.42), given the sample's size, mean value, and standard deviation among its scores.

The reason the t-table is used for smaller samples is because it will yield a slightly higher number to multiple the SEM by, compared to the z-table. This higher number, which creates a wider CI, reflects the greater uncertainty about the representativeness of smaller samples.

The construction of the CI is the foundation of the inferential statistics used in most quantitative scientific studies, as explained below.

4.3 INFERENCING WITH STATISTICS—THE ROLE OF PROBABILITY

Inferential statistical tests provide us a decision-making guide about the research study results. We express the statistical test results in terms of our confidence that the correlation seen is real (it exists in the population) and did not occur by chance, or that the difference in means between the two groups is real (exists in the population) and did not occur purely by chance, in a given study.

Studies investigating the association between two variables will be covered in Chapter 5, along with the various statistical tests to use in these studies.

Studies investigating the difference between two group means (usually: which intervention gave rise to a better outcome in the people in the group receiving that intervention) is used in this chapter as the model situation for statistical inferencing. Comparison of means of two or more groups and the statistical tests for these situations will be the content of Chapter 6.

4.4 INFERENCES BASED ON COMPARING GROUPS

Much research seeks to discover whether an **observed** difference between two (or more) groups is a REAL effect of some cause (usually, a new method of intervention) or whether the difference (in scores, or performance, or whatever it may be) is simply a result of random variation, or chance occurrence, in our **samples**.

We compose a **research hypothesis** that one intervention is better than another (or better than none at all, if we use a control group receiving no intervention). The research hypothesis can be directional (one-tailed) or non-directional (two-tailed). A two-tailed test is usually preferred, because it will detect whether the intervention group did better than the control, or the control group did better than the intervention group. A one-tailed test can only be justified if we have no interest in whether the control group did better than the intervention group. Such a study is usually not justified, because as health care professionals, we must remain concerned about whether our interventions are actually causing harm to clients (in the case where the control group performs better than the group that received the intervention).

The non-directional (two tailed) hypothesis is $\mu_1 \neq \mu_2$ (or $r \neq 0$, for a correlation), where μ is the mean value of the dependent variable in the population from which the sample was drawn.

The directional (one-tailed) hypothesis is $\mu_1 > \mu_2$ (or r is statistically significantly > 0, or statistically significantly < 0).

In order to conduct the statistical test, a "**null hypothesis**" is formulated, which is that there is no (REAL) difference between the populations the samples were drawn from.

The null hypothesis is $\mu_1 = \mu_2$ (or $r = 0$). *Stated in clinical research study*: There is no statistically significant difference between means (or no significantly statistical relationship between variables) in the study. Observed differences (or associations) are too likely to have occurred purely by chance.

Of course, when the performance of two groups is measured in a study, virtually every time the mean values of the two groups will not be the same. They may only differ by a little (25.8 in one group and 25.9 in the other), or they may vary by a great deal (25.8 in one and 75.2 in the other). The null hypothesis is set up as the claim that, no matter how much difference there is between the two group means, it isn't real, it just happened by chance. In other words, in the populations from which the samples were drawn, the actual mean values are the same, or put another way, the samples actually came from the same population.

Once the null hypothesis has been established, **inferential statistics** are used to quantify the probability (the p-value) that the groups had the differing mean values they did, even though they came from populations that weren't really different (put another way: even if they really came from the "same population," that is, the intervention wouldn't really work better for people in the population the samples were drawn from). If it turns out the two groups had results that are too different to have been that different by chance, we REJECT the null hypothesis. If they are not different enough to be convincing, we FAIL TO REJECT the null hypothesis. The outcome of the statistical test tells us which of these paths to take. If the calculated value of p is less than the alpha level (.05 or. 01), then the test statistic is telling the researcher to reject the null.

As you can imagine, this testing of the null hypothesis is going to hinge on **probabilities**. We can never **prove** or **disprove** the null hypothesis because there will always be a certain amount of sampling error—the chance occurrences leading to our getting the samples we ended up with. There will always be a certain amount of measurement error in studies, and an uncertain amount of systematic bias. Data cannot be extracted from people, by people, flawlessly. Thus, researchers can never be **certain** their findings are accurate or true. But they can be **confident**, either 95% confident (if we used an alpha level of .05, and $p < .05$), or 99% confident (if alpha was set at .01, and $p < .01$), or maybe even better (if the p-value was .005 or .001), when we reject the null hypothesis.

Because we can never be sure, there is a chance that we reject the null hypothesis when we **shouldn't** have (which represents a Type I error), just as there's a chance that we failed to reject it when we **should** have (a Type II error). The researcher can never know for a given study where the null was rejected whether a Type I error was made. Researchers can never know when they fail to reject the null in a given study whether they just made a Type II error. It is only known that in 100 studies, using a "95% confident" standard of statistical inference (an alpha level of .05) and where the null hypothesis is rejected every time, about 5 of those times would have been wrong. (But no one knows which 5!)

In any case, when the outcome of a statistical test indicates rejecting the null hypothesis, then it is said that the results are *statistically significant*. If the statistic was used to test the difference between the means of two samples, it would be said that their means were *statistically significantly different*. (In Chapter 5, the counterpart conclusion for an association test is if the test indicates rejecting the null, then the two variables were *statistically significantly correlated*, or correlated to a *statistically significant degree*.)

Even when there is statistical significance in the outcome of a statistical test, there remains the alpha or Type I error rate of 5% or 1%. This fact is **inescapable** when using statistics to analyze data.

It is important to keep in mind these "error probability constraints" when talking about the conclusions of research studies, especially as we try to translate them into plain English. Research findings should never be presented to clients or their families as certain or "proven." It is also important to understand that the size of $1 - p$ is NOT indicative of the degree of importance ("*significance*" in the plain English sense, not the statistical sense) of the results. How important the results are is an interpretation that considers personal, social, and environmental factors beyond the statistical test values. What $1 - p$ does signify is the degree of justifiable *confidence* in our claim about the group means. Thus, in strict statistical language, it makes no sense to talk of "highly significant results." A study's findings are either statistically significant or they are not.

In order to understand how valuable a quantification of our confidence in making a claim about the mean difference between two groups is, consider the following six graphs of the data distributions of two groups (see Figure 4–2). The researcher is interested in being able to make a persuasive claim about a difference in the means of the two groups being compared. In the first pair (labeled "A1" and "A2"), there is a very great difference between the means of the groups in graph A1, compared to the other, A2, where the difference in means is small. That is, one group did very much better on the outcome measure than the other group in A1, compared to A2. Other things (such as sample size and score variability) being equal, the picture in A1 is more persuasive of there being a real difference between the groups in the total population than the picture of A2. The magnitude of the difference between the means is important.

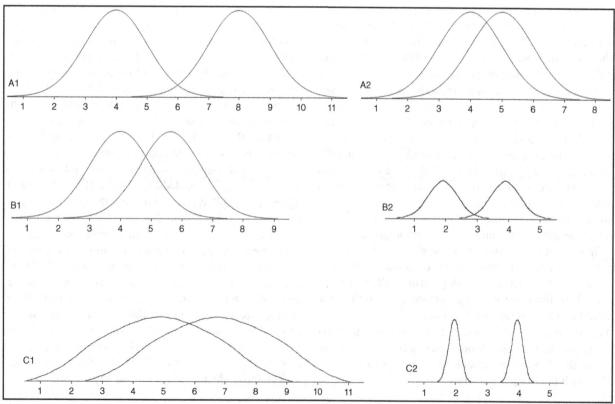

Figure 4–2 Mean differences between two groups under a variety of distributions.

Now consider the next two graphs (labeled "B1" and "B2"). In both, the mean difference is exactly the same, but the sample size is much greater in B1 than in B2. Graph B1 would be more persuasive that in the population there is truly a mean difference such as portrayed here. Graph B2, with its small samples, represents a situation that could have more easily happened by chance. Larger samples give rise to more persuasive claims.

Finally, consider graphs "C1" and "C2." In C2 the variability in scores within each group is small. In fact, it is so small that there is no overlap in data between the groups. Even the lowest scoring person in the group with the higher mean did better than the highest scoring person in the other group. That is more persuasive that a real difference exists, compared to C1. In C1 there is a great amount of score overlap. The mean difference is the same as in C2, but the variability alone in the picture of great data overlap weakens any claim that the mean difference is real in the population.

From these six graphs it can be deduced that in making any claim about the reality of a mean difference between two groups, three factors must be considered. First, the magnitude of the difference between the means; second, the size of the samples; and third, the variability of the scores within each group. A larger mean difference, larger sample sizes, and lower variability would combine to boost the confidence the researcher should feel in making a claim about the group means in the population from which the samples were drawn. If the three factors, though, are pulling in different directions (e.g., large mean difference, large samples, but also large variability in scores) the researcher would be less confident in making a claim. How much less confident should the researcher be? Quantifying how confident a researcher should be in making a claim about a mean difference between two groups is exactly what an inferential statistical test, such as the *t*-test, does. In fact, in the formula for a *t*-test appear the three factors noted above: the magnitude of the mean difference, the size of the groups, and the variability in the group scores. Their position in the formula for a *t*-test determines how confident the researcher should be.

To set the stage for determining this degree of confidence, the researcher selects the desired level of significance, called the alpha level. The alpha level is the degree of confidence we wish to have in making claims about the results of the statistical test. This confidence level is $1 - p$, where p is the probability that the results we got could have occurred purely by chance:

If 95% confidence is desired in our claims, then the alpha level is set at .05, and the *p*-value we seek is $p < .05$.

If 99% confidence is desired in our claims, then the alpha level is set at .01, and the *p*-value we seek is $p < .01$.

The alpha level should be pre-selected before the data are analyzed. The formula for each inferential statistical test gives a number, which is the observed value for that statistical test (for example, the "observed *t*"). For most tests, the greater this number, the less likely it was that these results could have happened by chance (that is, the greater the chance that the observed number exceeds a critical number for that statistical test, e.g., the "critical *t*"). If the observed value is greater than the critical value, that indicates the researcher should reject the null hypothesis, and be confident that the observed difference between the means of the two groups in the study also would be found in the whole population.

4.5 OUTCOMES OF TESTING THE NULL HYPOTHESIS: TYPE I AND TYPE II ERRORS

When conducting an inferential statistical test, there are four possible outcomes:

1. The null hypothesis is rejected when it should be: a real difference between groups (in the population) exists and that's our claim: a correct conclusion.

2. The null is rejected when it shouldn't have been: we claimed a real difference between the groups when there wasn't one. This outcome constitutes a Type I error. It will happen across research studies at the rate of the alpha level (5% or 1% of the times this experiment is done).

3. The researcher fails to reject null when the null should not have been rejected. There is no real difference between the groups and the researcher made no such claim of a difference: a correct conclusion.

4. The researcher fails to reject null when the null should have been rejected. There is a real difference between the groups but the researcher made no claim of a difference: a Type II error. This outcome will happen across research studies at a rate of 1 – statistical power of the test, or beta. See Table 4–1 showing the four possible outcomes of the statistical test in a 2-by-2 table.

It may be helpful in mastering the concept of Type I and Type II errors to consider the analogy with a medical test for the presence of a disease. It would be ideal if the test only indicated that someone had the disease if they truly did have it (a true positive result). It would also be ideal if a person did not have the disease, that the test would always indicate a negative result (a true negative). These two outcomes are comparable to the times a statistical test leads the researcher to drawing the correct conclusion (above). Suppose, though, that the person does not have the disease and the test indicates positive. That result is a false positive test result. It is analogous to rejecting the null when the null should not have been rejected (there is no real difference between the means, but the researcher claimed there was), or making a Type I error. The other scenario is that the person does have the disease, but the test indicates negative (a false negative). This outcome is

TABLE 4–1		
TYPE I AND TYPE II ERRORS IF THE STATED HYPOTHESIS PREDICTS A DIFFERENCE BETWEEN GROUPS		
	P-VALUE IS < ALPHA	*P*-VALUE IS > ALPHA
Effect truly exists	No error	Type II error
Effect does not exist	Type I error	No error

similar to not rejecting the null when it should have been rejected, or making a Type II error.

Note that if the two group means are exactly equal in a study, it will be impossible to reject the null hypothesis. Thus, there is no chance of a Type I error. One could say that in this case the researcher has not even a shred of evidence that the intervention is better than the control. Since the null was not rejected, there remains the possibility of a Type II error, that is, the intervention truly is better than (or worse than) the control in the population, but this experiment simply did not generate the evidence to allow us to confidently claim that difference exists.

If two group means are unequal (as they almost always will be)—an exploratory data check can be useful, before any inferential statistical test is conducted.

4.6 EXPLORATORY DATA ANALYSIS

As the researcher, it is essential to become very familiar with the data collected. As a research consumer (a reader of the research literature) it is important to become as sophisticated as possible in exploring the data and findings of a study. In either case, the items of exploratory data analysis, outlined below, can be of assistance.

1. Look at the raw data! Do any scores leap out as extremely high or exceptionally low? Were they perhaps measurement or data entry errors? Are all numbers within the possible range of the instrument? Should they be considered outliers? Look for clusters in the data distribution, which could indicate a lack of inter-scorer reliability.

2. Construct stem and leaf displays and box plots to show data distributions.

3. Establish some measures of central tendency in the data: in the overall group and in sub-groups, if any exist. Compare these measures (mean, median, mode) in the sample data to any known to exist in a whole population (such as with a standardized test that has been normed). This comparison can quickly tell you if the group's scores are above or below the population average.

4. Examine the distribution or dispersion of scores. There are two ways of doing this: pictorial and statistical. Graphing the data as, for example, a histogram, would be an example of the former. Calculating a standard deviation (or a range) is an example of the latter. Scores from different sub-groups may well have different data distributions. One may be more spread out than another, even though their means are the same, for example: the greater the standard deviation, the greater the dispersion (or spread) in the scores. By looking at a graph of the scores you can also see the amount of skew (asymmetry) in the data. You may also see the phenomenon called the "ceiling effect" or the "floor effect." An example of a ceiling effect would be if many members of a group are getting the highest possible scores, creating a skewed distribution of scores (this effect happens when the test is too easy for a group, or if the test was not designed to differentiate between people who are good at this skill and people who are VERY good at this skill). A floor effect is the opposite. All these effects may vary from sub-group to sub-group.

5. Calculate means and standard deviations of the groups—how far apart are the means, in terms of the SD? (the effect size; see below).

6. Compare the data to that of a normative group, if available. Did the group score higher or lower than the normative group (compare means)? Did the group have more or less dispersion in the data, compared to the normative group (compare standard deviations)? By calculating a z-score on the mean of the group it can be determined how much higher or lower those individuals scored, in "standard deviation units" (the units of a z-score), compared to the normed group.

7. When there are more than two groups, compare the comparisons! Maybe one sub-group got a higher mean than another sub-group, but also had a greater amount of dispersion (spread, or range) in scores, thanks to a few very low scores. Perhaps a sub-group does better than another and has a smaller standard deviation. Think about why these effects might appear. Of course, from descriptive statistics alone you cannot know why these effects occurred, but speculating may be helpful in designing later investigations.

8. Collapse data into ordinal categories ("blocks") and calculate a chi square test. Chi square will indicate if the distributions across the blocks are statistically significantly different between the two groups. Even when the two group means are not different, their dispersion across the categories (the blocks) may be different.

9. For association/correlation tests to be done: first, graph the data in scatterplots to show the relationship between the two variables across the ranges of both variables. Many interesting patterns can appear.

10. Finally, don't forget to look back over the raw data, once the group statistical characteristics have been established. See anything out of the ordinary?

For a detailed account of exploratory data analysis, see Hoaglin et al. (1991) or Tukey (1977).

4.7 Effect Size

Effect size is defined as the difference between the means of two intervention groups, divided by the standard deviation among their data. The formula for effect size (ES) is therefore

$$ES = \frac{(\mu_0 - \mu_1)}{SD}$$

where μ_0 *is the mean of one group,* μ_1 *is the mean of the other group, and SD* is the standard deviation in the pooled scores of both groups.

The advantage of using an effect size to describe group differences in a study is that it can be used to compare effects across studies. The raw difference in means between one group and another in a study is dependent on the type of measuring scale used. If a scale from 1 to 1,000 were used, and the two group means differed by 500 points, how could that be fairly compared with a group difference of 7 in a study where the scale was from 1 to 10? Using the effect size is a way to standardize group mean differences.

Note that the effect size is a pure number (.2, .5, or .8, for example). This will always be true, because the standard deviation in a set of scores is in the same units as the scores themselves, and as the mean of those scores. With the same units in the numerator and in the denominator of the fraction for calculating the ES, the units cancel out, leaving a pure number. This number can be compared across studies, even those using different dependent variables to measure the effect of the intervention.

The effect size is expected to be zero when the null hypothesis is true (Cohen, 1988). Of course, due to sampling error and measurement error, it is likely, even when the null is true, that the means of the two groups in a study will not be exactly the same. The difference between them, however, will usually be small. If the study were to be replicated many times, the small effect sizes, positive and negative, would tend to cancel out. Thus, the expected ES in the long run would be zero.

The effect size serves as an index of the degree of departure from the null hypothesis. For example, a large effect size can be interpreted to mean that the study had higher statistical power for correctly rejecting the null hypothesis. By scientific convention, a small effect size would be .2, a medium effect size .5, and a large effect size .8 or above (Cohen, 1988). With an ES of .8 (other features in the studies being equal), that study will have a higher probability of finding a difference if there really is one in the populations, compared to a study where the ES is .5 or .2. This fact will be elaborated in section 4.8 below.

4.8 Statistical Power

Definition: Statistical power is the likelihood that an inferential statistical test will result in rejecting the null hypothesis when there is a real difference between the groups in the study. It is expressed as a percentage (usually 70% or 80% or 90%), or as a decimal number less than one: .70, .80, .90.

Statistical power is affected by:

1. the chosen alpha level—the more stringent (i.e., $p < .01$), the less power in the test

2. the effect size between the groups (the greater the effect size, the more the power)

3. the size of the groups (other things being equal, larger groups means greater power)

4. the variability of the scores in each group (the more variance, the less power).

Obviously, then, if being able to claim that there is a real difference between the groups (when there is a real difference) is very important (such as when there is an urgent search for any intervention that may be effective), and it is not dangerous to make a Type I error (claim there is a more effective intervention when there really isn't), then the study should be designed to maximize power in all the following ways:

1. Select an alpha level with a higher Type I error rate (i.e., pick $p < .05$, not .01).

2. Provide the strongest possible "dose" of intervention to maximize the effect size between the groups (e.g., provide therapy 5 times a week for one hour, rather than 3 times a week for 30 minutes).

3. Enroll the greatest number of volunteers for the study that can feasibly be taken through the study protocol in the time available and can be afforded by the funds for the study (i.e., maximize *n*).

4. Select homogeneous groups (e.g., exclude people with a dual diagnosis, focus on a narrower age range, select one level of severity for the disease or condition: mild

or moderate or severe), and reduce error variance to a minimum (ensure all raters are well calibrated, control the conditions so as to be nearly identical for all participants, use standardized procedures for data collection, and check for accuracy of the data gathering methods throughout the study to prevent observer drift or instrument de-calibration).

Then if a real difference does exist between the populations that the sample groups were drawn from, the researcher will have the best possible chance of finding it and being justified in claiming confidently that the difference really exists.

There is a formula that takes all four factors affecting power into account that is called "Lehr's Equation" (Lehr, 1992). It can be used by research designers to calculate how many participants are needed in a given study:

$$n = \frac{16}{\left(\frac{\mu_0 - \mu_1}{\sigma}\right)^2}$$

Where
  n = number of participants needed in each group
  μ_0 = the mean of the first group and
  μ_1 = the mean of the second group
  σ = the variance of the scores of the people in both groups, pooled.

The number 16 is a constant and is part of Lehr's Equation. This version of Lehr's Equation assumes α is set at .05 and β is set at .2, that is, the researcher wants to have a chance of 1 – 0.2 = 0.80, or 80%, that the statistical test will indicate a difference between the groups when there really is one in their respective populations.

In order to use this equation, it is necessary to have access to some prior data, in order to have values for μ_0, μ_1, and σ. These prior data can be derived from pilot testing, where a researcher obtains some preliminary data, or it could come from other prior studies that have investigated similar dependent and independent variables. For example, consider a study investigating the efficacy of two types of splints (a hard splint and a soft splint) on the ability to grasp clothes pins for hanging clothes out to dry after an extensor carpi ulnaris tear. Assume the mean of the hard splint group functional score was 11 and the mean of the soft splint group was 17. Assume the variance among the two groups' scores is 8. Lehr's Equation would give the following:

$$n = \frac{16}{\left(\frac{11-17}{8}\right)^2}$$

Carrying out the arithmetic yields
$n = 28.44$

According to Lehr's formula, and the prior data assumed, the researcher would need to recruit 29 participants for each condition, that is, 58 for the entire study, in order for the statistical test on the group means to have an 80% chance of indicating a statistically significant difference between those group means when there truly was a difference between the two populations the two samples were drawn from.

BOX 4-1. STEPS IN A STUDY USING INFERENTIAL STATISTICS

Step 1. *State the hypothesis.* A null hypothesis is stated unless the researcher is replicating a previous study or has research evidence to support a directional hypothesis.

1. The null hypothesis is $\mu_1 = \mu_2$ or $r = 0$. *Stated in research study*: There is no statistically significant difference between the means of the groups in the study.
2. The non-directional hypothesis is $\mu_1 \neq \mu_2$.
3. The directional hypothesis is $\mu_1 > \mu_2$.

Step 2. *Select a level of significance.* In the social sciences, the researcher usually selects the .05 level of significance (α = .05). This means that the researcher accepts a Type I error rate of 5%. The researcher can also state that at α = .05, when the null is rejected, that there is a 95% confidence level that results are not due to chance (that the group means truly are different).

Step 3. *Select a parametric or a non-parametric statistical test.* Which type of inferential statistic to use is based on the assumptions underlying the test such as normally distributed data, equal variance in the groups, equal sized groups, large enough groups, and whether the data as collected were ratio or interval, versus ordinal or nominal. (Often it can be justified using parametric statistics with ordinal data.)

Step 4. *Obtain the critical value* from the appropriate table for statistical tests based on whether it is a one-tailed or two-tailed test, the level of statistical significance, and the degrees of freedom (df) in this comparison. (For most statistical tests, the df is $n – 1$.)

(continued)

Box 4-1. Steps in a Study Using Inferential Statistics (continued)

Step 5. *Calculate the value of test statistics,* such as *t*-observed, *F*-observed, chi-square or correlation coefficient through a mathematical formula. The statistics application the researcher is using performs steps 4 and 5. It behooves the researcher to be familiar with the process, however, in order to catch errors in the procedures.

Step 6. *Reject or fail to reject the null hypothesis,* depending on the relationship between α and *p*.

Step 7. *Interpret the implication of this finding from the statistical test in the context of the original study.* Compare this finding to those from similar studies.

4.9 Summary

In this chapter, the difference between descriptive and inferential statistics was discussed. This differentiation was articulated by expressing the respective definitions of the two types of statistics. Additionally, the concept of sampling was explored which reinforced the notion of the Central Limit Theorem as it pertains to statistical degrees of freedom and its implications upon Type I and Type II errors. Effect sizes, which involve the notion of the influence or size of the effect without regard to the degrees of freedom, were explored. Lastly, power analysis was defined and discussed with respect to research study planning.

5

Correlation and Regression

When we see a strong correlation, and the matter at-hand is something with major health or safety or security implications, then we are behooved to at least begin taking preliminary precautions in case the correlation proves to be causative.

David Brin (n.d.)

OPERATIONAL LEARNING OBJECTIVES

By the end of this chapter, the learner will be able to:
1. Define correlation
2. Discern the difference between associational relationship and causality
3. Describe a correlational matrix
4. Differentiate the Pearson correlation with the Spearman rank order correlation
5. Articulate how to interpret the correlation coefficient
6. Discriminate the differences between correlation and linear regression
7. Define coefficients of a regression model
8. Define the formulary components of a regression line
9. Articulate what the R^2 represents in terms of variance of the regression model

What is correlation? What is the difference between an associational relationship and causality? How do we graph the relationship between variables? What is a correlational matrix? What is a regression line? What is the difference between the Pearson correlation coefficient and the Spearman rank order correlation coefficient? All of these questions relate to the correlational model in statistics and will be discussed in this chapter.

5.1 Definition of Correlation

Correlation is the reciprocal relationship between two variables. It is a general concept that assumes that variables can be measured and correlated. The index of the degree of relationship between two variables is the correlation coefficient. This index can range from zero, which indicates no relationship, to + 1.00 or – 1.00, which indicates a perfect correlation between two variables. For example, a correlation coefficient of .30 indicates a low correlation, whereas .90 is a high correlation. The symbol for correlation is *r*. A correlational relationship indicates an association between variables; it does not indicate a causal relationship.

Many studies published in occupational therapy are primarily correlational and retrospective. This research is similar to experimental research in that the investigator tests a hypothesis. However, unlike the experimental researcher, the investigator neither manipulates the independent variables, nor simulates a cause-effect relationship. In correlational research, the investigator compares the relationships between variables by measuring how one measured behavior or phenomenon changes in relation to another behavior or phenomenon. It is applied frequently to areas in the social sciences because the very nature of the problem limits the experimenter from inducing causal effects. If, for example, a researcher's purpose is to correlate characteristics in an individual who is alcoholic with causative factors, then the investigator is limited to an ex-post-facto design where it is not possible to induce experimentally the onset of alcoholism. The researcher in this example is limited to a retrospective analysis of the assumed causes of alcoholism. Kerlinger (1986), in discussing the value of non-experimental research, concluded that "social, scientific, and educational problems do not lend themselves to experimentation, although many of them do lend themselves to controlled inquiry of the non-experimental kind" (p. 359).

A sequential analysis of correlational research is diagramed in Figure 5–1. These steps are reviewed in the section below.

The majority of occupational therapists work with clients who have some sort of diagnosis. A common question arises regarding the etiology of many of these diagnoses. For instance, why did this client become schizophrenic? Why did this individual develop learning problems? What factors led to arthritis? What environmental factors contributed to juvenile delinquency? These questions regarding etiology and relationships between variables are feasible for correlational research.

5.2 Pyramid Orientation/ Connection

Correlation is located on the third rung on the descriptive side of the Research Pyramid for evidence-based OT practice. It is found above case-series, normative and below descriptive systematic reviews. As mentioned below, correlation research, while descriptive in nature, is also driven by hypothesis testing focusing on the relationship between two data sets.

5.2.1 Study Design Including Applicability/Features and Inherent Limitations

The first step in correlational research is to identify the variables in a target population to be studied. These variables are presumed causative factors and may be genetic, neurophysiological, psychosocial, or cultural. The variables are identified from clinical observations, by examining previous studies or theoretical papers, or through deductive reasoning. The presumed independent variables and presumed dependent variables are identified. Because the researcher does not actively induce the independent variables, an associational or statistical relationship can only be assumed. Commonly, the two variables are assigned as "X" and "Y," respectively, but it doesn't matter which is which when running the correlation statistic because the same result will occur regardless of how the variables are labeled.

Correlation tests the direction and the strength of relationships between two variables. As outlined below, the parametric correlation statistic is the Pearson correlation whereas the non-parametric is the Spearman correlation. These tests use the coefficient "*r*" and will also yield a *p*-value. It is important to note that correlation test only provide the strength and direction of the relationship, they are not tests of causation. For example, just because an *r* of .9 is both positive and nearly perfect, this doesn't mean that one variable caused the other variable to increase at almost the same rate. A good example of this is the incidence of measles and marriage rates in the United States, where there is a close correlation but almost certainly no causation (see www.statology.org/spurious-correlation-examples/). Another important aspect is that correlational statistics generate a *p*-value. This *p*-value has to do with the statistical integrity of the calculated *r* coefficient. That is, if the *p*-value is smaller than the stated alpha

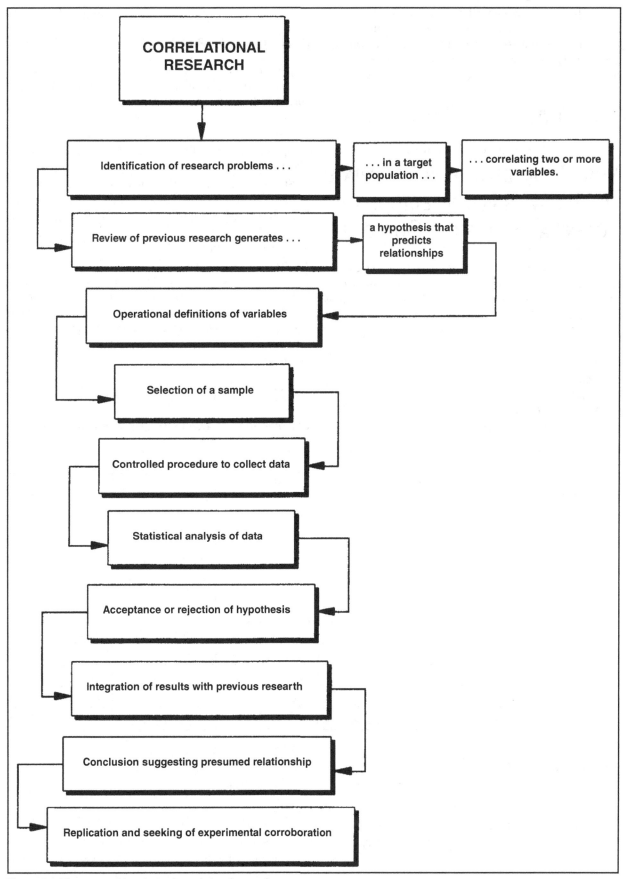

Figure 5–1 The sequential analysis of correlational research.

level (which is usually.05), then the research investigator can interpret the *r* coefficient with confidence. If the *p*-value is larger than the stated alpha, then the researcher cannot make any statement of interpretation other than the correlational statistical analysis was inconclusive.

5.3 AFFILIATED STATISTICS, PARAMETRIC AND NON-PARAMETRIC AS APPROPRIATE ALONG WITH INTERPRETATION OF POTENTIAL STATISTICAL OUTCOMES

As mentioned above, the Pearson correlation is the parametric correlation statistic whereas the Spearman correlation is a non-parametric statistic. When interpreting correlation coefficients, the following guideline is used (Hinkle et al., 2003):

$r \geq .9$ (Very high)
$r \geq .7$ and $r < .9$ (High)
$r \geq .5$ and $r < .7$ (Moderate)
$r \geq .3$ and $r < .5$ (Low)
$r \geq .0$ and $r < .9$ (No Correlation to Very Low)

5.3.1 Procedure for Calculating Pearson Correlation

Step 1. *State the research hypothesis.* For example, there is no statistically significant relationship between variable *X* and variable *Y*. (Null hypothesis, *r* =.00 or below predetermined level of correlation.)

Step 2. *Determine the level of significance acceptable to interpret the calculated correlation coefficient, for example, alpha = .05.*

Step 3. *Calculate the Pearson r correlation coefficient.* The Spearman (rank order) is a good screening test for the Pearson (product-moment), which is a more accurate test because the Pearson *r* computes raw scores, whereas the Spearman r_s computes ranks that are transformed scores. The reader shall note that the Pearson *r*, which is a parametric test, should be applied to interval or ratio scale data. The Spearman r_s is a non-parametric statistical test that can be used with ordinal scale data. As the reader will note, interval scale data can be transformed to ranks (ordinal scale data).

The formula for the Pearson *r* product-moment correlation is:

$$r = \left[N\Sigma XY - (\Sigma X)(\Sigma Y) \right] \Big/ \sqrt{\left[N\Sigma X^2 - (\Sigma X)^2 \right]\left[N\Sigma Y_2 - (\Sigma Y)^2 \right]}$$

Calculation for Pearson *r* Product-Moment Correlation

SUBJECT	X	X²	Y	Y²	XY
01	31	961	45	2025	1395
02	22	484	58	3364	1276
03	19	361	57	3249	1083
04	16	256	48	2304	768
05	78	6084	61	3721	4758
06	3	9	36	1296	108
07	93	8649	18	324	1674
08	78	6084	88	7744	6864
09	23	529	9	81	207
10	15	225	12	144	180
	378	23642	432	24252	18313
	$\Sigma X = 378$	$\Sigma X^2 - 23,642$	$\Sigma Y = 432$	$\Sigma Y^2 = 24,252$:	$\Sigma XY = 18,313$

$N = 10$ $\Sigma X^2 = 23,642$
$\Sigma XY = 18,313$ $\Sigma Y^2 = 24,252$
$\Sigma X = 378$ $(\Sigma X)^2 = 142,884$ t
$\Sigma Y = 432$ $(\Sigma Y)^2 = 186,624$

$r = [(10)(18313) - (378)(432)] \Big/$

$\sqrt{(10)(23642) - (142884)][(10)(24252) - (186624)]}$

$= [183130 - 163296] \Big/$

$\sqrt{(236420 - 142884)(242520 - 186624)}$

$= 19834 \Big/ \sqrt{(93536)(55896)}$

$= 19834 \Big/ 72317$

$r = .274$

The Pearson *r* of .274 is similar to the Spearman r_s of .29. In both computations, the correlation is low and will not be clinically significant because only a small portion of the variance is accounted for.

5.3.2 Procedure for Calculating Spearman Correlation

Step 1. *State the research hypothesis.* For example, there is no statistically significant relationship between variable *X* and variable *Y*. (Null hypothesis, *r* = .00 or below predetermined level of correlation.)

Step 2. *Determine the level of significance acceptable to interpret the calculated correlation coefficient, for example, alpha = .05.*

Step 3. *Collect data and arrange raw scores into a table.* For example:

SUBJECTS	VARIABLE X RAW SCORE	RANK	VARIABLE Y RAW SCORE	RANK	D (DIFFERENCE IN RANKS BETWEEN X AND Y)	D² (DIFFERENCE SQUARED)
1	31	7	45	5	2	4
2	22	5	58	8	–3	9
3	19	4	57	7	– 3	9
4	16	3	48	6	– 3	9
5	78	8.5	61	9	– 0.5	0.25
6	3	1	36	4	– 3	9
7	93	10	18	3	7	49
8	78	8.5	88	10	– 1.5	2.25
9	23	6	9	1	5	25
10	15	2	12	2	0	0
	$\Sigma X = 378$		$\Sigma Y = 432$		$\Sigma d = 0^a$	$\Sigma d^2 = 116.5$

Note: d = difference in ranks between X and Y; d2 = difference squared.

[a]Note that in computing the differences (*d*), the sum of the rank differences should equal zero when taking into consideration the negative and positive signs.

Step 4. *Rank order each raw score, with lowest score being assigned rank of 1. Note: for tied ranks, take the midpoint of the rank. For example, a raw score of 78 occupies ranks 8 and 9 and becomes rank of 8.5.*

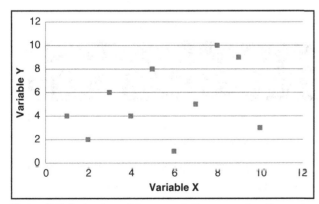

Figure 5–2 Exploratory data on a scattergram using the ranks of the scores. Notice that each point is a coordinate value. There appears to be a low to moderate correlation between the two variables.

Step 5. *Do exploratory data analysis.* Note in Figure 5–2 that each point in the scatter diagram is a coordinate value. It appears from the scatter diagram that there is a low to moderate correlation between the two variables.

Step 6. *Calculate Spearman rank correlation coefficient and estimate degree of relationship between the two variables (X and Y). The formula for Spearman r_s is:*

$$r_s = 1.00 - [\ (6)\ (\Sigma d^2)\ /\ (N^3 - N)\ ]$$
$$= 1.00 - [(6)\ (116.5)\ /\ (1{,}000 - 10)]$$
$$= 1.00 - [699\ /\ 990]$$
$$= 1.00 - .71$$
$$r_s = .29$$

The exploratory data analysis indicates that there is a low correlation between the *X* and *Y* variables.

Step 7. *Calculation of Regression Line.* A regression line describes the relationship between variable X and variable Y. The formula for the regression line is:

$$Y = a + bX$$

Where
Y is a predicted variable from the known *X* value
b is the slope of the line
a is the Y intercept.

The regression line that is calculated assumes that if a perfect correlation 1.00 exists between two variables, then one could predict the Y value if the X value is known. For example, suppose we derive the formula for a specific regression line to be:

$$Y = 1.50 + .30X$$
and $X = .500$
$$Y = 1.50 + .30(.500)$$
$$= 1.5 + .15$$
$$Y = 1.65$$

Therefore, if X = 5.00, then Y = 1.65 in this example. The calculation of a regression line is useful when there is a high correlation between two variables. On the other hand, a low correlation of r =.29 would not warrant constructing a regression line.

The computational formula for the slope is:

$$b = [N (\Sigma XY) - (\Sigma X)(\Sigma Y)] / [N \Sigma X^2 - (\Sigma X)^2]$$

The formula for the Y intercept is:
$$a = Y - bX$$

Step 8. *Identify the critical values for the Spearman Rank Order Correlation Coefficient.*
   a. Determine number of subjects (*N*)
   b. Significance level, such as α = .05, .01
   c. Directional or non-directional hypothesis

For example, with $N = 10$, α = .05, non-directional test, $r_{s(crit)} = .648$. (See Table C–6 in the appendices.) In the example above, $r_{s(obs)} = 29$. In this result, the researcher will accept the null hypothesis and conclude that there is no statistically significant relationship between the two variables.

Step 9. *Identify the critical values for the Pearson Product-Moment Correlation.*
   a. $df = N - 2$
   b. Significance level
   c. Directional or non-directional hypothesis

In the example as shown, $df = 8$, α = .05, non-directional test. $r_{crit} = .6319$ (See Table C–6 in the appendices.) Because $r_{obs} = .27$, the null hypothesis is accepted, and the researcher concludes that there is no statistically significant relationship between the two variables.

The reader should note that as the *N* increases, the $r_{crit} =$ decreases. For example, for 100 *df*, α = .05 level of significance, $r_{crit} = .1966$, while for 20 *df*, $r_{crit} = .4227$.

While the above explanation of how to manually calculate a correlation between two variables, it is not uncommon for studies to correlate more than two variables together. Some researchers will include many variables simultaneously. For example, in a hypothetical example, a researcher may correlate many variables to performance on an intelligent quotient test. Such variables could include age, height, weight, and years of education. When correlating all of these variables at the same time using a statistical software program like IBM's SPSS, the software's output will include a correlational matrix. Table 5–1 is a hypothetical example of a correlational matrix output using the above stated variables. Note that, while the investigator was only interested in the correlation between IQ and each of the other variables (which can be found in the top row of the matrix as well as the first column), the matrix provides the correlation coefficient between all possible combinations of all of the variables. Another thing to note is that there is a perfect correlation going down from the top left to the bottom right of the matrix where the variable "IQ" is correlated with itself. Additionally, the coefficients below the diagonal "1"s are a mirror of the coefficients above the diagonal "1"s. Lastly, statistically significant coefficients are denoted with an * with a note at the bottom of the table explaining its associated significance level.

TABLE 5–1					
CORRELATIONAL MATRIX					
	IQ	**AGE**	**HEIGHT**	**WEIGHT**	**YEARS OF EDUCATION**
IQ	1	0.45*	0.03	0.14	0.69*
Age	0.45*	1	0.77*	0.8*	0.82
Height	0.03	0.77*	1	0.79*	0.53
Weight	0.14	0.8*	0.79*	1	0.67
Years of Education	0.69*	0.82	0.53	0.67	1
*p<.05					

5.4 JOURNAL ARTICLE EXAMPLE REFLECTING CHAPTER DESIGN AND STATISTICS: CORRELATION STUDY

Rapolienė et al. (2018) investigated the relationship between the level of motivation and the effectiveness of occupational therapy in a population of 30 participants who suffered a stroke and who were being treated at a rehabilitation clinic. These investigators used the Multidimensional Health Locus of Control (MHLC) to measure motivation and performance in performing activities of daily living using the Functional Independency Measure (FIM) as the variable measuring effectiveness of occupational therapy. Measurements on these two instruments were recorded at initial intake and at discharge. These researchers found that both the participants' motivation and their ADL performance improved from intake to discharge. A Pearson's correlation was calculated which yielded a positive, moderate correlation with $r = 0.72$ ($p < .05$). The authors interpreted the results by stating that as the participants' motivation increased, so too did the performance in ADLs. They were careful not to state that the one variable caused the other to increase, but rather that a moderate relationship existed between these two variables.

5.5 REGRESSION

Regression is mathematically related to correlation in that both are about relationships. Moreover, regression uses the same correlation coefficient r, in that it squares the r to represent the variability for which the regression model accounts. There are different types of regression, notably, linear and non-linear. Linear regression will be the focus of this text and statistically "predicts" the value that one variable has upon another based on a calculated straight line, that is, the linear regression line. Non-linear regression does essentially the same thing, only is based upon a non-linear line, that is, a curved line. While both types of regression use one predicted variable (Y), they can use one or more independent variables (X). The latter would include the term "multiple" in its description, for example, *multiple linear regression*. These types of regression models are parametric and use continuous data. Non-parametric examples include logistical regression models which can accommodate dichotomous and nominal data. These specific types of regression are beyond the scope of this text. Regardless, the utility of regression (parametric and non-parametric), is that within a given variable's set of values, the value of another variable can be estimated. For linear regression, this prediction is based upon a linear equation, mentioned in the previous section on correlation, notably,

$$Y = a + bX$$

Where
Y is a predicted variable from the known X value
b is the slope of the line
a is the Y intercept

Similar to correlation, simple linear regression is based upon two columns of data, denoted by an X and a Y variable. X-Y scatter plots are often helpful in visualizing the data. A regression line is then calculated and placed upon the scatter plot. This regression line, $Y = a + bX$, is calculated using a residual least square's method. What is a residual you ask? For any given data point on the scatter plot, it is the vertical distance to the regression line. See Figure 5–3 as an example. Regression models with large residuals have high variability and decreased precision. On the contrary, regression models with small residuals have low variability and high precision.

The degree of precision is represented by squaring the correlation coefficient, r, denoted by r^2. Specifically, r^2 represents the amount of variability that the regression model accounts for. Said another way, models with a large r^2 have high internal validity, meaning relatively low statistical error. Models with a small r^2 have low internal validity, meaning relatively high statistical error. That is, unknown variables are influencing the predicted Y variables which are beyond the X variable, hence *error*. The analysis of variance (ANOVA) calculation behind the regression model tests to see if there is a statistically significant relationship. Thinking about it another way, if the regression line's slope was zero, there would be no relationship between X and Y. The regression's ANOVA tests whether the model's regression line's slope is significantly different from zero. Amongst other things, the statistical output for a regression analysis includes an r^2, the y-intercept, the slope (the latter two are referred to as coefficients in many types of statistical outputs), and an ANOVA table. If the p-value from the ANOVA is less than

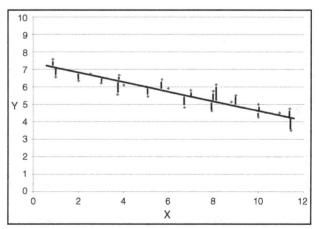

Figure 5–3 *X-Y* scatter plot showing the residuals denoted by the black vertical lines spanning the distance between the data point and the regression line.

the stated alpha, commonly set at .05, then one can assume that the model is statistically significant. The r^2 value will speak to the level of variability that the regression model accounts for. r^2 values range from 0, which means nothing in the regression model accounts for the model's variability, to a perfect 1, which means that the model accounts for all of the model's variability; this latter example rarely happens. Ideally, the p value will be small and the r^2 value will be large in order to confidently assume the model statistically predicts Y based upon X. Figure 5–4 demonstrates a scatter plot with low variability amongst the data along with a regression line, its equation, and a large r^2. Conversely, Figure 5–5 is a scatter plot with high variability amongst the data along with a regression line, its equation, and a small r^2. The variables contributing to the statistical outcome include the variability within the data, how many data points there are, and how they are distributed on the X-Y scatter plot. The less the variability, the easier it is for the model to find a relationship, the larger the data set, the more statistical power, hence the "easier" it is to find statistical significance, and the way the data are distributed will speak to the direction (positive or negative) of any given relationship.

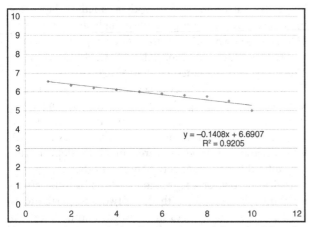

Figure 5–4 *X-Y* scatter plot showing data with low variability, the equation for the regression line, and the associated r^2 value.

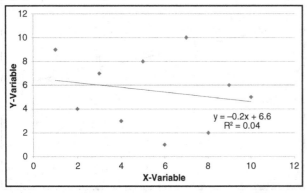

Figure 5–5 *X-Y* scatter plot showing data with high variability, the equation for the regression line, and the associated r^2 value.

Things to consider regarding the difference between the coefficients of r and b include the following points (and it doesn't have anything to do with rhythm and blues):

- r and b always have the same sign which shows whether the variables are positively or negatively associated.
- r deals with how close the observations are to the predicted best-fitted line.
- b deals with how steep the line is (i.e., slope).
- The sign "–" or " " deals with the relationship being negative or positive (i.e., inverse or proportional).
- r^2 deals with the variance accounted for by the regression model.

In summary, linear regression is a useful statistical tool that can provide information about the predictive relationship, its strength, and whether the relationship is proportional or inversely proportional, between two variables.

5.5.1 Example of a Study Using Linear Regression

Magnusson et al. (2021) investigated the relationship between sleep and occupational balance in women. These researchers measured the quality and quantity of sleep using the Karolinska Sleep Questionnaire (KSQ) and the occupational balance using the Occupational Balance Questionnaire (OBQ). In this survey-based study, data from 157 community dwelling women were included in the study. The survey was delivered using the internet via Survey Monkey. These researchers found a relationship between the quality of sleep and the ability to manage a balance in occupational engagement. In particular, the linear regression model found that sleep, sleepiness, and fatigue were significant contributors to the number of occupations in which participants were able to engage over the course of a week; that is, the better the quality of sleep, the better the occupational balance. The researchers concluded that it is important for occupational therapists to consider sleep and the quality of sleep when evaluating a client's ability to balance occupations in daily life.

5.6 CHAPTER SUMMARY

This chapter focused on correlation and regression with respect to the descriptive side of the Research Pyramid. Correlational statistics provide information about relationships including whether they are proportional or inversely proportional. Additionally, they indicate the strength of relationships from being a perfect 1.0 or –1.0 to where there is no relationship, that is, 0.0. Correlations are not statistics of causation. The Pearson correlation is parametric, and the Spearman correlation is a commonly used non-parametric statistic. Linear regression has similarities to correlation in that both calculate a correlation coefficient, but regression involves the calculation of a regression line. This regression line can be used to "predict" with a certain level of confidence the value of a dependent variable from an independent variable, or in the case of multiple regression, multiple independent variables. Associated with regression is the r^2 statistic, which provides information about how effective the regression model is in accounting for the variance. Linear regression calculates an ANOVA, which determines whether the slope of the regression line is statistically significantly different from zero. This chapter focused on linear regression, but there are other forms of regression including, but not limited to, non-linear and logistical regression.

6

Experimental Research

Statistical interpretation depends not only on statistical ideas, but also on "ordinary" thinking. Clear thinking is not only indispensable in interpreting statistics, but is often sufficient even in the absence of specific statistical knowledge.

Wallis et al. (2014)

OPERATIONAL LEARNING OBJECTIVES

By the end of this chapter, the learner will be able to:

1. Differentiate between experimental designs; namely one-sample, independent group comparison, and multiple comparison (> 2) group designs

2. Articulate common assumptions associated with inferential statistics

3. Associate parametric and non-parametric inferential statistics appropriate for various types of experimental research designs

4. Understand when to apply specific statistical test to clinical research designs

DOI: 10.4324/9781003523154-6

6.1 Introduction to the Topic/ General Overview

This chapter introduces experimental research. The word "experimental" is common in the English lexicon, as is the word "research," each carrying a variety of definitions, but put the two words together (i.e., "experimental research") and this has a specific definition. It denotes a research design that in its simplest form uses two groups: one is the experimental group and the other is a control group. This two-group design is used to test the independent variable in that the experimental group receives the intervention, treatment, or experimental manipulation whereas the control group receives a placebo. Both groups are measured on the same test instrument and are statistically compared for differences. Inferential statistics are commonly used to test the study outcome. Statistical tests pertinent to common experimental designs are the focus of this chapter. Starting with the aforementioned simple experimental design, the chapter will progress to multifactorial designs, with common parametric and non-parametric statistical tests, respectively. Also included in this chapter is a discussion on an expansion of the simple experimental design to include multiple levels of the independent variable(s).

6.2 Pyramid Orientation/ Connection

As the chapter title suggests, this chapter highlights the "experimental" side of the pyramid as denoted at the bottom. Single Case Experimental Design (SCED), the first level of the experimental side of the pyramid is discussed at length in Chapter 7. On the pyramid directly above SCED is controlled clinical trial and above that is randomized controlled trial. Both of these will be included in this current chapter. Meta-analysis is at the top of the experimental side of the pyramid and will be discussed in Chapter 10.

6.3 Experimental Designs

Prior to introducing specific statistics common to experimental research designs, it is apropos to continue the discussion about experimental research designs, particularly the clinical controlled trial and randomized controlled trial varieties. As mentioned above, the basic characteristic of a simple experimental design is that there are two groups, one involves the experimental manipulation of the independent variable and the other is a control group. The independent variable manipulation is derived from the experimental hypothesis. Participants are randomly recruited from a target population and are again randomly assigned to either the experimental or the control group. Ideally, neither the research investigator nor the participant knows the participant group assignment; this is known as a double-blind study. This describes necessary components of a randomized controlled trial. The major difference between this design and a clinical controlled trial is the group assignment. With a clinical controlled study, the randomization of group assignment may be impossible because of the likelihood that a medical diagnosis is linked to the experimental condition and the control group participants do not have the experimental group diagnosis. While the clinical controlled trial does not have this essential component required for a randomized controlled trial, other controls are still employed to protect the internal and external validity to the greatest extent possible. For instance, the participants may be matched on a number of demographic characteristics such as age, gender, socioeconomic level, and education levels.

Beyond the simple experimental design are experimental design characteristics that increase the complexity of the design, but that still have the essential components delineated above. Studies may involve more than just two groups and there may be more than one level of independent variable manipulation, but the design will still have a control group which is an absolute essential component to maintain internal validity. These designs are often referred to as "k-independent samples" designs which involve a multilevel independent variable manipulation. Such an example would be a study investigating multiple approaches to stroke rehabilitation and may involve a comparison of the Neurodevelopmental Treatment (NDT) approach and the Modified Constraint Induced (MCI) approach. Such a hypothetical experiment would randomly recruit post-stroke participants and randomly assign them to one of three groups, the NDT, MCI, and control groups. Possible dependent variables may include performance in activities of daily living and motor performance. These may be taken as a baseline before any treatment is given, then again after an 8-week period intervention. The control group would receive no therapy. The post-treatment measurement across all three groups would then test the hypothesis that one of the three groups outperformed the other two groups. Proper ethics would also dictate that if there was a clear adventitious treatment group that the other two groups would then receive the same 8-week interval of the best treatment approach. The statistical design for this type of study is known as a one-way analysis of variance (ANOVA). ANOVA designs can be one-way as highlighted in the above example, or they can be considered to be multifactorial. A common multifactorial example would be where there are two independent variables being tested at the same time. Whereas the one-way ANOVA example above had one associated independent variable with three levels (i.e., NDT, MCI, and control), an example of a multifactorial design might also include an independent variable of limb dominance, specifically to ascertain if limb dominance would have an influence in the efficacy of the various treatment approaches. Such a multifactorial design would be referred to as a 3 × 2 ANOVA with the first factor representing the treatment conditions and the second factor representing limb dominance. Multifactorial designs are not limited to two factors; they can include as many as the imagination can conceive. However, there is practical side restraining the proliferation of factors not the least of which is the multiplicative need for an increased number of participants to generate an adequate level of statistical power to match every possible factor and level combinations. For example, if an a priori power analysis revealed that at least 30 participants would be needed in each group to anticipate statistical significance, and there were 3 levels to the first factor and 2 associated with the second, that would require 90 to cover the first factor with each being multiplied by 2 to satisfy the second factor, this study would need 180 participants for a fully balanced study. Recruiting this many participants from a special population can be challenging unless great resources can be pooled across a large health care network or networks.

What the reader can expect for the remainder of this chapter are examples of statistics, both parametric and non-parametric, that are commonly associated with experimental-type research designs.

6.4 ONE-SAMPLE PROBLEMS

The first statistical model presented here does not actually fit the "experimental design" in that it doesn't actually have a control group; in a one-sample design, the experimental group is compared to a previously measured population, usually a norm-referenced population. Regardless, the one-sample design is included here because the one-sample *t*-test is similar to the statistical models associated with the experimental side of the pyramid.

As mentioned above, the purpose of this statistical model is to compare data collected from a representative sample of a population and then to compare the obtained value with a parameter value that is known or estimated or to a standard value. One-sample *t*-tests are applied to research studies in which the investigator is testing whether a sample mean is equal to, less than, or greater than a given value. An example from environmental science is the sampling of air or water to determine if the air or water is polluted. Scientists concerned with the quality of air and water use one-sample *t*-tests to compare samples with parameter values. These parameter values are health standards that have been predetermined by scientific evidence to be at acceptable health levels. At which point is the air considered to be polluted? What are the accepted levels of bacteria for water consumption? These are problems for one-sample *t*-tests. We can also use one-sample *t*-tests for screening populations. For example, is a group sample above or below normal values in height, weight, cholesterol level, blood pressure, heart rate, and hearing

acuity? The procedure for applying a one-sample *t*-test is to compare the sample mean with a hypothetical parameter value.

An inherent limitation to the one-sample design is that the normative data being compared has been collected at some point in time in the past, perhaps years ago. This difference in time introduces possible error because, as the cliche suggests, things change with time. Comparing measurements taken on Gen-Z participants with a normative sample based upon Baby Boomers is a potential example of an ill-matched comparison.

6.5 HYPOTHETICAL EXAMPLE FOR TESTING FOR STATISTICALLY SIGNIFICANT DIFFERENCES BETWEEN SAMPLE MEAN AND PARAMETER MEAN VALUES

Step 1. *State the research hypothesis.*
1. *Null Hypothesis:* There is no statistically significant difference between the height (μ) of adult Japanese-American men and the standard height (μ_0) of all adult American men.

$\mu = \mu_0$ (mu, parameter mean value)
$N = 10,000$

2. *Alternative Hypothesis:* There is a statistically significant difference between the height (μ) of adult Japanese-American men and the height (μ_0) of all adult American men.

$\mu \neq \mu$ (mu, parameter mean value)

Step 2. *Select the level of statistical significance:* $\alpha = .05$
Step 3. *Select test statistics.* Use *t*-test.
The formula for a *t*-test is

$$t = \frac{\overline{X} - \mu_o}{s / \sqrt{N}}$$

(Note: *s* divided by square root of *N*)
Step 4. *Identify the* t_{crit} *from the t distribution table.*
a. significance level: a = .05
b. two-tailed test of significance
c. $df = N - 1 = 10,000 - 1 = 9,999$
$t_{crit} = .196$[1]

Step 5. *Calculate the test statistic value.* From a random sample of 10,000 adult Japanese-American men

---
[1] Because *df* = 9999, which is larger than 120, t_{ctit} may be obtained from Table C–2.

living in the United States, the following data were collected. An $\overline{X}$ is used rather than a μ because only a sample of the total number is used. In this case, the $\overline{X}$ is a value obtained from a representative sample of the population (μ).

$$\overline{X} = 64 \ in.$$

standard deviation (sd) = 1.8 in.

Step 6. *Identify parameter values.* The parameter values[2] for the average adult American men are:

$$\mu_0 = 69 \ in.$$
$$sd = 1.9 \ in.$$

In this case, μ is used because the total population is being considered.

Step 7. *Graph normal curve for parameter value.* Because the parameter values are a constant, we can use the normal curve to describe the distribution of parameter values. This is shown in Figure 6–1. For a normal distribution with a mean of 69 and a standard deviation of 1.9, we will expect 68% of adult American men to have heights between 67.1 and 70.9 inches.

Step 8. *Graph normal curve for sample.* This is shown in Figure 6–2. For the sample distribution with a mean of 64 and a standard deviation of 1.8, we will expect 68% of the adult Japanese-American men to have heights between 62.2 and 65.8 inches.

---

2   These are hypothetical values set to explain concepts.

Step 9. Calculate the t_{obs} using the formula for *t*-test (see Step 3).

$$t = \frac{\overline{X} - \mu_o}{s / \sqrt{N}}$$

Where
$\overline{X}$ = sample mean equals 64
sd = sample standard deviation equals 1.8
μ_0 = parameter mean equals 69
N = sample number of subjects = 10,000

$$t = (64 - 69) / 1.8 \sqrt{10,000}$$

$$= (-5) / (1.8 / 100)$$
$$t_{obs} = -5 / .018$$
$$t_{obs} = -277.78$$

Step 10. *Compare* t_{obs} *with* t_{crit}

$$t_{obs} = -277.78$$
$$t_{crit} = 1.960$$
$$t_{obs} > t_{crit}.$$

Due to this being a 2-tailed test of significance, it is the absolute values that are considered here.

6.6 One Sample: Interpretation of Potential Statistical Outcomes

Thus, the researcher rejects the null hypothesis and concludes that there is a statistically significant difference

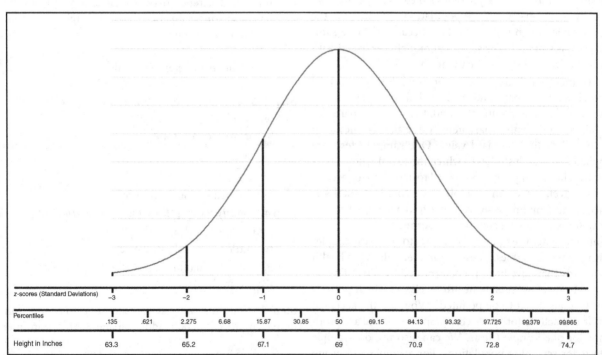

Figure 6–1 Hypothetical data for typical adult American men depicting a normal distribution in which the mean height is 69 inches and the standard deviation is 1.9; 68% of the adult population should fall between +1 and −1 standard deviations, or heights of 67.1 and 70.9 inches.

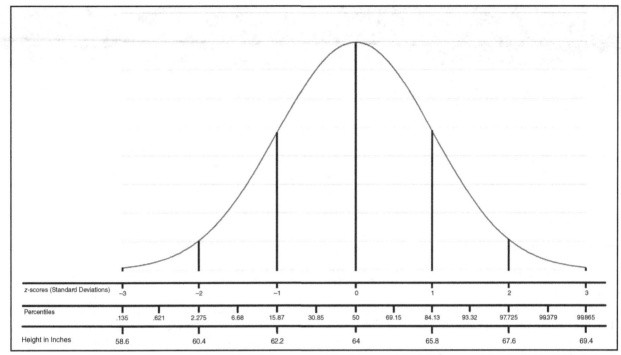

Figure 6–2 Hypothetical data for a sample of 10,000 adult Japanese and American men depicting a normal distribution in which the mean height is 64 inches and the standard deviation is 1.8; 68% of the adult population should fall between +1 and −1 standard deviations, or heights of 62.2 and 65.8 inches.

between the height of adult Japanese-American men compared with the average heights of all adult American men.

6.6.1 One Sample: Journal Article Examples Reflecting Chapter Design and Statistics

Prowd et al. (2020) investigated the 9-Hole Peg Test performance and the Purdue Peg Board performance of 20 male and female adults with mild to moderate Parkinson's disease with published normative data, respectively, for these two fine-motor dexterity tests. Using one-sample t-tests, these researchers found that the male and female participants with Parkinson's disease performed significantly poorer with both the dominant and non-dominant limbs than the normative age-matched sample on both dexterity tests with the exception of the non-dominant limb performance for women on the 9-hole peg test. The researchers' conclusion reflected these differences and suggested that when evaluating fine motor performance in a similar population, that decreased performance from the "norm" can be expected.

6.7 INDEPENDENT *T*-TEST

The purpose of this statistical model is to test whether there is a statistically significant difference between the means of two independent samples. This frequently is used to test the differences between two clinical techniques applied to an experimental group and a control

or comparative group. For example, if a researcher is examining the comparative effectiveness of two treatment techniques in two independent groups, such as *Progressive Relaxation Exercise* versus *Transcutaneous Electrical Nerve Stimulation* in reducing pain, then an independent t-test will be applied to the outcome measure for pain (dependent variable). The t-test is also applied when the researcher examines whether there is a statistically significant difference in the characteristic abilities of two groups. For example, in a hypothetical experiment, authors compared performances of a group of stroke survivors who were randomly assigned to an experimental or a control group. The experimental group was enrolled in an enhanced occupation-based training regime whereas the control group was enrolled in a traditional exercise regime. The outcome variables (i.e., dependent variables) included the Sock Test, the 9-Hole Peg Test, and the Get Up and Go Test. The independent t-test analysis compared pre-test/post-test change score between groups for each of the outcome variables. Table 6–1 contains the hypothetical outcome means for these variables.

Of the three variables tested, only one did not reach statistical significance with $\alpha = 0.05$. The researchers used an independent two-tailed t-test for determining the critical level of significance with a total n of 30 subjects (15 in each group), at a df of $n - 2$. In a two-tailed test with 28 df, the critical value of t is 2.0484. (See Table C–3 in the appendices.) The observed t was above 2.0484 in two of the three variables tested. The t values reflected the differences between the group means and the comparative homogeneity of the two independent sample standard deviations. In

TABLE 6–1				
COMPARISON OF PRE-TEST/POST-TEST CHANGE SCORE				
OUTCOME VARIABLES	ENHANCED OCCUPATION-BASED GROUP PRE-TEST/POST-TEST CHANGE SCORE *N*=15 *M (SD)*	TRADITIONAL EXERCISE GROUP PRE-TEST/POST-TEST CHANGE SCORE *N*=15 *M (SD)*	*T*-SCORE	*P*-VALUE
Sock Test	1.8(1.2)	1.1(.9)	2.08	.047
9-Hole Peg (seconds)	15.7(9.9)	13.5(8.8)	0.64	.525
Get Up and Go (seconds)	3.5(1.8)	2.3(.7)	2.41	.023

general, a *t* value is statistically significant when there is a relatively large difference between the group mean and a small difference within the groups. On the other hand, if the differences within the groups are larger than the differences between the groups, then there will likely not be a statistically significant difference between the groups as reflected in the observed *t* value. For example, in examining the first variable, Sock Test, the enhanced occupation-based group mean was 1.8 and the traditional exercise group mean was 1.1. The mean difference between the groups was 0.7. The standard deviations of 1.2 and.9 were comparatively homogeneous. With the calculated *t* score of 2.08 being larger than the *t*-critical score of 2.0484 along with a *p*-value of 0.047 being less than the stated α = 0.05, there was a statistically significant difference between the two groups. However, in examining the 9-Hole Peg Test outcome scores, the calculated *t-score* of 0.64 is smaller than the *t*-critical score of 2.0484, the *p*-value is larger than the stated α = 0.05; there is not a statistically significant between the two groups.

Operational Procedure for Testing for Statistically Significant Differences Between Two Independent Samples:

Step 1. *State the research hypothesis.*

1. Null Hypothesis: There is no statistically significant difference between the mean of group 1 versus the mean of group 2:

$$H_0: \mu_1 = \mu_2$$

2. Directional Hypothesis: Mean 1 is significantly statistically different from mean 2 in a stated direction:

$$\mu_1 > \mu_2$$

3. Alternative Hypothesis: Mean 1 does not equal mean 2, and there is a statistically significant difference between the two means (non-directional):

$$H_1: \mu_1 \neq \mu_2$$

Step 2. *Select the level of statistical significance.* In social sciences research, the.05 level of significance is traditionally selected.

Step 3. *Select the statistical test.* Use independent *t*-test.

Step 4. *Decide whether to use a one-tailed or two-tailed test for statistical significance.* A two-tailed test is used with a null hypothesis to determine if there are statistically significant differences in either direction of the tail. The model for a two-tailed test are the tails in a normal curve (Figure 6–3). A one-tailed test is used with a directional hypothesis when the researcher predicts that the experimental group mean will be either statistically greater or lesser than a comparison mean.

Step 5. *Look up the critical value (t_{crit}) from the published statistical table.* The critical value is determined by:

a. the degrees of freedom (*df*)

b. the level of significance (α < .05 or < .01)

c. the direction of the test (one-tailed or two-tailed)

d. the value of t_{crit} as indicated in the statistical table. (See Table C–3 in the appendices.)

Step 6. *Calculate the group means and standard deviations.*

Step 7. *Do an exploratory data analysis* to determine if the differences between the two means are clinically significant and that the standard deviations in both groups are approximately equal.

Step 8. *Plot a graph.* Use the graph mean and raw scores of group 1 and group 2 to visualize whether there seems to be a statistically significant difference between the group

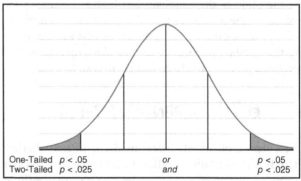

Figure 6–3 Model for a two-tailed test. A one-tailed test would use only one of the two marked areas and the alpha would be adjusted accordingly.

means. (See Figure 6–4.) If there appears to be a difference between the two group means, then go to Step 9 and calculate the values.

Step 9. Calculate the t_{obs} using the formula.

The formula for t_{obs} is:

$$t_{obs} = \frac{\overline{X_1} - \overline{X_2}}{\sqrt{\{[(n_1-1)(s_1^2) + (n_2-1)(s_2^2)]/(n_1+n_2-2)\}\left[\left(\frac{1}{n_1}\right)+\left(\frac{1}{n_2}\right)\right]}}$$

Where
$\overline{X_1}$ = mean value of group 1
$\overline{X_2}$ = mean value of group 2
n_1 = total number of cases in group 1
n_2 = total number of cases in group 2
s_1^2 = variance (the standard deviation squared) for group 1
s_2^2 = variance for group 2

Step 10. *Compare the two values:* t_{obs} *and* t_{crit}.

a. Accept the null hypothesis if t_{obs} is less than t_{crit}
b. Reject the null hypothesis if t_{obs} is equal to or greater than t_{crit}
c. Accept the directional hypothesis if t_{obs} is greater than or equal to t_{crit} in the direction that is hypothesized
d. Reject the directional hypothesis if t_{obs} is less than t_{crit} or if the mean value that is predicted to be greater is less than the mean value of the control or comparative group. For example, a researcher predicts that cognitive training is more effective than

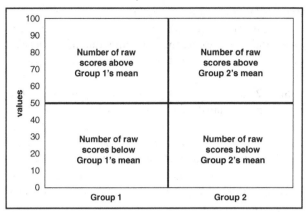

Figure 6–4 Graph to visualize values of scores as a way to estimate possible statistical significance between the group means.

behavioral therapy in increasing attention span. The results show a statistically significant difference between the two means, but behavioral therapy is more effective. Because the researcher predicted that cognitive therapy is more effective than behavioral therapy, the directional hypothesis is rejected.

6.8 TWO INDEPENDENT GROUPS EXAMPLE

Is there a statistically significant difference between stress management and group psychotherapy in reducing anxiety scores in patients with clinical depression?

HYPOTHETICAL POST-TEST SCORES ON THE STATE-TRAIT ANXIETY INVENTORY*					
STRESS MANAGEMENT GROUP			PSYCHOTHERAPY GROUP		
SUBJECT	SCORE (X_1)	X_1^2	SUBJECT	SCORE (X_2)	X_2^2
01	35	1225	01	51	2601
02	41	1681	02	48	2304
03	38	1444	03	52	2704
04	42	1764	04	43	1849
05	43	1849	05	49	2401
06	36	1296	06	54	2916
07	32	1024	07	61	3721
08	40	1600	08	56	3136
09	41	1681	09	54	2916
10	43	1849	10	60	3600
11	42	1764	11	48	2304
12	34	1156	12	46	2116
$\Sigma X_1 = 467$ $\Sigma X^2 = 18333$ $\overline{X_1} = 38.9$			$\Sigma X_2 = 622$ $\Sigma X_2^2 = 32568$ $\overline{X_2} = 51.8$		
Grand Mean $= (\Sigma X_1 + \Sigma X_2)/24 = (467+622)/24 = 45.37$					

* Smaller score indicates less anxiety

Step 1. *State the research hypothesis.* There is no statistically significant difference between a stress management group and a psychotherapy group in reducing anxiety in a sample of depressed patients. The hypothesis is stated in null form ($\mu_1 = \mu_2$).

Step 2. *Select the level of statistical significance.* The $\alpha = .05$ level of statistical significance will be accepted.

Step 3. *This is a non-directional two-tailed test for statistical significance because a null hypothesis was stated.* Decide the test statistic. Independent *t*-test will be used.

Step 4. Determine the critical value for *t* from published statistical tables. (See Table C–3 in the appendices.)
a. $df = n_1 + n_2 - 2 = 22$
b.   level of significance $\alpha = .05$
c. $t_{crit} = 2.0739$

Step 5. *Calculate the mean and standard deviations.*

STRESS MANAGEMENT GROUP	PSYCHOTHERAPY GROUP
$\overline{X_1} = \Sigma X_1 /$	$\overline{X_2} = \Sigma X_2 /$
$n = 467/12 = 38.9$	$n = 622/12 = 51.8$
$\overline{X_1} = 38.9$	$\overline{X_2} = 51.8$
$s_1 = 3.80$	$s_2 = 5.45$

Computational Formula for Standard Deviation

$$s = \sqrt{\left[n\Sigma X^2 - (\Sigma X)^2\right] / \left[n(n-1)\right]}$$

$$s_1 = \sqrt{\left[(12)(18333) - (467)^2\right] / \left[12(12-1)\right]}$$

$$s_1 = \sqrt{(219996 - 218089) / \left[12(12-1)\right]}$$

$$s_1 = \sqrt{1907 / 132}$$

$$s_1 = \sqrt{14.44}$$

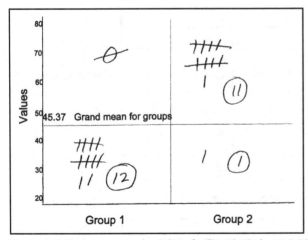

Figure 6–5 Exploratory graph analysis for hypothetical post-test scores on the *State-Trait Anxiety Inventory*. The graph shows the difference between scores between two independent groups of patients with clinical depression receiving either stress management training or group psychotherapy. The test being performed is an independent *t*-test.

$s_1 = 3.80$

$$s_2 = \sqrt{\left[(12)(32568) - (622)^2\right] / \left[12(12-1)\right]}$$

$$s_2 = \sqrt{(390816 - 386884) / \left[12(12-1)\right]}$$

$$s_2 = \sqrt{3932 / 132}$$

$$s_2 = \sqrt{29.78}$$

$$s_2 = 5.45$$

Step 6. *Exploratory data analysis.*

$$\overline{X_1} - \overline{X_2} = 38.9 - 51.8 = 12.9$$
$$s_1 = 3.80$$
$$s_2 = 5.45$$

The mean difference is greater than the standard deviation for group 1 or group 2. Standard deviation difference between the two groups is 1.65. There is a relative homogeneity of variance for the two groups.

Step 7. *Exploratory graph analysis.* Figure 6–5 shows the graph obtained from the analysis. There appears to be a significant difference between the two groups.

Step 8. *Calculate t_{obs}.*

$$t_{obs} = \frac{\overline{X_1} - \overline{X_2}}{\sqrt{\{[(n_1 - 1)(s_1^2) + (n_2 - 1)(s_2^2)] / (n_1 + n_2 - 2)\}\left[\left(\frac{1}{n_1}\right) + \left(\frac{1}{n_2}\right)\right]}}$$

Where

GROUP 1	GROUP 2
$\overline{X_1} = 38.9$	$\overline{X_2} = 51.8$
$n_1 = 12$	$n_2 = 12$
$s_1^2 = (3.80)^2 = 14.44$	$s_2^2 = (5.45)^2 = 29.70$

$$t_{obs} = \frac{38.9 - 51.8}{\sqrt{\{[(12-1)(14.44) + (12-1)(29.78)] / (12+12-2)\}\left[\left(\frac{1}{12}\right) + \left(\frac{1}{12}\right)\right]}}$$

$$t_{obs} = \frac{-12.9}{\sqrt{[(158.84 + 327.58)/22][1.667]}}$$

$$t_{obs} = \frac{-12.9}{\sqrt{[(486.12)/22][1.667]}}$$

$$t_{obs} = -12.9 / \sqrt{3.685}$$

$$t_{obs} = -12.9 / 1.9196$$

$$t_{obs} = -6.72$$

Step 9. *Compare* t_{obs} *and* t_{crit}.

$t_{obs} = -6.72$
$t_{crit} = 2.0739$

The examination shows $|t_{obs}|^3 > t_{crit}$. Reject the null hypothesis. There seems to be a statistically significant difference between the two means, indicating that the stress management group was significantly more effective that the psychotherapy group in the reduction of anxiety in patients with clinical depression.

6.9 Mann-Whitney *U* Test

Rationale

The Mann-Whitney, a non-parametric alternative to the independent *t*-test, is used to test whether two independent groups have been drawn from the same population. In practice, the Mann-Whitney is used with ordinal scale data.

1. The null hypothesis states that the two independent groups have the same population distribution.

2. An alternative, directional hypothesis is that there is a significant difference between the group means (when the distributions are approximately the same).

---

3 $|t_{obs}|$ is an absolute value that disregards the sign. The parallel lines indicate absolute value.

Assumptions

1. Random selection of each group.
2. Two mutually independent groups are compared.
3. The measurement scale is at least ordinal.
4. *n* for each group is less than 20.

Computation

1. Rank order every raw score combining the two groups (e.g., lowest score in both groups is assigned the rank of 1).
2. When two or more raw scores are the same, average the ranks.
3. Add the ranks for one group, obtaining T_A value.

Formula for Mann-Whitney *U* Test

$$U_{obs} = (n_A n_B) + [(n_A)(n_A + 1) / 2] - [T_A]$$

Where
n_A = number of subjects in 1st group
n_B = number of subjects in 2nd group

Example

Language intelligibility scores were compared between an experimental and control group after a six-month treatment period. There was no significant difference between the groups on the pre-test. (Two-tailed test α = .05.)

The following data were collected:

EXPERIMENTAL GROUP A			CONTROL GROUP P		
SUBJECT	SCORE	RANK	SUBJECT	SCORE	RANK
101	33	12	201	35	13
102	30	10	202	32	11
103	25	8	203	27	9
104	24	6.5	204	24	6.5
105	22	5	205	21	4
106	19	3	206	18	2
			207	16	1
$T_a = 44.5$ $n_A = 6$			$T_b = 46.5$ $n_B = 7$		

$U_{obs} = [(6)\,(7)] + [6\,(6 + 1) / 2] - [44.5]$
$U_{obs} = 42 + 21 - 44.5$
$U_{obs} = 63 - 44.5$
$U_{obs} = 18.5$

Obtain U_{crit}: from table for Mann-Whitney *U* test. (See Table C–7 in the appendices.)

$n_A / n_B = 6 / 7$
$U_{crit} = 6 / 36$

If U_{obs} is between 6 and 36, do not reject null hypothesis.

Conclusion

Null hypothesis is not rejected because $U_{obs} = 18.5$, which is between 6 and 36. Thus, the researcher concludes that there is no statistically significant difference in the experimental and control groups in language intelligibility post-test scores.

6.10 *k*-INDEPENDENT SAMPLES

If the researcher is comparing the means of more than two independent samples, then he or she applies an analysis of variance (ANOVA). The ANOVA is similar to the independent test when two independent samples are compared. If the results of the ANOVA are statistically significant, then the researcher employs post-hoc tests to determine which groups are statistically different from each other. Examples of these post-hoc tests (similar to *t*-tests) include the Scheffé, Duncan multiple analysis, or Tukey tests. The non-parametric alternative to ANOVA is the Kruskal-Wallis statistical test.

6.11 ANALYSIS OF VARIANCE

ANOVA is a widely used statistical test equivalent to the independent *t*-test when testing for significant differences between two means. ANOVA is applied to statistical data when two or more independent group means are being compared. The statistic for the ANOVA is *F*. (*k* refers to the number of independent groups or conditions in the study.)

F = variance between groups / variance within groups

The concept of the ANOVA is that if there are large differences between the group means compared with relatively small differences within the variances or scores within the group, then a statistically significant result is evident. ANOVA answers the question: Is there a statistically significant difference between the independent groups being tested? For example, does $\mu_1 = \mu_2 = \mu_3 = \mu_k$? ANOVA is always tested by a null hypothesis. When there is a statistically significant result, the researcher then carries out a post-hoc analysis, such as the Scheffé, Duncan Multiple Range, Neuman-Keuls, and Tukey's procedures. These post-hoc tests are similar to *t*-tests for independent measures, applied to the data after attaining a significant *F*.

6.12 ONE-WAY ANOVA

A one-way ANOVA simply analyzes the group means for statistically significant differences. The hypothetical table of results that follows is a typical example of a one-way ANOVA for comparing the effectiveness of three handwriting programs among 19 children with handwriting problems.

ANOVA SUMMARY TABLE FOR COMPARING TWO TREATMENT GROUPS

SOURCE OF VARIANCE	df	SS	MS	F
Between treatment groups	2	16	8	4.0*
Within treatment groups	16	32	2	
Total	18			

*$p = <.05$, $F_{crit} = 3.63$

Where
SS = sums of squares
MS = mean squares
k = number of treatment groups
N = total number of subjects in all groups

F is a derivative value equivalent to F_{obs} that is compared with the F_{crit} derived from a statistical table of values. For example, the F_{crit} for 2 *df* (treatment groups −1) and 16 *df* [number of subjects (19) − number of groups (3)] with 2 / 16, α =.05 is 3.63. Degrees of freedom (*df*) is derived from between treatment groups (*k* −1) and within treatment groups (*N* − *k*).

The result in this hypothetical example shows that there is a statistically significant difference between the three treatment methods for handwriting disorders. F_{obs} 4.00 is > F_{crit} 3.63. Thus, the researcher will reject the null hypothesis.

Example of Two-Factor ANOVA From the Literature

A one-way ANOVA analyzes the group means for statistically significant differences. The two-factor ANOVA looks at the variables from a two-dimensional perspective. It analyzes interactive effects, such as treatment method and therapist personality or treatment method and patient diagnosis. Lin et al. (2015) investigated upper extremity motor control under challenging versus easier cognitive tasks. The design involved a 2 × 2 (Condition × Group) design with the Condition factor being either the single task or the dual task and the Group factor being either participants with Schizophrenia or health controls. Results are shown in the following table.

SUMMARY TABLE OF ANOVA ON CONDITION AND GROUP

SOURCE OF VARIANCE	df	F	p VALUE
Condition (single, dual task)	1	33.49	<.001*
Group(schizophrenia, control)	1	47.59	<.001
Condition × Group	1	6.15	.02

*$p < .05$ significant

The results show that there was a significant different in upper extremity motor performance between the single and dual tasks conditions, between the two population groups, and there was a significant interaction between the Condition and Group factors, meaning that the differences between the single and dual task performances were significantly different depending on the population.

6.13 STEPWISE PROCEDURES FOR ONE-WAY ANOVA (HYPOTHETICAL EXAMPLE)

Step 1. *State the research hypothesis.* The hypothesis is always stated in the null form when using ANOVA. For example, there is no statistically significant difference between electrical stimulation (ES), acupuncture (A), and proprioceptive neuromuscular facilitation (PNF)

in improving upper extremity function in patients with chronic hemiplegia.

$$H_0 = \mu_1 = \mu_2 = \mu_3$$

Step 2. Select the level of statistical significance.

$\alpha = .05$

Step 3. *Identify F_{crit} from table.* (See Table C–4 in the appendices.)
 a. *df* for the numerator = 2 (three treatment groups – 1) *df* for the denominator = 15 (number of subjects minus the number of groups:
 18 – 3 = 15), *df* = 2 / 15
 b. $\alpha = .05$
 c. $F_{crit} = 3.68$

Step 4. Calculate means and standard deviations.[4]

---

[4] The *Fugl-Meyer Poststroke Motor Recovery Test* scores were used for the example. (Range is from 0–60.)

ES GROUP			A GROUP			PNF GROUP		
SUBJECT	SCORE (*X*)	$X_1{}^2$	SUBJECT	SCORE (*X*)	$X_2{}^2$	SUBJECT	SCORE (*X*)	$X_3{}^2$
0l	23	529	01	13	169	01	33	1089
02	31	961	02	19	361	02	42	1764
03	16	256	03	19	361	03	30	900
04	27	729	04	25	625	04	38	1444
05	32	1024	05	18	324	05	44	1936
06	18	324				06	41	1681
07	38	1444						
$\Sigma X_1 = 185$	$\Sigma X_1{}^2 = 5267$		$\Sigma X_2 = 94$	$\Sigma X_2{}^2 = 1840$		$\Sigma X_3 = 228$	$\Sigma X_3{}^2 = 8814$	
$\overline{X_1} = 26.4$			$\overline{X_2} = 18.8$			$\overline{X_3} = 38.0$		

$$s = \sqrt{\frac{N\Sigma X^2 - (\Sigma X)^2}{N(N-1)}}$$

$$s_1 = \sqrt{\frac{7(5267) - (185)^2}{7(7-1)}}$$

$$s_1 = \sqrt{2644 / 42}$$

$$s_1 = \sqrt{62.95}$$

$$s_1 - 7.93$$

$$s_2 = \sqrt{\frac{5(1840) - (94185)^2}{5(4)}}$$

$$s_2 = \sqrt{364 / 20}$$

$$s_2 = \sqrt{18.2}$$

$$s_2 = 4.26$$

$$s_3 = \sqrt{\frac{6(8814) - (228)^2}{6(5)}}$$

$$s_3 = \sqrt{(900 / 30)}$$

$$s_3 = \sqrt{30.00}$$

$$s_3 = 5.48$$

Step 5. *Exploratory data analysis.*

$\overline{X}_1 = 26$	$s_1 = 7.93$
$\overline{X}_2 = 18.8$	$s_1 = 4.26$
$\overline{X}_3 = 38.0$	$s_3 = 5.48$
$\overline{X}_1 - \overline{X}_2 = 7.6$	$s_1 - s_2 = 3.67$
$\overline{X}_1 - \overline{X}_3 = -11.6$	$s_1 - s_3 = 2.45$
$\overline{X}_2 - \overline{X}_3 = -19.2$	$s_2 - s_3 = -1.22$

There appears to be a statistically significant difference between the means and a relatively homogenous variance.

Step 6. *Exploratory graph analysis.* This graph is shown in Figure 6–6.

$$\text{Group mean} = (\Sigma \overline{X}_1 + \Sigma \overline{X}_1 + \Sigma \overline{X}_1) / (N_1 + N_2 + N_3)$$
$$= (185 + 94 + 288) / (7 + 5 + 6)$$
$$= 507 / 18$$
$$= 28.17$$

There appears to be a statistically significant difference between group 2 and group 3.

Step 7. *Calculate F.*

SUMMARY TABLE FOR ONE-WAY ANOVA

SOURCE OF VARIANCE	df	SS	MS	F
Between groups (BG)	2	1039.98	519.99	12.99
Within groups (WG)	15	600.52	40.03	
Total	17			

Formulas for ANOVA:

a. $F = MS$ between groups / MS within groups

b. df between groups (df_{bg}) = Number of groups minus 1 = (3 – 1) = 2

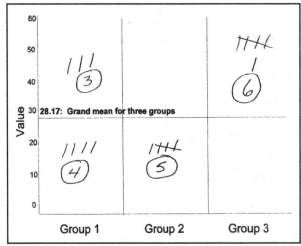

Figure 6–6 Exploratory graph for ANOVA using hypothetical data. The graph shows differences in scores between three different groups.

df within groups (df_{wg}) = Total number of subjects in all groups minus the number of groups = 18 – 3 = 15

c. Mean Square between groups = SS_{bg} / df_{bg}

Mean Square within groups = SS_{wg} / df_{wg}

d. Sum of Squares between groups:

$$SS_{bg} = \Sigma \left[(\Sigma X_1)^2 / n_1 \right] + \left[(\Sigma X_2)^2 / n_2 \right] + \left[(\Sigma X_3)^2 / n_3 \right] - \left[(\Sigma X_1 + \Sigma X_2 + \Sigma X_3)^2 / \Sigma N \right]$$

Group 1
$(\Sigma X_1)^2 = (185)^2 = 34225$
$n_1 = 7$
$(\Sigma X_1)^2 / n_1 = 4889.29$

Group 2
$(\Sigma X_2)^2 = (94)^2 = 8836$
$n_2 = 5$
$(\Sigma X_2)^2 / n_2 = 1767.2$

Group 3
$(\Sigma X_3)^2 = (228)^2 = 51984$
$n_3 = 6$
$(\Sigma X_3)^2 / n_3 = 8664.0$

Total = (4889.29 + 1767.2 + 8664.0) = 15320.49
$(\Sigma X_1 + \Sigma X_2 + \Sigma X_3) / \Sigma N) = 257049 / 18 = 14280.5$
$SS_{bg} = [(4889.29 + 1767.2 + 8664.0)] - [(257049) / 18]$
$SS_{bg} = 15320.49 - 14280.5$
$SS_{bg} = 1039.99$

e. Sums of Squares within Groups

$SS_{wg} = \Sigma (\Sigma X_2^2 + \Sigma X_2^2 + \Sigma X_3^2) - 15320.49$
$SS_{wg} = \Sigma (5267 + 1840 + 8814) - 15320.49$
$SS_{wg} = 15921 - 15320.49$
$SS_{wg} = 600.51$

Mean Square between groups
$SS_{bg} / df_{bg} = 1039.99 / 2 = 519.99$

Mean Square within groups
$SS_{bg} / df_{wg} = 600.51 / 15 = 40.03$
$F = MS_{bg} / MS_{wg} = 519.99 / 40.03 = 12.99$

Step 8. *Compare F_{obs} with F_{crit}*

$F_{obs} = 12.99$ $F_{crit} = 3.68$

Thus, we reject the null hypothesis and conclude that there is a statistically significant difference between the three groups. This confirms our exploratory data analysis.

Step 9. *Conduct a post-hoc test.* If there is a significant F, meaning that the mean values are statistically significant, then the researcher carries out a post-hoc analysis. This analysis is parallel to doing independent t-tests and determines which pairs of means have statistically significant differences.

There are a number of post-hoc tests that are available to the researcher, such as:

- Tukey's Honestly Significant Differences (HSD)
- Neuman-Keuls
- Duncan Multiple Range
- Scheffé

Example of a Post-Hoc Analysis.

In the previous example, it was found that F_{obs} is statistically significant when

$$\overline{X_1} = 26.4$$
$$\overline{X_2} = 18.8$$
$$\overline{X_3} = 38.0.$$

H_0: Null hypothesis is rejected and we conclude that all the means are not the same. We can now compare each pair of means, such as:

$$\overline{X_1} \text{ compared to } \overline{X_2}$$
$$\overline{X_1} \text{ compared to } \overline{X_3}$$
$$\overline{X_2} \text{ compared to } \overline{X_3}$$

A significant F means that at least one pair of means are significantly different, that is, the highest and lowest mean. Therefore, $\overline{X_2}$ compared to $\overline{X_3}$ has a statistically significant difference. We do not know whether there is a statistically significant difference between $\overline{X_1}$ and $\overline{X_2}$ and/or $\overline{X_1}$ and $\overline{X_3}$. A post-hoc analysis tests for statistically significant difference in these two situations.

In this example the Tukey (*HSD*), a widely used post-hoc analysis, was selected. The formula for the Tukey is (Gravetter & Wellnau, 2016):

$$HSD = q\sqrt{\frac{MS_{wg}}{n}}$$

Where

q = a derived table value (See Table C–9 in the appendices: The Student Range Statistic.) In this case, $q = 3.67$

MS_{wg} = the value calculated for mean squares within groups and is taken from the ANOVA table. In the above example this value is 40.03.

n = the average of the number of cases in each group. In the above example $n_1 = 7$, $n_2 = 5$, and $n_3 = 6$. The average is 6.

k = number of groups (k) = 3
df for MS_{wg} = 15
$\alpha = .05$

$$HSD = q\sqrt{\frac{MS_{wg}}{n}}$$
$$HSD = 3.67\sqrt{\frac{40.03}{6}}$$
$$HSD = 9.479$$

Therefore, the mean difference between any two group scores must be at least 9.48 to be statistically significant.

a. $\overline{X_1} - \overline{X_2} = 26.4 - 18.8 = 7.6$. Therefore, the null hypothesis is accepted and $\overline{X_1} = \overline{X_2}$

b. $\overline{X_1} - \overline{X_3} = 26.4 - 38.0 = 11.6$. Therefore, the null hypothesis is rejected and $\overline{X_1} \neq \overline{X_3}$

c. $\overline{X_2} - \overline{X_3} = 18.8 - 38.0 = 19.2$. Therefore, the null hypothesis is rejected and $\overline{X_2} \neq \overline{X_3}$

In conclusion, a post-hoc analysis test determines the pairs of means that have statistically significant differences.

6.14 KRUSKAL-WALLIS TEST FOR K SAMPLE

The Kruskal-Wallis test is a non-parametric alternative to the one-way ANOVA when comparing three or more independent groups.

Assumptions

a. Random selection or random assignment of subjects to each independent group
b. Ordinal scale measurement
c. Each group should have at least five subjects

Example of Applying Kruskal-Wallis

Step 1. The investigator hypothesizes that there is no statistically significant difference between the three groups.

GROUP 1		GROUP 2		GROUP 3	
SUBJ	RAW SCORE	SUBJ	RAW SCORE	SUBJ	RAW SCORE
101	10	201	14	301	12
102	8	202	12	302	14
103	6	203	10	303	7
104	10	204	8	304	6
105	12	205	9	305	10
106	14				

Step 2. *Rank order every raw score, combining all groups (in this example, three groups) with the lowest score assigned a rank of 1. In this example, the raw score of 4 made by Subject 303 raw score of 4 is assigned the rank of 1.*

SUBJECT	RAW SCORE	RANK	
101	10	8.5	
102	8	4.5	
103	6	2.5	
104	10	8.5	
105	12	12	

106	14	15	$\Sigma_{\text{ranks}} = 51$
201	14	15	
202	12	12	
203	10	8.5	
201	8	4.5	
205	9	6	$\Sigma_{\text{ranks}} = 46$
301	12	12	
302	14	15	
303	4	1	
304	6	2.5	
305	10	8.5	$\Sigma_{\text{ranks}} = 39$

Note: n = 16

Step 3. *Sum the ranks for each group.*

GROUP 1	GROUP 2	GROUP 3
8.5	15	12
4.5	12	15
2.5	8.5	1
8.5	4.5	2.5
12	6	8.5
15		
$\Sigma_1 = 51$	$\Sigma_2 = 46.0$	$\Sigma_3 = 39.0$
$n_1 = 6$	$n_2 = 5$	$n_3 = 5$

Step 4. *Calculate the formula for Kruskal-Wallis (H_{obs})*

$$H_{\text{obs}} = 12 \; / \; [N \, (N + 1)] \; [(T_1^2 \, / \, n_1) + (T_2^2 \, / \, n_2) + (T_3^2 \, / \, n_3)] - [3 \, (N + 1)]$$

Where

$N = n_1 + n_2 + n_3 = 16$

$T_1^2 = (\Sigma_{1\text{-ranks}})^2 = 51^2 = 2601$

$T_2^2 = (\Sigma_{2\text{-ranks}})^2 = 46^2 = 2116$

$T_3^2 = (\Sigma_{3\text{-ranks}})^2 = 39^2 = 1521$

$H_{\text{obs}} = 12 \, / \, [16 \, (17)] \, [(2601 \, / \, 6) + (2116 \, / \, 5) + (1521 \, / \, 5)] - [3(17)]$

$= [12 \, / \, 272] \, [433.5 + 423.2 + 304.2] - [51]$

$= [.044][1160.9] - [51]$

$= 51.08 - 51$

$= .08$

Step 5. *Calculate H_{crit} for $\alpha = .05$, df = number of groups (k) – 1 = 2.*

$H_{\text{crit}} = 5.99$. (Use chi-square, Table C–10, in the appendices to test for statistical significance.)

Step 6. *Compare H_{obs} (.08) with H_{crit} (5.991). If H_{obs} is equal to or more than H_{crit}, reject the null hypothesis.* In this example the null hypothesis is accepted and we conclude that there is no statistically significant difference between the three groups tested.

6.15 Experimental Model

For example, a researcher is interested in testing two therapeutic interventions for students with moderate intellectual disability who have difficulty in self-care activities. The experimental model is used in this study. The diagrammatical relationship between variables is depicted in Figure 6–7.

- In this hypothetical example, the guiding question is, "Is the cognitive approach more effective than the behavioral approach in increasing self-care abilities among individuals with moderate intellectual disability?"

- An operational definition of moderate intellectual disability is required (IQ score obtained on an individual test between 40 and 55, or sub-average adaptive behavior skills in two or more areas [e.g., leisure, communication, social skills] and occurrence in the developmental years). Age, gender, ethnicity, and socioeconomic status should be considered.

6.16 Describe a Controlled Clinical Trial (E2)

In its simplest form, a controlled clinical trial, noted at the E3 level on the experimental side of the Research Pyramid, involves pre-existing groups of participants with each group receiving different interventions. Often this involves being assigned to either an experimental or a control group. With all possible experimental controls in place, experimental designs at this level lack true random assignment into one group or the other. For instance, researcher in China recruited 20 children aged three to six years diagnosed with autism spectrum disorder who were enrolled already enrolled in a research protocol and were receiving transcranial magnetic stimulation and who were receiving treatment and education of autistic and related communication for handicapped children (TEACCH). The control group included 20 gender and age-matched children with ASD who were recruited from a welfare institution who were just receiving the TEACCH protocol. After a six-month follow up the investigators assessed the two groups on communication, body movement, language ability, and self-care and found that the group receiving the transcranial magnetic stimulation performed better on these outcome variables. They concluded that the transcranial magnetic stimulation coupled with the TEEACCH protocol could improve developmental outcomes within this population of children (Yanlin et al., 2018).

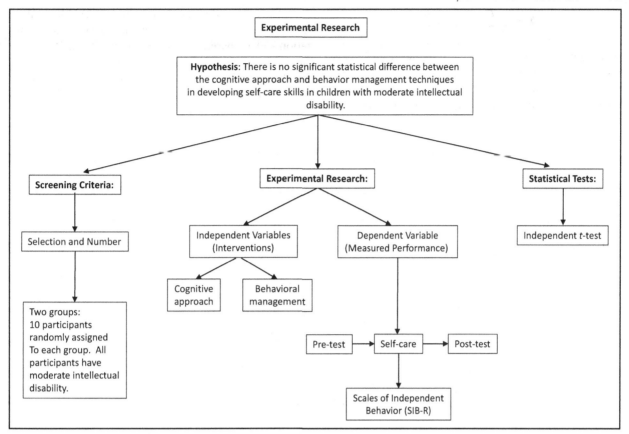

Figure 6–7 Diagrammatic relationship between variables in experimental research.

6.17 DESCRIBE A RANDOMIZED CLINICAL TRIAL [E2]

As mentioned in Chapter 2, the randomized clinical trial (RCT) is the classical prospective, scientific research method. Distinguishing it from other levels on the Research Pyramid, RCTs include the random selection of a sample of participants from a pre-defined population, random assignment of participants to at least two different groups, a testing of an independent variable, usually in the form of an experimental design (e.g., intervention versus no intervention or a placebo group). Additionally, participants and research personnel collecting the data are unaware of the group assignments (referred to as a double-blind study). The most distinguishing factor unique to RCTs is that attempts to control for *all* extraneous influences on the outcome variables, including researcher and participant biases, and environmental (temperature, stimuli) and chronological (time of day, day of week) artifacts. When control is implemented effectively, claims can be made about a cause-and-effect relationship between the independent and dependent variables with greater confidence than when these controls are not in place. In other words, a claim could be made that a certain intervention caused a better outcome in the group of people that received that intervention compared to the group that didn't.

As an example, Madhoun et al. (2020) investigated mirror therapy as a strategy for functional improvement for stroke survivors. These researchers recruited 30 stroke survivors and randomly assigned them to either the intervention ($n = 15$) or the control group ($n = 15$). While both groups received conventional occupational therapy, part of the therapy time for the intervention group involved task-based mirror therapy (TBMT). After 25 days of occupational therapy, the two groups were assessed on several outcome measures including the Fugl-Meyer Assessment, the Brunnstrom Assessment, the Modified Barthel Index, and the Modified Ashworth Scale. The results were that the group receiving the TBMT training performed significantly better on the Fugl-Meyer and certain upper extremity function as measured by the Modified Ashworth Scale including elbow flexion, wrist flexion, wrist extension and finger extension. The authors concluded that combining TBMT with conventional occupational therapy is an effective strategy to enhance function improvement in survivors of stroke.

6.18 SUMMARY

This chapter focused on study designs and related statistics associated with the experimental side of the Research Pyramid. Included in the chapter is a discussion on one-sample designs, experimental designs, multifactorial designs, controlled clinical trials, and RCTs. Most inferential statistics have assumptions that inform their utilization and are based upon the experimental controls and data characteristics. These assumptions help determine whether parametric versus non-parametric statistics are the best choice.

7

Single Case Experimental Design

Every clinical therapist providing service, however, has the responsibility to document, in a systematic manner, the effectiveness or non-effectiveness of the service provided to any given client... The primary tool advocated for achieving this goal is the small-N or "intensive" design.

Ottenbacher (1986a)

OPERATIONAL LEARNING OBJECTIVES

By the end of this chapter, the learner will understand:

1. The unique contribution of single case experimental design (SCED) studies to evidence-for-practice in occupational therapy
2. The most common terms used in SCEDs
3. SCED as a type of controlled experimental design, and thus its place in the Research Pyramid (E4)
4. The process of operationally defining the intervention (independent variable), and the measurement of the outcome (dependent variables) in a SCED
5. The types of demonstrable changes in performance in a SCED (level, slope, variability) through figures
6. Approaches to an analysis of the results through visual and statistical methods and through interpretation of the findings
7. The strengths and limitations of SCEDs pertaining to measurement, statistical, and generalizability issues
8. The historical contributions of SCEDs in the occupational therapy literature and its application to professional practice

7.1 INTRODUCTION

Imagine an occupational therapist providing services to a client with an inability to dress independently after a stroke. First the therapist will evaluate the client to determine current functioning. The therapist notices an inability to close buttons, due to a lack of fine motor coordination in the affected hand. The therapist decides on the intervention of providing a buttonhook. During the intervention, the therapist keeps track of the client's performance with the buttonhook each day to monitor progress. After two sessions, the client can dress independently, including using fasteners in a blouse or shirt.

The evaluation was equivalent to collecting baseline data (called Phase A), and the intervention was like the treatment phase (called Phase B). Although the client improved, was it because of the therapy? Consider the two extremes of possible situations: in one scenario, the therapist just treated the client without an evaluation (performed Phase B only). Suppose the client does better after a couple of sessions. The therapist claims it was the treatment that caused the improvement. Wouldn't you be skeptical?

In the second scenario, the therapist evaluates the client and establishes the client's stable functional performance level (Phase A). Then the intervention is applied and the client's performance improves (Phase B). Then the therapeutic effect is removed (the buttonhook is taken away), and the performance declines to what it was before (return to Phase A). The intervention is reapplied and the performance improves again (second Phase B). Removal, decline, reapplication, improvement (A, B, A, B)—after a few cycles anyone would be persuaded that the intervention does indeed cause the improved performance. Furthermore, the client is convinced and refuses to have the therapeutic intervention removed again.

This scenario is meant to illustrate the essence of a SCED and to show how much it resembles the occupational therapy process itself.

A clear distinction needs to be made among terms that are similar sounding and often confused. A SCED is not the same as a *case report*, a *case study*, or a *case series*, which are considered to be basic **descriptive** research (D4 or D3) in the Research Pyramid model (Tomlin & Borgetto, 2011). SCEDs represent a type of controlled experimental design, specifically level E4 in the pyramid model (Tomlin & Borgetto, 2011). Synonyms for SCED are single case research, single subject research, single system research, and an N-of-1 study.

7.2 TYPOLOGY: SCED AS A TYPE OF EXPERIMENTAL RESEARCH

SCEDs have many similarities to traditional group experimental designs:

- They are inspired by an important research question that can be applied to a single client or a small group of clients, such as "Do alternative seating devices lead to greater classroom attention by children with autism spectrum disorder (ASD)?"
- They seek to justify the claim of a likely causal relationship between an intervention and an improved outcome in the client, such as, "Does constraint induced movement therapy (CIMT) bring about greater functional use of the affected upper extremity in an individual who has had a stroke?"
- They identify demographic characteristics of the research participant(s), such as age, sex, diagnosis, performance challenges, and the occupational profile.
- Their design involves the manipulation of conditions to isolate a causative factor (i.e., what is the effect of the independent variable, or intervention, on the dependent variable, or outcome?).
- They contain an operationalization of the independent and dependent variables, of the procedure used for delivering the intervention, for collecting the data, and of the conditions under which data are collected.
- They are concerned with procedural reliability (i.e., fidelity) in the application of the designated intervention.
- They are concerned with procedural reliability of measurements of the dependent variable in the baseline and intervention phases, as well as intra- and inter-rater reliability.
- They often triangulate data collection by measuring multiple types of dependent variables, such as a physiological measure, a standardized test of skills/performance/behavior, and a self-evaluation.
- Experimental control can be applied in SCEDs by participants acting as their own control (in the baseline phase or phases).
- Control of confounding variables (e.g., history effects) or their documentation is incorporated into the design to enhance the accuracy of the interpretation of results.
- Blinding of evaluators or test administrators is sometimes possible, even if blinding of participants and therapists may not be possible.
- Outcomes are often appropriate for statistical analysis.
- Analysis, interpretation, and generalization of the results and their limitations are stated and the occupational implications are projected.
- Conclusions can suggest a possible cause-and-effect relationship between the independent variable and the dependent variable. In most cases the study should be replicated to strengthen the dependability of the conclusions and their generalizability.

SCEDs can be used as pilot projects to explore the relationship between variables and to test intervention protocols for later revision. In addition, whenever it is too costly, too time-consuming, or simply infeasible to conduct a study using group experimental design because a sufficient number of individuals with like challenges is not available in a setting, much can be gained through a SCED (Ottenbacher, 1986b). Their minimum recommended structure (Lane et al., 2017; Tate et al., 2016) now is a baseline phase followed by an intervention followed by a return to baseline followed by another phase of intervention (ABAB; see below). In this structure they closely mimic the sequence of the occupational therapy process itself (ABAB: evaluation, intervention, re-evaluation, adjusted intervention; AOTA, 2013). SCEDs can present a feasible means for therapists to scientifically evaluate the effects of their work with individual clients.

7.3 STRUCTURE OF SINGLE CASE EXPERIMENTAL DESIGNS: DESIGN CONSIDERATIONS TO STRENGTHEN CAUSAL CLAIMS

7.3.1 AB Structure

The simplest SCED has the structure A, that is, a baseline (A) phase of a certain length of time, followed by an intervention (B) phase, also of a certain length of time. Each phase involves multiple measurement occasions to provide confidence that the researcher has an accurate estimate of the client's actual performance level during this phase. Typically, data are measured 3 to 8 times per phase, each time on a different day (see Figure 7–1). Statistically speaking, a minimum of 6 is recommended so that any one data point does not overly influence the findings. For example, Mulcahey et al. (1995) studied the hand dexterity before and after tendon transplant surgery of an 11-year-old boy with tetraplegia due to a spinal cord injury. The surgery, post-operative care, and 4 weeks of hand therapy coincided with an immediate and steady improvement in hand function and ADL performance (Mulcahey et al., 1995). Sufficient data were assembled in this study to provide persuasive evidence that the surgery and therapy caused the improvement in function.

Whenever a marked difference in performance is apparent after the intervention is started (the transition to the B phase), then the researcher could formulate the claim that the intervention caused the improved performance. However, it is possible that something else may have happened just at the phase change that was the actual cause of the improvement. This actual cause might be another intervention being started by a different practitioner, a developmental milestone being naturally reached by the client, or an event in the living situation of the client (changing residence, absence or return of a family member, or recovery from an illness).

7.3.2 ABA Structure

Thus, a stronger causal claim could be made if data were further collected during a return-to-baseline phase, where the client's performance sharply returns to that in the original baseline phase when the intervention is removed. This design would be called an ABA (Figure 7–2).

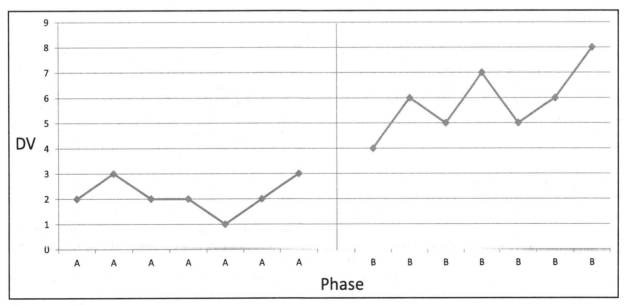

Figure 7–1 AB design.

Note: DV = dependent variable; each "A" is a data collection occasion in baseline; each "B" an occasion during intervention; A and B phases are separated slightly for clarity.

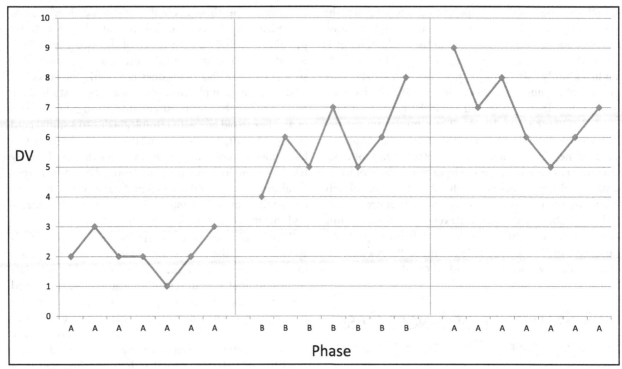

Figure 7–2 ABA: Withdrawal design.

Note: DV = dependent variable; each "A" is a data collection occasion in baseline; each "B" an occasion during intervention; phases are separated slightly for clarity.

For interventions providing a non-permanent effect, one expects the dependent variable to decline when the intervention is stopped, such as in the provision of assistive technology. Alternatively, if the intervention seeks to make a permanent change in the client, then one would expect the better performance to be maintained in the return to baseline (the second Phase A). For example, Dickerson and Brown (2007) studied the effects of CIMT on upper extremity use and quality of functional movement in a 24-month-old child with hemiparesis. Upon application of a constraint on the unaffected arm of the child (Phase B), performance improved in six of seven outcome variables. After the constraint was removed, performance was better than baseline in seven of eight recorded variables (Dickerson & Brown, 2007).

7.3.3 ABAB Structure

Stronger yet would be if data were measured in a second Phase B (ABAB; Figure 7–3). If performance improvement was observed both times there was an A-to-B transition, then the researcher could be much more confident that the change was caused by the intervention. Hence, the SCRIBE (Single Case Reporting Guideline in Behavioral Interventions) recommendation for contemporary SCEDs to have a design at least as thorough as ABAB. For example, Watling and Dietz (2007) studied the classroom behaviors of four 3- to 4-year-old boys with ASD

before and after providing two separate phases of Ayres Sensory Integration intervention. Although no immediate clearly beneficial changes were observed in undesired behavior or task engagement, parents noted more positive behaviors at home and therapists documented new, positive behaviors for each boy during therapy (Watling & Dietz, 2007).

7.3.4 ABC/ABAC Structure

Phase pairs AB could be repeated further, but more common is the introduction of a second, different intervention, called C. The simplest design with a Phase C would be ABC. Here, the baseline phase is followed by a period of intervention B followed by a period of intervention C. Performance during B might not show an improvement over that in A, but perhaps with the onset of C it does show improvement. For example, Gustafson et al. (2016) examined whether compression bandaging (Phase B) and compression gloves (Phase C) could reduce edema in the stroke-affected upper limb of four individuals. They found the bandaging was accompanied by reduced edema at all five measured anatomical sites for each of the four participants; however, edema in Phase C rebounded in most sites for most participants, calling into question the effectiveness of a glove that was not custom fitted (Gustafsson et al., 2016).

It would have been better if Phase C had been preceded by a return to baseline, or ABAC. Stronger still would be

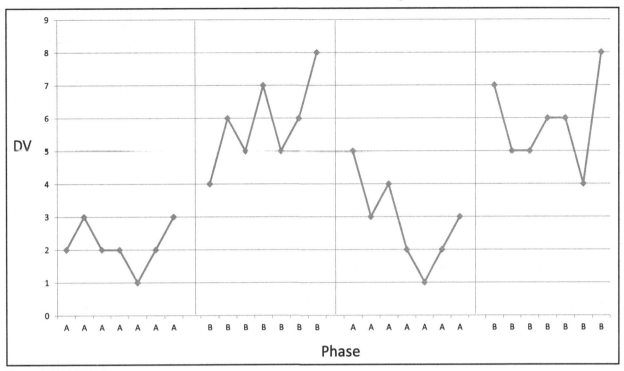

Figure 7-3 ABAB design.

Note: DV = dependent variable; each "A" is a data collection occasion in baseline; each "B" an occasion during intervention; phases are separated slightly for clarity.

the design ABACA, where a final return to baseline tests whether the intervention of C was actually effective. That is, what happens when it is removed? Does the client's performance drop back to that of the original baseline? It is also sometimes possible to design a study where interventions are applied separately, and then together (ABACA, then B+C simultaneously). Each additional comparison made between phases offers the opportunity to make a stronger causal case because coincidences are even more unlikely to have caused the noted pattern of changes in performance.

7.3.5 Alternating Treatment Design Structure

A different approach is used in the SCED called *alternating treatment design* (ATD). In this design, two interventions are compared on several occasions (usually at least six). On each occurrence of measurement, one intervention is applied first and then the other is applied; the resulting performance level of the client is measured. If one intervention is clearly superior to the other, the plotted lines will diverge and remain separate. Tanta et al. (2005) used an ATD design (with a preparatory Phase A) to determine whether five children with developmental play delays showed more initiation and more response during play when paired with a higher functioning child or a lower functioning child (Figure 7-4). The three boys

and two girls (3- to 6-years-olds) had play ages of 2.5 to 4.4 years. Generally, the initiation and response of all five participants was greater when they played with a higher-level playmate, in contrast to the findings of some earlier research (Tanta et al., 2005).

7.4 Multiple Baselines

To enhance the portrayal of a client's performance and to strengthen the internal validity of the study, another addition is undertaken in some SCEDs: multiple baselines. This term refers to the presence of more than one dependent variable on which the research participant is tracked. The differential effect of the independent variable on the various dependent variables can be carefully weighed in the interpretation of findings. For example, Watling and Dietz (2007) tracked both undesirable behavior and task engagement in four children with ASD receiving Ayres' Sensory Integration therapy. They also staggered the transition from baseline phase to intervention phase across the children to control for history effects. A single dependent variable might also be measured in multiple settings (e.g., home, school, neighborhood park), and thus under different contextual conditions. Multiple baselines (settings) can show how widely applicable the performance improvement is, strengthening the external validity (generalizability) of the findings to more aspects of the participant's life.

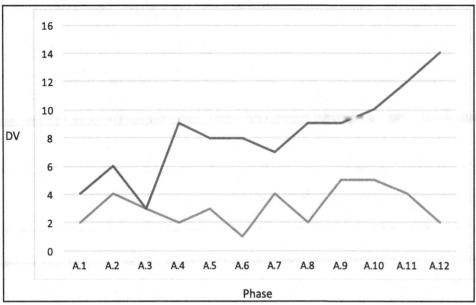

Figure 7–4 Alternating treatment design (ATD).

Note: DV = dependent variable; each "A" is a data collection occasion; blue line standard intervention; red line, new intervention.

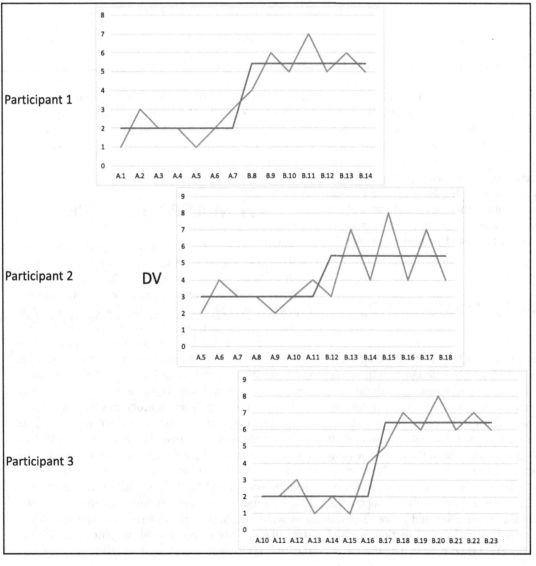

Figure 7–5 Offset start of baseline phases, N of 3.

Note: Numbers after "A" or "B" represent calendar dates. A and B are phases of baseline and intervention, respectively. Blue lines represent data. Horizontal red lines are mean levels in each phase. Diagonal red lines represent jump in level. The jumps occur not on the same calendar day but as intervention is begun, on different days for each participant.

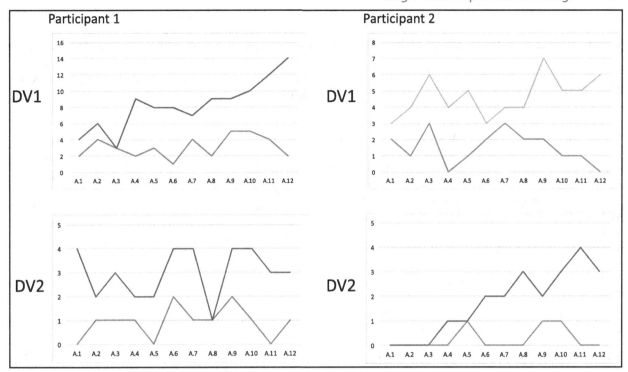

Figure 7–6 Alternating treatment design, two participants, two dependent variables (DV)

Another example of multiple baselines is the inclusion of more than one participant in a SCED. In recent years a higher proportion of published SCED in the *American Journal of Occupational Therapy* (*AJOT*) contain data from more than one participant. (The average number of cases per SCED in *AJOT* has risen from 2.5 in the 1990s, to 3.0 in the 2000s, and to 4.7 in the 2010s, and 5.8 in the first 3.5 years of the 2020s.) If each participant is started into their Phase A on a different calendar day and then transitioned to Phase B on a different day, possible history effects are strongly mitigated (see Figure 7–5). A multiple-case SCED can sometimes suggest patterns that help explain why the intervention worked for some but not for others (McGruder et al., 2003). The essence of such a comparison is shown in Figure 7–6. Comparing data from multiple participants can allow for the discovery of the effects of various demographic or clinical characteristics or hidden differences on the outcome variables.

7.5 OPERATIONALIZATION OF VARIABLES

Just as a precise description of the protocols in group experimental studies is crucial for future replication, so it is for SCEDs. This precise definition of the applied intervention (e.g., amount, frequency, by whom, conditions) and of how the outcomes are measured is called *operationalization of variables*.

7.5.1 Operationalization of the Independent Variable

To replicate or generalize a SCED, readers must be informed about the exact nature of the intervention that was delivered to the participant. First, to ensure that the intervention was delivered as intended to the participant, procedural reliability is monitored. Typically, this monitoring is done via a checklist of every pertinent detail of the set-up and delivery of the therapy, as well as of the surroundings. Is furniture exactly in its intended place? Are supplies laid out exactly the same each time a data measurement occurs? Are seating, lighting, temperature, and background noise standardized from session to session? Is the intervention provided in exactly the intended manner (also called *treatment fidelity*)? The demands of fidelity can run the gamut from a precisely specified protocol (e.g., "ABA therapy for a child with ASD") to a globally outlined procedure ("intervention was applied according to the professional judgment of the treating therapist"). If the intervention is provided under requirements more similar to the latter description, then the representativeness of the occupational therapy practitioner providing the intervention becomes of greater importance. Would the average therapist implement such an intervention in approximately the same way? To the extent the answer to this question is "no," the generalizability of the findings to other places is correspondingly weakened.

Of course, if the SCED protocol includes the provision of more than one type of intervention (either separately or combined), then each intervention must be operationalized.

7.5.2 Operationalization of the Dependent (Outcome) Variables

See Chapter 6 for information on operationalizing outcome variables in a group experimental study.

Just as crucial as operationalization of the independent variable is the precise definition of how the outcome variable (dependent variable) was collected. When were measurements taken (what time of day, day of week, intervals, any interruptions; what were conditions before, during, and after)? By whom were the measurements made (occupational therapist, parent or caregiver, teacher, paid graduate student, the researcher)? Did the research protocol include provisions for controlling observer drift (i.e., maintenance throughout the study of intra-rater reliability)? If more than one data gatherer or rater were involved, did the researcher take steps to establish, measure, and maintain inter-rater reliability? These reliabilities are all the more important in SCED due to the repeated measurement of the same individuals in the generation of the data. If observer drift occurs, then an apparent change in the performance displayed by the data might not have been caused by the intervention, but rather could be attributable to the drift (systematic measurement error) instead.

7.6 Specific Considerations for Collecting Data in Single Case Experimental Design

Often in SCED, the dependent variable is a repeatedly occurring behavior or performance of a task. Whether such a behavior or performance can be reliably observed and measured is influenced by the following considerations.

7.6.1 Counting

If the outcome is a behavior to be counted, what is and what is not an occurrence? a separate occurrence? a double occurrence? For example, suppose a SCED is testing whether a specific sensory approach in the classroom is effective for reducing the biting behavior of a child with a developmental disorder. What, exactly, counts as a bite? Bear in mind, this definition of *bite* must be such that a bite can be observed in a reliable way. Part of the operationalization of a bite must be to describe when a bite occurs as opposed to a non-bite or a near-bite. What counts as two bites, versus a double-bite? The operationalization is not as simple as it might at first appear.

One possible operationalization would be to define a bite as happening when the teeth visibly touch the skin of the child (easy to observe), regardless of how much pressure may be applied (which would be difficult to judge

reliably by observation alone). The bite ends when the teeth cease to have contact with the skin. If contact is made with the skin immediately thereafter, then that counts as two (separate) bites. If, however, after contact the jaws seem to clamp down on the skin twice, with the teeth never breaking contact with the skin, then that counts as only one bite. A motion toward the skin with the mouth open, but where the teeth never touch the skin, does not count as a bite.

In this way the counting of bites can be made more reliable among raters, or within a single rater over many data collection occasions. This reliability is crucial for the internal validity of a SCED due to the multiple times of measurement. The researcher and the reader must both be confident that plotted changes in the dependent variable are due to actual changes and not to spurious variability introduced by less reliable measurement.

7.6.2 Timing

The researcher has several alternatives when employing timing of behaviors in a SCED. Is the total amount of time the participant is engaged in a behavior to be measured? Or is the longest single occurrence of the behavior what is most important in the study? Perhaps it is the average length of engagement in a behavior over a given span of time that is of greatest functional importance. It might also be that the frequency of the behavior is most important: how many times did it occur in a 5-minute period? a 45-minute classroom session? during recess? (in which case, see section 7.6.1, Counting). How is the timing exactly to be done? When does the timing of the behavior start? When does it stop? The more precisely these moments can be defined in advance, including all the complicating contingencies that might occur, the more thoroughly operationalized the dependent variable is, the more accurate the data will be, and the greater the internal validity and replicability of the study.

In some SCEDs the behavior of interest occurs too rapidly for a timing of it or an accurate frequency count. In this case, a time sampling of behavior may be indicated. For example, exactly every 5 minutes the data gatherer looks to see whether the participant is engaged in the behavior. The outcome is recorded as a 0 (no) or a 1 (yes). If observations take place each day for an hour, then 12 5-minute intervals will be sampled, yielding a possible total score of 0 to 12. An occupational therapy practitioner might have a set performance as the client's long-term goal (e.g., 10 times of every 12 opportunities the behavior is manifested). The SCED researcher is interested in documenting whether the independent variable brings about any reliable improvement in the dependent variable over the duration of the study.

Time sampling is often used when the participant is engaged in a group activity. Can the observer reliably pick the participant out of the group? Can the observer reliably observe the participant's behavior, or do others block the view? These questions are best answered empirically through a pilot data collection session (often with similar individuals not in the study itself to avoid contamination). Based on the findings from the pilot test, the operationalization of the dependent variable collection of the SCED can be adjusted.

7.6.3 Graphing the Data

The report of results from a SCED almost always includes one or more graphs of the data. The multiple times of measuring the dependent variable per participant, separated into phases where the phase transition is of great importance, lend themselves to a pictorial display. In a simple AB study, the appearance of the plotted data points and of how they differ from Phase A to Phase B provides a direct avenue for a visual interpretation of the results. (See Ottenbacher, 1986b, and the following for how visual analysis alone under certain circumstances can be misleading.)

Setting up the Axes of the Graph

By convention, moving along the x-axis (horizontal axis) from left to right represents the passage of time. Each time an outcome behavior or performance is collected, it is noted on the graph as a single point. The amount of the variable that was measured at this time x is plotted along the y-axis (vertical axis). This axis represents the dependent variable (see Figure 7–1). Almost always the y-axis indicates a linear (equal interval) scale. Most commonly the x-axis also shows a scale of equal intervals, where each measurement occasion is an interval. However, these equal intervals may not represent equal intervals of time. That is, if measurements are made on a Monday/Wednesday/Friday schedule for three weeks, then nine data points will appear on the graph. They are plotted at equal distances horizontally from one another, however, the points representing a Friday and the subsequent Monday have two non-data days between them (Saturday, Sunday), whereas those collected during the week are only separated by one day (Tuesday or Thursday). This simplification in the graph may have implications for the findings as explained below. In addition, by convention adjacent data points are connected by a solid line. Connecting the points through time indicates an assumption of an underlying potential to produce this behavior or achieve this performance that is continuous or ongoing. The actual data points represent the results when this potential is sampled at discrete points in time. If an intended data collection point is missing (e.g., due to illness in the participant), then some researchers advocate breaking the data line, or indicating it by a dotted line between the data points on either side of the missing point.

With an ATD, both conditions (with or without adaptive equipment, as in McGruder et al., 2003; or playing with child A or child B, as in Tanta, 2005) are typically plotted on the same graph so that a visual comparison can easily be made. In standard SCED designs (e.g., ABA, ABAB) there is usually only one dependent variable per graph plotted, although more are possible, as in Dickerson and Brown (2007). However, a single figure of the published article may contain two or more graphs aligned for easier visual comparison by the reader (Figure 7–6). These graphs may show an alignment of all dependent variables from one participant, the results on one dependent variable from more than one participant, or the dependent variable data from one participant measured in different settings.

The researcher should unambiguously state for each graph whether up (more of y) represents better. For example, when functional behaviors or positive performance is plotted, up is better and a rising graph is what the researcher hopes for. In contrast, in the case of dysfunctional behaviors, the hope is that what is plotted will decline. Likewise, if "time taken to perform a task" or "number of errors committed" or "amount of assistance needed" is how the dependent variable was operationalized, then a decline in scores is desirable. Care must be taken when a study measures multiple dependent variables and for some of them "up" is better and for others "down" is better.

Indicating the Phases

Even the simplest design in a SCED has a phase change between the Phase A (baseline) and Phase B (intervention). This change is usually displayed as a vertical dashed line at the point of phase change (halfway between the last baseline data point and the first intervention phase data point). In an ABA design, there would be two vertical dashed lines separating A from B and B from the return to Phase A. In an ABAB design, there will be three phase transitions (see Figure 7–3).

Ordinarily, each phase would be an equal length of time. For any statistical analysis, having an equal or near-equal number of data points in the phases to be compared is advantageous. However, there is one circumstance where equal length of phases is not sought. If the participant's behavior or performance in the baseline phase is extremely variable, some researchers continue Phase A until the behavior stabilizes. The measurement logic of this elongation of phase is based on sampling theory. A sample will be a more accurate representation of the actual capabilities of the participant if it is larger and less variable. For example, if you only observed a child on the playground twice and one time the child played with classmates appropriately and the other time the child withdrew from them and hid, you could not feel confident stating that the regular experience of the child at recess was to hide 50% of the time. If, however, you had observed the child 20 times during recess and the child hid twice, you could be more

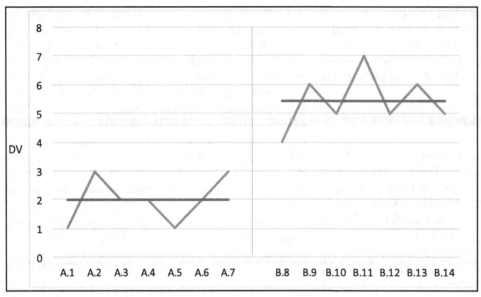

Figure 7–7 Change of level in an AB design.

Note: DV = dependent variable; each "A" is a data collection occasion in baseline; each "B" an occasion during intervention; phases are separated slightly for clarity.

confident in saying that the worrisome behavior occurred about 10% of the time.

Thus, the goals of the study are to enable the researcher to make some inferences about the relationship between the independent variable and the dependent variables, and to draw some conclusions about the effectiveness of the interventions. Because the data analysis rides on the picture the data points form, the reliability in their determination is crucial. Accuracy in plotting the points is also of vital importance. In the section following, the three types of changes between phases that can be identified will be discussed, along with the various techniques (statistical and non-statistical) of quantifying these changes in a dependable way.

7.7 VISUAL AND STATISTICAL ANALYSIS

A valuable aspect of SCEDs is that three types of changes between phases can be detected: change in level, change in slope, and change in variability. These changes could occur one at a time, two at a time, or all three at once. Note that in traditional **group** experimental design, the main attention is placed upon changes in level (i.e., a difference in the means of the two groups being compared). Much less often is attention placed in a group design on differences in slope (differences in the change in the dependent variable over time) between the groups or on differences in variability between the two groups. There is nothing that prevents a researcher from building these analyses into a group design. However, a SCED more readily lends itself to examining both level and slope, and sometimes in addition variability, given the way data are collected and displayed.

7.7.1 Change in Level

A change in level of the dependent variable from one phase to the next would be indicated by a bump in the graphed line upward or downward (Figure 7–7). Assuming that up is better in this case, the researcher would want to know two things about this bump. First, could it have happened purely by chance (through random variation in the behavior or performance of the participant), and not be due to the independent variable? Second, if the level change upward seems to be the new norm for the participant, is the performance now at a level that is functional, akin to normal, or meeting a criterion for task completion, habit consistency, or maintenance of a routine? In other words, as with group experiments, the researcher must appraise both the statistical validity and the clinical or occupational validity of the change. Statistical procedures adapted for SCEDs can help answer the first question. Only knowledge of human occupation and of the goals of the participant and family can help answer the second. Tools for the analysis of level will be discussed in section 7.7.5.

7.7.2 Change in Slope

During the baseline phase there could be any of three types of slope in the data points. They could show essentially no change in level over time (i.e., a zero slope); they could slope upward (assuming still that up is better); or they could be sloping downward. Now assume the intervention has begun and data are being collected during Phase B. For each of the slopes of Phase A (−, 0, +) there could arise a negative, zero, or positive slope in the subsequent Phase B. Consider what the importance of each of these combinations might be. If the baseline slope is zero and the intervention slope is also zero (with no change

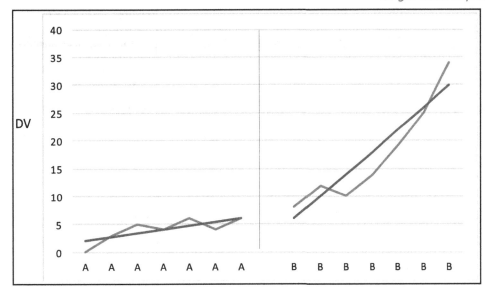

Figure 7–8 Change in slope.

Note: DV = dependent variable; each "A" is a data collection occasion in baseline; each "B" an occasion during intervention; phases are separated slightly for clarity; red lines are slope for that phase.

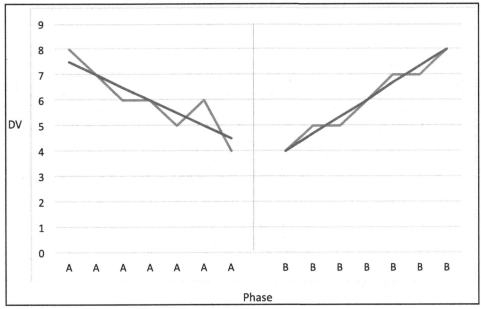

Figure 7–9 No change in level, change in slope.

Note: DV = dependent variable; each "A" is a data collection occasion in baseline; each "B" an occasion during intervention; phases are separated slightly for clarity; red lines are slopes for that phase.

in level), we would tend to conclude that the intervention had no effect. If the baseline slope is zero and the intervention was accompanied by an upward slope, then we might conclude that the intervention probably had a positive effect on the participant's outcome. If the baseline slope was already upward, it would take a sharp ramping up of that slope to persuade us that the intervention had a beneficial effect (Figure 7–8). After all, in this case the participant was already performing better over time in the baseline phase before any intervention began. If the baseline slope were downward, we might consider it a victory for the intervention to have changed that slope to zero (that is, help a person whose behavior was in decline to level off). Of course, the researcher would be most happy if a negative baseline slope were changed by the intervention into a positive, upward slope (Figure 7–9). Tools to help the researcher determine whether these

changes in slope could have merely happened by chance are discussed later in this chapter.

7.7.3 Change in Variability

Variability itself is not often a concern in therapy situations; however, it may sometimes be the key consideration. Suppose a young man or a young woman had a flat affect due to an emotional trauma. Showing little to no variation in facial expression could lead to notable disadvantages in social communication and participation. The goal for therapy, and thus the focus of analysis in a corresponding SCED, would be to increase the variability of facial expression. A different situation would be where a person is experiencing marked role dysfunction due to alternating periods of mania and depression. Here, the therapist, and likewise the SCED researcher, would seek

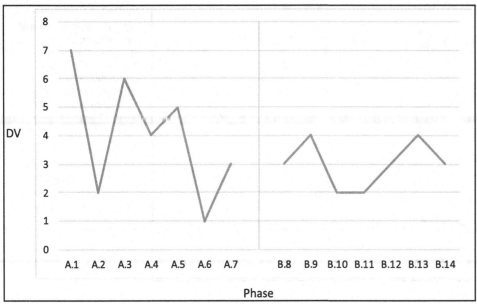

Figure 7–10 Change in variability.

Note: DV = dependent variable; each "A" is a data collection occasion in baseline; each "B" an occasion during intervention; phases are separated slightly for clarity.

to dampen the variability of mood experienced by the person (Figure 7–10). Thus, depending on the condition and the situation, it may be beneficial in some studies for the variability of behavior to be increased and in others decreased. In either case, a SCED, with its repeated measurements, could be the means for persuasively demonstrating that the intervention probably had the desired effect.

7.7.4 Change in Level with a Positive or Negative Baseline Slope

Assume the slope in the data during baseline phase is upward, and the intervention was accompanied by a positive bump to the natural healing, learning, or developmental process, without the slope changing. That would probably indicate that the intervention was at least to some extent successful. If the baseline slope was downward (as in a chronic, progressive disease) and the intervention gave a decline-stalling bump to the process, that could also be considered a positive effect, even if the long-term downward trend continues.

Occasionally an intervention will temporarily have a negative effect on a client's performance but will result in greater benefits in the long run. Ayres (1972) claimed that traditional Ayres Sensory Integration therapy for children with learning disabilities would sometimes cause an immediate disorganization in the child's movement (Ayres, 1973). However, after some weeks of therapy, the child would have improved at such a pace (despite the momentary bump downward) that the current performance was superior to where it would have been without therapy. In a SCED graph, this scenario might resemble Figure 7–11.

Changes in level, slope, and variability must be interpreted in light of the salient factors pertaining to the particular situations studied in the SCED. Furthermore, when multiple graphs are available, either because of multiple participants or because of multiple baselines, there are more opportunities to examine and interpret similarities and differences or to point out where the data fulfilled the expectations of the researcher and where they did not. Such detailed "narratives" interpreting client changes in functional performance with respect to level, slope, and variability—within a participant as well as across participants—virtually never occur in a group experimental design study, with its focus on the comparison of group mean scores.

7.7.5 Statistical Analysis

Despite some early objections to using statistical approaches for the analysis of SCED data, doing so is now widely accepted. Some mathematical assumptions of the statistical procedures are not met; thus, it is prudent to conduct any statistical analysis cautiously, with a recognition of where limitations may exist.

There are three basic statistical approaches to the analysis of data in SCEDs: (a) the two-standard deviation (2-SD) band method (when there is a zero slope in the baseline phase); (b) the split-middle/binomial test (when the baseline data do show a slope up or down); and (c) the C statistic (showing whether there is a trend in the baseline phase and, if not, whether the intervention data in the subsequent Phase B differ from the baseline data; Portney & Watkins, 2009). There are additional, less common statistical methods that are not covered in this chapter, such as the non-overlap techniques described by Parker et al. (2011).

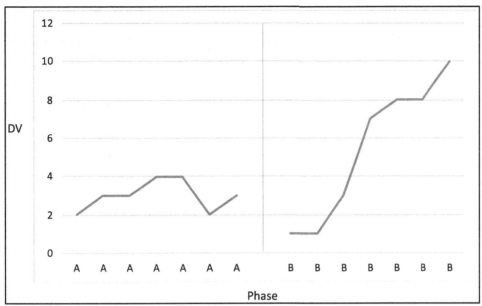

Figure 7–11 Drop in level with increase in slope.

Note: DV = dependent variable; each "A" is a data collection occasion in baseline; each "B" an occasion during intervention; phases are separated slightly for clarity.

Two Standard Deviation Band Method

If the data in the baseline phase are stable (have a zero slope) and are about six or more in number, then the 2-SD band method may be used. The analysis is based on the logic of the null hypothesis, which would declare that any difference in level seen between the baseline phase and the intervention phase data is due solely to chance (random variation). If the data of Phase B show enough difference that it is improbable it would have happened by chance, then we can reject the null hypothesis and claim that the difference seen is probably real.

To use the 2-SD band method, the mean value for the points in the baseline phase is found (add the value of the points together and divide by the number of points). A solid line is drawn across Phase A at this level on the graph, then the SD of the Phase A points is calculated. Only include the Phase A data points (not A and B) when calculating the SD. The size of the SD is then doubled, and this amount is added to and subtracted from the mean value found earlier. Dashed or dotted lines are drawn at these two levels across Phase A, forming a band. This band is 2 SDs above the mean and 2 SDs below the mean (or actually 4 SDs wide). The dashed lines of the 2-SD band are now drawn across Phase B. If two consecutive data points from Phase B fall outside the band, then one can reject the null hypothesis of there being no real difference between Phases A and B. Having two consecutive points outside the band is held to be too unlikely for the null to be retained. If the points outside the band are outside in the desired direction, then one may claim that the Phase B performance level is better than the Phase A level (Figure 7–12).

Split-Middle/Binomial Test Method

If there appears to be a slope in Phase A then using the 2-SD band method is not valid, because the slope, left alone as it continues across Phase B, would result in higher data points. Even if the conditions in the 2-SD band method for rejecting the null hypothesis were triggered, it would not enable a valid claim that Phase B performance was higher due to the intervention. The Phase A slope indicated that the participant was already improving before the intervention began. Under this condition, a difference in the level between Phases A and B would not be evidence of an effective intervention.

In this case, the split-middle/binomial test method can be used. Here, the null hypothesis is employed once again, but this time with respect to the existing slope in the data across Phase A. If the intervention had no effect, then this slope would be expected to continue unchanged across Phase B, except for random variation. However, if the Phase B points show enough of a deviation from this expectation, then we can reject the null and claim that a change probably did take place when the intervention was instituted.

To find the line representing the overall slope of Phase A, count the number of data points in the baseline. Divide this number in half. Draw a dashed vertical line between the two adjacent points between the first half of points and the second half of points. (If the baseline had an odd number of points, then draw the vertical line through the middle point, leaving an equal number of points to the left and right of it.) Within each of these half-phases, find the median value on the y-axis of the points in that half-phase. Plot this median value at the position on the x-axis representing the mid-point of time in this half-phase. Repeat for the second half-phase of Phase A. Draw a solid line connecting these two points. If necessary, adjust this line upward or downward (but keeping it parallel to its original alignment) so that there are an equal number of Phase A points above and below the line. (This adjustment is often not necessary.)

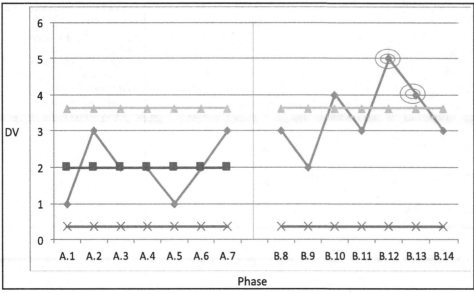

Figure 7–12 Two standard deviation band method of analysis.

Note: DV = dependent variable; each "A" is a data collection occasion in baseline; each "B" an occasion during intervention; phases are separated slightly for clarity; two consecutive circled points mean performance improved in B phase (p <.05).

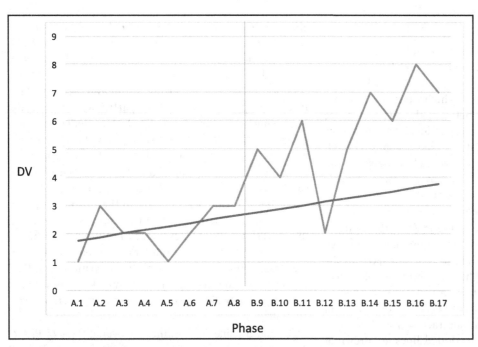

Figure 7–13 Celeration line with binomial test.

Note: DV = dependent variable; each "A" is a data collection occasion in baseline; each "B" an occasion during intervention; red line is slope of data in A projected across B phase; with eight points above red line and one point beneath, one can conclude the B phase performance is improved (p <.05).

Now extend this solid line into and across Phase B. Phase B points will lie on either side of this line (Figure 7–13). If the null hypothesis is true, 50% of the points would appear above and below the line (the intervention made no difference). However, it would also not be unlikely if the points divided 60/40%, or even 70/30% in cases where there are not many data points in Phase B. Indeed, with only 4 to 8 data points in Phase B, they would all need to be above the solid line drawn from the baseline phase in order to reject the null. If there are nine points in Phase B, then one of them could be below the solid line and we could reject the null at an alpha of .05. For 12 points in Phase B, two of them could be below the solid line and we could still reject the null hypothesis at alpha = .05. These decisions are based on the probability values in a binomial test statistical table (see Table C–11).

If the evidence is present to reject the null, then the claim can be made that we are 95% confident that performance in Phase B is better (or worse, if the points went that direction) than in Phase A—and probably not from pure chance. The strength of any argument that the intervention itself caused this difference would need to be built up with supporting evidence. For example, if a return to baseline conditions was accompanied by a decline in performance, and then a reapplication of the intervention caused an increase, the researcher could feel more confident that indeed the intervention is causing the increases. Nonetheless, this evidence does not constitute proof that the intervention was the cause. It just makes it more plausible that the intervention caused the change.

C-Statistic

A less-often used alternative analytic method for SCED data is the C-statistic. The C-statistic estimates trends in a time series. It needs a minimum of eight data points in Phase A (Tryon, 1982). First it determines whether there is no trend in the baseline. Then if there is not, it determines whether there is a difference between the baseline (A) and the treatment (B) phases. For more detail on the C-statistic, see (Ottenbacher, 1986b; Tryon, 1982).

All three of the approaches described above can be equally used to test for changes from Phase B to a return to baseline, or from the second Phase A to the second Phase B, and so on. Most authors explicitly warn that these analyses should only be used to compare adjacent phases in the data stream. The most important reason for this warning is that the logic of the null hypothesis only applies between a given phase and the immediately proceeding phase of data.

The Phenomenon of Serial Dependency (or Autocorrelation)

In many group statistical comparisons, one assumption of the statistical test is that the data points are independent of one another (e.g., in an independent *t*-test or analysis of variance). An example of non-independence of data would be if children were given a motor test where those waiting their turn could see the children being tested before them. The performance of one child could influence the performance of another, contaminating the independence of the data. In a SCED, since the entire data stream is derived from the same individual, it is likely that the assumption of independence of data is violated. If it is, there could exist the situation of serial dependency or autocorrelation. Ottenbacher (1986b) and others recommend testing for autocorrelation in any data set in SCED. Its presence would not affect the C-statistic, but could affect the accuracy of the 2-SD band method or the split-middle/binomial test method.

Therefore, although it is advisable to use statistical analyses to avoid some of the pitfalls of a pure visual analysis, these analyses have their own limitations. They should always be interpreted in context and with caution.

7.8 Interpretation of Results in Single Case Experimental Design

7.8.1 Immediate Interpretation

Applying visual and statistical analyses to the data points of a SCED puts the researcher in a position to make justifiable inferences about what the experiment has shown. These inferences should only be made while keeping in mind the following possible limitations.

Did the measuring instrument for the dependent variable (or the operationalization of the dependent variable) have noteworthy limitations? Larger than desirable random measurement error in the dependent variable might manifest itself as larger than expected variability in the plotted data. If the 2-SD band method of analysis was used, then the larger variability in Phase A would result in a wider SD band. This greater width would have made it less likely for any improvement to have produced two consecutive Phase B points outside the band. This disadvantage is analogous to greater variability in a group experimental design, lessening statistical power.

According to the scale used for the dependent variable, it might display a floor or ceiling effect. A *floor effect* means that the dependent variable scale cannot measure below a certain performance or behavior level. Suppose the researcher is seeking to show statistically that the intervention diminished a negative behavior. The plotted data from Phase A give rise to a 2-SD band that is below the lowest possible score on the dependent variable. It would then be impossible for Phase B to produce two consecutive data points outside the SD band. It will appear that the intervention had no noteworthy effect. If the change sought is upward, then a *ceiling effect* could likewise prevent the researcher from using a 2-SD band method to demonstrate the intervention's effectiveness.

Another interpretive limitation comes about when there are missing data points. The participant may be ill one day and no data were collected. Should the x-axis be collapsed across that missing day? Whether the researcher compresses the x-axis could have an effect on the outcome if a split-middle/binomial test is used in the analysis. Similarly, if there are only a few data points in Phase A, then the 2-SD band will be based on such a small number of points that confidence in its accuracy will be weakened. Likewise, the split-middle/binomial test method, when used with only a few data points in Phase A, may become unstable and thus be potentially misleading. When there are few points in Phase B (fewer than nine), it is difficult or impossible to reject the null hypothesis.

Mid-phase changes in level, slope, or variability pose additional challenges for interpretation. First there arises the question, what could have caused this change? It is convenient to think that only the independent variable could cause a change in the dependent variable, but we know that for matters of human performance, this assumption is far too simple. Such mid-phase changes also create the following dilemma. Should only the data after the change be used to examine subsequent changes between Phases A and B? Or should all the A phase points still be averaged together to form a representative SD band or sloped line? There is no mathematical answer to these questions. The researcher must make the case logically, with reference to the context of the participant being studied.

7.8.2 Long-Term Interpretation

Once the decision has been made whether Phase A to Phase B transition is accompanied by improved performance, no change, or a decline in performance, and once parallel decisions have been made for every other phase transition (e.g., B to A, A to B), there remains the need to interpret the meaning of the SCED as a whole. In a multi-participant SCED, this task would also involve considering why the intervention seemed to work for some individuals but not for others (McGruder et al., 2003; see Figure 7–6). Having demographic and diagnostic information about the participants in order to hypothesize about possible causes of a difference can be helpful here.

7.9 GLOBAL/SOCIAL/ECOLOGICAL VALIDITY

Even clear and persuasive inferences from the experimental data of SCED, with their selected, operationalized outcomes, do not automatically translate to the actual contextualized, occupational life of the individual participant. One way to improve external validity is to collect data in multiple settings and from several participants. A final inference needs to be made, ultimately, about whether the intervention holds promise for similar individuals in their own unique naturalistic settings.

7.10 STRENGTHS

The strengths of SCED are multiple. The intervention usually takes place in naturalistic (non-contrived) settings, such as a school, the community, or the home. The intervention is individualized, which accords with client-centered practice. In some SCEDs, the intervention is graded up or down as necessary. They offer the possibility of enlisting multiple cases or collecting data in multiple settings or under multiple conditions to reveal how variables may interact. Indeed, by focusing attention on a single individual case a SCED can reveal some of the cumulative and complex interactions among all variables that are measured, giving rise to new insights, hypotheses, or theories.

A particular strength of SCEDs is their ability to display changes in the level of the dependent variable, in the change in the dependent variable over time (slope), and in the variability of the dependent variable during control (A) and experimental (B) phases. This detail allows for a more sophisticated investigation of the relationship between the independent and dependent variables in the context of existing knowledge about them. Further illustration of this relationship follows.

Historically, SCEDs have been criticized for lacking generalizability. Of course, as an N-of-1 study, a SCED cannot have the type of statistical generalizability that a group experiment can have when its sample has been randomly selected from a population. Such a claim is rarely made by the authors of SCEDs. However, these authors themselves often underestimate the strength of generalizability that a SCED can have. That is, one therapist achieving a positive outcome with one client using a specified intervention demonstrates that it is at least a possibility that other therapists can achieve this same result by applying the insights gained. The knowledge that a possibility exists can be particularly valuable for intervention decisions for clients who have a rare or new condition, multiple diagnoses, unusual impairments or challenges, or for whom standard approaches have not been successful.

Some SCED designs (e.g., ATD) offer a fast, reliable comparison of equipment options, tool options, postural or technique options, or options in environmental conditions or modifications, allowing for a persuasive argument to be made for the superiority of one over another.

Finally, SCEDs can suggest why an intervention works with one individual and not with another, or which intervention works better for which individuals. This aspect of discovering knowledge for customized therapy is often not pursued in group experimental studies.

7.11 WEAKNESSES

Nonetheless, there are certain inherent weaknesses in SCEDs. Chief among them is a challenge with external validity. Is the participant in a SCED representative of other clients? The random selection of a sample, sometimes possible in group experimental studies, strengthens the external validity of group studies. As mentioned previously, SCEDs do not have the statistical models of traditional group experimental designs with adequate degrees of freedom and statistical power to support those aspects of internal validity. Additionally, the influence on the outcome of the therapeutic relationship between the independent variable provider and the client may be difficult to assess. Indeed, practitioner bias should be addressed in SCEDs but is difficult to control in this design. Measurement limitations may also exist. Although not exclusive to SCEDs, these consist of floor and ceiling effects, insensitivity of the dependent variable to small but important changes, an unknown relationship of the outcome performance or behavior to the norms in society, or an unknown amount of the dependent variable that would be the criterion for independent performance in a population.

In the analysis of SCED data, there is often a bending of certain statistical assumptions, especially independence among data points. The data display of SCED is vulnerable to graphing contingencies, such as missing data.

Finally, a dependable argument for the causal relationship between the independent variable and the dependent variable can be complicated. It is often built upon several component inferences, unlike in a group experiment. In the latter, rejecting the null via a single statistical test can be taken as a sufficient reason to confidently claim that the intervention caused the better outcome in the clients receiving it, compared to the control group. Due to the possible honeymoon, or short-term Hawthorne effect in the client upon receiving a novel treatment, SCEDs need to be replicated in order to strengthen any causal claim.

For these and other reasons, SCED researchers have recently issued the SCRIBE Guidelines (Tate et al., 2016), to protect against some of the possible flaws in SCEDs and to provide better detail and transparency so that replication by other researchers is more straightforward.

7.12 When Is a Single Case Experimental Design Applicable?

It is feasible to undertake a SCED when:
- Maintaining a baseline period is ethical and can be done long enough to establish a relatively stable picture of the typical range of performance on the dependent variable for this individual before intervention begins.
- The desired outcome performance is measurable.
- Repeated measurements of the individual are feasible and not contra-indicated by limited endurance or a measurement tool that is affected by repeated administration.
- Intervention creates an immediate or a near-immediate effect on outcome.
- The case can be followed long enough to establish a persuasive pattern in the data.
- Constructs of interest (whether occupation-based or client factors) are feasible to quantify.

7.13 When Is a SCED Not Applicable?

A SCED is not applicable for studying a case when:
- The baseline measures show great instability.
- It is not feasible, ethical, valid, or safe to measure the dependent variable repeatedly.

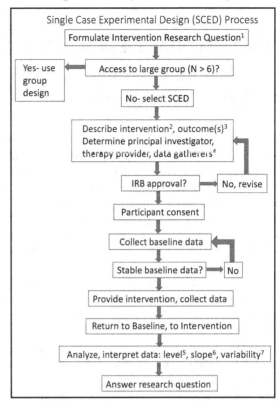

Figure 7–14 SCED process.
1. For example, "Is two weeks of 23 hours/day constraint-induced movement therapy effective in improving affected upper extremity function in a six-year-old child with high tone cerebral palsy?"
2. Operationalize the intervention so that it could be replicated.
3. Identify outcome measures that are reliable and valid to the greatest extent.
4. Design greatest degree possible of blinding of intervention providers, outcome data gatherers.
5. Analyze level change with 2-SD band method, if baseline data are not sloped.
6. Analyze change in slope with split-middle/binomial test method
7. Examine change in variability with Levene's Test or equivalent.

- There is a long or unknown lag time between the intervention and a demonstrable effect.
- An interaction of the intervention studied with other simultaneous interventions may be present.
- Uncontrollable outside events or dramatically changing external conditions occur.
- Only a brief period is available for intervention and measuring its effect (except for SCEDs using the ATD).
- The selected occupation based constructs are difficult to measure through repeated data collection.

See Figure 7–14 for a flowchart illustrating the design and implementation of a SCED.

7.14 ROLE OF SINGLE CASE EXPERIMENTAL DESIGN IN THE PROFESSION: CONTRIBUTIONS TO RESEARCH AND PRACTICE

Of 59 SCED published in *AJOT* during the period 1990–June 2023, 39 (66.1%) pertained to pediatric clients and 20 to adults. Of the total, 10 (16.9%) were concerned with sensory integration intervention, 7 (11.9%) with classroom seating and weighted clothing, 6 (10.2%) with computers, 5 (8.5%) with pediatric splinting, 4 (6.8%) with vision, 3 (5.1%) with oral function in young children, 3 (5.1%) with edema treatment, 2 (3.4%) with pediatric constraint-induced movement therapy, 2 (3.4%) with intervention for adults with traumatic brain injury, 12 (20.3%) with miscellaneous pediatric topics, 3 (5.1%) with the elderly, and 3 (5.1%) with miscellaneous adult topics.

These SCED made notable contributions to knowledge in the field in many ways. As their participant selection was rarely anything other than a convenience sample, one cannot make a statistical projection about the generalizability of their findings to the larger population. However, their findings do offer other evidence about practice that is of value to therapists. First, some SCED allow a generalization from one or a few cases to a hypothesis—that is, why a certain intervention was effective for a person, or why there was a difference in response among different individuals. For example, in McGruder et al. (2003), wearing a weighted wrist cuff was accompanied by taking less time to self-feed in 4 of 5 participants with a static acquired brain lesion. In 2 of 5 participants, the tremors themselves occurred at a statistically reduced rate during feeding. However, the mechanism of reduction for one participant seemed to be greater proprioceptive input but was greater biomechanical inertia for the other. The participant who showed no statistically significant improvement on any outcome variable had had surgery to remove a brain tumor. Other symptoms seemed to mask her tremors (McGruder et al., 2003). From these differences among participants, several hypotheses about the complex effects of using weighted cuffs could be devised. Such insights could then inform practitioners making decisions about the type of intervention to try with future clients.

Other SCEDs provide the opportunity to generalize from a case to the idea of an innovative possibility. For example, Casby and Holm (1994), discovered that in 2 of 3 elderly individuals with dementia, playing music via personal earphones was accompanied by a significantly diminished number of disruptive vocalizations. Even if this intervention was effective for only a minority of a larger group of clients, its ease and low cost would indicate that practitioners should certainly consider it.

It is also possible for a SCED to demonstrate how occupationally-important variables can be operationalized and reliably measured (Watling & Dietz, 2007). The authors defined *undesired, interfering behavior* and *engagement* for four 3- to 4-year-olds who were video-recorded during structured play sessions. Inter-rater reliability for these two constructs was 95% and 91%, respectively. Although the provision of sensory integration treatment did not result in immediate statistically significant effects in the children, their parents and their treating therapists reported greater social interaction and easier transitioning between activities after the treatments (Watling & Dietz, 2007).

Just as group experimental studies, SCEDs can indicate what amount of improvement in client performance might be expected from a given intervention over a certain period of time. DeVries et al. (1998) demonstrated that in two clients with a spinal cord injury, neither a mouth-stick nor a head-mounted pointer allowed word processing speeds at a vocationally competitive rate for text entry. Gutman et al. (2012) demonstrated that the greatest amount of learning of social skills in 15- to 17-year-olds with ASD occurred in the first phase of the program—namely, a 150% increase in the appearance of targeted positive behaviors. Mulcahey(1995) documented how an 11-year-old boy improved from 0 lateral pinch to 3.5 pounds of pinch after 1 year, subsequent to tendon transfer surgery and occupational therapy intervention. In all three cases the SCED showed what is possible in magnitude of outcome following the intervention.

SCED can be very effective in showing how durable improvements may be over time. Gustafsson et al. (2016) presented findings that indicated the reduction in post-stroke edema accompanying the use of finger to axilla compression bandages for seven days was not maintained after bandage removal. Furthermore, when circular-knit compression gloves were used after bandage removal, success was mixed. Only at the mid-proximal phalanx of the third digit were edema reductions sustained; at the other four more proximal points of the upper extremity the reductions were reversed. Such SCEDs inform practitioners about which interventions are likely not to provide client benefit.

Another important purpose of SCED is to serve as a pilot project, where promising results would justify further research. Crocker, MacKay-Lyons, and McDonnell (1997) found that after three weeks of splinting the less-involved upper extremity, a two-year-old girl with cerebral palsy had better quality, quantity, and variety of use in the more involved extremity, persisting at a six-month follow up. Dickerson and Brown (2007) discovered that gains in spontaneous reach, pushing a button for sound, and pulling a toy in the more involved upper extremity of a two-year-old boy with prenatal stroke accompanied three weeks of constraint induced movement therapy. Most of the gains were sustained at a one-month follow-up. In the ensuing ten years at least five group experimental studies on pediatric CIMT were published in *AJOT*. The SCED showed the feasibility, operationalization of procedures, and promising outcomes from this approach, enabling the later, larger studies.

Also of value, SCEDs can inform practitioners of the possibility that a certain intervention gives rise to no measurable effect in the type of client studied. Ross (1992) found that early versions of visual scanning computer applications, popular at the time in rehabilitation facilities, were not actually accompanied by increased performance in functional tasks by three adults with a traumatic brain injury. Umeda and Deitz (2011) found no measurable improvements in classroom behaviors of two kindergarten pupils with ASD when therapy cushions were used for seating. Nonetheless, because they were simple to use and showed no noticeable negative effects, the classroom teacher involved in the study wanted to keep them available. He reported that the cushions sometimes appeared to help the students' attention to task. These SCEDs serve as a reminder that findings might become outdated (given the increase in sophistication of software between 1992 and now), and that an intervention with no known harmful effects can be perceived as useful to have at hand.

A SCED can be used to demonstrate the positive effects of a newly-invented intervention. Babik et al. (2021) investigated the effects of an exoskeletal device on 17 young children with arthrogryposis. They noted increased active ROM, expanded reach, better grasp, and greater object exploration when the children were wearing the exoskeleton. Note the *N* of 17 did not preclude the study design being a SCED, as the data were plotted and analyzed individually, not as a group.

Finally, SCEDs can serve as a model for collaboration between practitioner and academician where the practitioner provides the clinical case and the academician assists in the research methodology improving the control over confounding variables (Sharpe & Ottenbacher, 1990). In fact, given the thin coverage of the 59 SCED published in *AJOT* over the past 33 years reviewed, one could cogently advocate for far more collaboration between researchers and practitioners in documenting these small-scale but important advances in occupational therapy practice.

7.15 SUMMARY

In this chapter, the authors described various components of a single case experimental design (SCED). SCEDs can be used in occupational therapy research to provide evidence for assessing the effectiveness of an intervention. As a type of experimental design, SCED studies apply a research hypothesis, operationally define an independent variable (intervention), control extraneous variables, and measure outcomes (dependent variable) by using reliable and valid assessments with one or a small number of participants. Their design structures range from the simple (AB) to the complex (ABABAB). Internal validity of the findings of a SCED can be strengthened by multiple phase changes, multiple baseline starting times, multiple outcome measures, and multiple contexts of investigation. One of the distinct advantages of a SCED is that it can be used to portray changes in level, slope, and variability in the data, a more detailed analysis than usually available with other methodologies. Another advantage is that with one or two participants, it can serve as a pilot study to justify further research. The 59 SCEDs reviewed for this chapter, appearing in *AJOT* from 1990 through June, 2023, have made several distinctive contributions to the occupational therapy literature. They identified interventions that may be effective, even in individuals with severe or complex conditions. They have suggested why a particular therapy works for some individuals and not for others. Last, they have documented the magnitude of effect that an intervention may have.

As occupational therapy strengthens itself as an evidence-based health care profession, there is good reason to generate SCEDs. They can involve more practitioners in research and generate more evidence to support interventions in practice.

8

Outcome Studies

The aim of scientific research is to produce generalizable knowledge about the real world. Without high external validity, you cannot apply results from the laboratory to other people or the real world.

Pritha Bhandari (2023)

OPERATIONAL LEARNING OBJECTIVES

By the end of this chapter, the learner will be able to:

1. Differentiate between outcomes research and experimental research
2. Distinguish between retrospective and prospective studies
3. Define the term covariate
4. Discern the difference between independent and repeated measures
5. Differentiate levels of outcomes-based research in terms of scientific rigor

8.1 INTRODUCTION TO OUTCOMES STUDIES

Traditional experimental methodology puts a premium on maintaining internal validity of the study. That is, was the experiment conducted with sufficient controls to leave the researcher confident that the results did not occur due to a confounding factor. The applicability in professional practice, however, of such highly controlled studies is sometimes problematic. Usually, controlled experiments do not replicate the conditions of real-life health care and educational settings.

Outcome studies, on the other hand, the topic of this chapter, have as their strength the realistic conditions under which the study is conducted. Their relative weakness in internal validity is made up for by their strong external validity or generalizability. Outcomes of therapy achieved in one realistic setting may reasonably be expected to be repeatable in another realistic setting. Outcome studies also usually display stronger external validity by virtue of the heterogeneity of their study participants. Whether they are conducted prospectively or retrospectively, they typically draw upon the clients who are seen in a given practice or set of practices.

The outcome study side of the Research Pyramid contains steps that indicate increasing rigor of methodology as one moves toward the top, as explained in detail below. Structurally, this stepping up of rigor is similar to that seen on the experimental side and indeed as seen in the descriptive base of the pyramid. Without giving up external validity, the features of outcome studies added as one steps up the side strengthen the internal validity of the studies.

The term "quasi-experimental" is a synonym for outcome studies. Characteristics that influence whether a study is placed on the outcome side of the pyramid include (a) that the participants were not randomly selected from a larger population, (b) that the participants were not randomly assigned to a group condition, but rather they belonged to pre-existing groups, and (c) the researchers were unable or chose not to control the experience of participants during the study, but rather allowed the course of therapy to proceed under those natural conditions as it normally would. Often outcome studies are conducted in the field and it is not practical or ethical for the researcher to randomly recruit potential participants, particularly when the population of interest contains too few individuals fitting the inclusion criteria. Random assignment to a control group that receives no intervention despite having a need, would be seen as improper. An example of this might be a study involving persons with progeria, also known as Hutchinson-Gilford progeria syndrome, which is a rare genetic disorder resulting in a rapid aging process beginning in childhood. For instance, as of March 31, 2023 it was estimated that there were 193 children with progeria in 51 countries around the world (Progeria Research Foundation, 2023). Since the incidence is so low in any one geographical location, it is unlikely that a traditional experimental design sample size complete with an experimental and control group sample size could be realistically recruited.

Another example occurs when the study is retrospective. In this type of outcome study, the researchers may investigate the health outcomes of one particular group that was provided an intervention, and compare those outcomes to those of another group who received a different intervention, or perhaps through unfortunate circumstances (e.g., a pandemic lockdown) received no intervention. In this latter example, while it appears that there is a control group, it is not "controlled" in the same manner as it would be in a prospective experimental study where researcher has a greater ability to manage potentially confounding variables. As mentioned above, a retrospective study is one that involves investigating data that has already been collected. Often this type of data are found in medical record and databases. For example, the study may investigate the health of one particular group that was exposed to a unique event or experience and compare that group to another particular group who, presumably, was not exposed to the same event or experience. An example of this type of study was done by Ding and Logemann (2000), who investigated the medical records of 378 persons who were at least six months post stroke. From this sample, participants were divided into one of two groups; with pneumonia or without pneumonia. Through exploring health-related factors within the database the researchers determined through chi-square analyses that those people in the pneumonia group had a higher incidence of multifocal strokes, had a higher incidence of aspiration during videoflouroscopy, had a greater incidence of hypertension and diabetes than the non-pneumonia group. In this example, while it appears that there is a control group, it is not "controlled" in the same manner as if it were a prospective study where the investigator has a greater ability to manage any potential confounding variables. In a retrospective study, it can only be assumed that there is a certain level of difference between the two groups.

Yet another reason for studies being categorized on the outcome side of the pyramid is if there is a repeated factor in the study design. Any study involving a pre- and post-test would violate the assumption for experimental studies that state that all comparisons are made between independent groups. As such, repeated measures that involve comparing multiple measurements at different times on the same individuals would, by design, place the study on the outcome side of the pyramid.

8.2 Evidence Hierarchy on the Outcome Side of the Research Pyramid

As mentioned above, the outcome study side of the pyramid has a similarity with the experimental and descriptive sides, in that they all use quantitative data and display progressively more rigor for internal validity (soundness of conclusion) as one progresses up that side of the pyramid.

8.2.1 One-Group Pre-Post Intervention Study [O4]

To begin, the lowest rung on the outcome side (O4) is a one group pre-post study. For example, one group of therapy clients is given a baseline measurement (the pre-test), is provided with an intervention, and at the completion of the intervention is measured again (the post-test). This type of study is one with a repeated measures design where there is no control group. A weakness in this design is that even if the post-test measures indicate improved performance by the group as a whole, they remain a multitude of reasons besides the intervention why the group improved: the mere passage of time (natural recovery/healing), an outside event accidentally occurring (an improvement in diet), or even a concurrent therapy, not the studied therapy, was the cause for the improvement. An advantage of this type of study is that it can be conducted in any therapy setting where a meaningful group can be defined. For example, Vanderkay et al. (2019) investigated the efficacy of an online educational format for ethics training in occupational therapy clinicians. In their study, 33 clinicians took a pre-test, on ethics in occupational therapy, then they took the online ethics training, after which, they took a post-test over the same material as the pre-test. Paired *t*-tests indicated a statistically significant increase in knowledge and a commitment to change their practice. The researched concluded that this online module was effective as a learning tool for ethics-related topics for occupational therapy clinicians. In this example, the same group of participants were tested before and after an intervention, but there was no control group that was also tested pre- and post-test at the same interval. While the results of this study appear to support the hypothesis and it is likely the improvement was because of the training, but because there was no control group, it is possible that another factor was at play that facilitated the learning beyond the online training. If the study did include the control group, then this would qualify it to be at the next higher level (O3)

because this study would have relatively more rigor than its counterpart at the O4 level.

Whether retrospectively or prospectively, it is a design that can be implemented quickly. For example, during the COVID-19 pandemic early information about outcomes from therapy for people with severe COVID could have great value for other practitioners, even though the results come from a quasi-experiment lacking some of the controls of a full-fledged experiment.

8.2.2 Two-Group Intervention Comparison Study [O3]

If a study compares the outcomes of two groups then it would qualify as the next higher level (O3) because this study would have relatively more rigor than its counterpart at the O4 level. That is because now if one group had a better outcome than the other group, the researcher could assume that both groups experienced the same amount of self-healing, thus removing that factor as a possible confound.

Another type of study that is considered to be at the O3 level is the case-control study involving pre-existing groups. These types of studies compare a group that has a certain health condition with a group of people who are free of the health condition. In this type of study, researchers "look back" to investigate the exposure to a suspected culprit and statistically compare that group to the group that was not exposed. An example of this type of retrospective study was done by Harper et al. (2023) who examined records of 109 patients admitted to the hospital, regardless of diagnosis, who experienced a fall within the first 48 hours of hospital admission, and 109 patients who did not fall. A multivariate regression analysis identified significant predictors of falling including attempts at independent mobilization (i.e., unsupervised mobilization), poor balance, reduced muscle strength, and impulsivity with the latter having the highest odds ratio. Further analysis revealed that patients receiving occupational therapy decreased their risk of falling by 81%.

It is also possible to investigate groups in outcome studies prospectively. Even if the groups are pre-existing, the researcher's ability to control for some sources of error or confounding (less reliable measurements, bias due to knowledge of group membership) can eliminate possible contamination of the results. These steps strengthen the internal validity of the study. There remains, without random assignment to group, the possibility that the groups differed in some important way that affected their response to the intervention provided. Showing that the groups have similar demographic factors (age, sex, severity of diagnosis, support system) goes part-way in demonstrating that the two groups were essentially equivalent. It does not address, though, those variables that are unknown or hidden on which the groups may differ.

8.2.3 Two-Group Intervention Comparison Study with Covariate Investigation [O2]

Even when participants cannot be randomly assigned to the study group conditions, it may be possible to lessen the effects of other variables on the performance comparison. If it is known or discovered that data were collected on a third variable (neither independent nor dependent variable), and that third variable affects the outcome (dependent) variable, then a statistical adjustment, or re-leveling, of the two groups can be performed. This third variable is called a covariate. Statistics such as the analysis of covariance (ANCOVA) correct for the differing presence of the third variable in the two groups. In a sense, it "levels the playing field" so that the groups' performance on the dependent variable can be more fairly compared. This comparison would contain more rigor and would be placed at the next higher level on the outcome side of the pyramid (O2). Obviously, the advantage of this type of study, where one or more covariates can be identified and dealt with, is a stronger internal validity. The possible confounding effect of one or more covariates has been removed. Unfortunately, there remains the possible confounding effects of all other variables—known or unknown.

8.2.4 Meta-Analysis of Outcome Studies [O1]

The highest level (O1) on the outcome side of the pyramid consists of meta-analyses which involve a compilation of outcome studies that have examined the same independent variables and ideally, similar dependent variables. The more similar the dosing of the intervention (how much was given, how often, for how long) the better for the accuracy of the overall comparison. An analysis is performed to determine the overall effect size (defined in section 4.7 in Chapter 4), based upon the pooled samples sizes and variances of the respective groups or conditions. For example, Ikiugu et al. (2017) completed a meta-analysis that examined the effectiveness of theory-based occupational therapy in improving mental health. These researchers included 11 randomized controlled trials with a combined total of 520 participants with a mental health diagnosis. The dependent variables (i.e., outcomes) included occupational performance and well-being. The results revealed theory-based occupational therapy had a medium effect for improvement in occupational performance and a small effect for an improvement in well-being.

8.3 STUDY DESIGN STATISTICS TO USE

8.3.1 One Group Pre-Post Intervention Designs [O4]

Repeated measures designs can incorporate varying levels of complexity, but at the simplest level is the one group pre-test, post-test study design. In this design, measurements are taken from one group of participants at two points in time. The first, known as the pre-test, is a baseline measurement and it acts as a control, of sorts. After this baseline measurement, an intervention that constitutes the independent variable is delivered. There may be some learning that is required during the intervention, depending on the independent variable. Once the intervention is completed, a second measurement is taken, known as the post-test. In its simplest form, the repeated measures design has a pre-test, an intervention phase, and a post-test. An advantage of this design is that each participant acts as their own control. This reduces variability, and it reduces the number of participants needed to acquire the desired statistical power, as no separate control group needs to be recruited. A disadvantage attributed to this design is the multitude of factors that any progress on the post-intervention measure could be attributed to. Nonetheless, because of its feasibility with special populations already undergoing treatment, the one group pre-post has been a popular design in therapy studies. Common statistics associated with this design include the correlated t-test, also known as the paired or dependent t-test, or its non-parametric counterpart, the Wilcoxon test. These statistics will be discussed below.

The correlated t-test, also called a paired or dependent t-test, is applied to data when a researcher compares a group's performance or characteristic across two times of measurement. For example, a researcher compares the difference between pre-test and post-test scores on an observed variable (the desired therapy outcome). The difference between the correlated t-test and the independent t-test is that the correlated t-test is applied with one independent group and two measurement events, whereas the independent t-test is applied to scores on one measurement for two independent groups.

An example of a correlated t-test can be found in Van Heest et al. (2017), titled "Effects of a One-to-One Fatigue Management Course for People with Chronic Conditions and Fatigue." The authors compared the difference in the score on the same test between a pre- and post-test performance on several measures (outcome or dependent variables), including energy conservation, fatigue, self-efficacy, and quality of life. The table below describes the means, mean differences, and values for t_{obs}.

CORRELATED *T*-TESTS BETWEEN PRE-TEST AND POST-TEST SCORES				
SUBTESTS	PRE-TEST MEAN (SD)	POST-TEST MEAN (SD)	FOLLOW UP MEAN (SD)	PRE-POST FOLLOW-UP *p*-VALUE
Facit FS	22.7 (8.2)	29.5(10.4)	29.4 (11.0)	<.001;.315
Fact-G	69.0 (16.8)	77.7 (16.6)	77.8 (17.6)	<.001;.085
Physical well-being[a]	17.1 (4.8)	20.2 (4.9)	20.2 (5.4)	<.001;.237
Social well-being[a]	19.4 (6.1)	20.1 (6.3)	20.0 (6.6)	.186;.361
Emotional well-being[a]	16.2 (4.0)	18.3 (3.8)	18.5 (4.0)	<.001;.164
Functional well-being[a]	16.5 (5.2)	19.1 (4.9)	19.2 (5.1)	<.001;.108
SEPECSA	7.2 (1.7)	8.3 (1.1)	8.4 (1.1)	<.001;.439

Note: For pre-test versus post-test, *n* = 49; for post-test versus follow-up, *n* = 36. FACIT FS = Functional Assessment of Chronic Illness Therapy–Fatigue Scale; FACT–G = Functional Assessment of Cancer Therapy–General; SD = standard deviation; SEPECSA = Self-Efficacy for Performing Energy Conservation Strategies Assessment.
[a]Subscales of the FACT–G.

There was a statistically significant difference between pre-test and post-test means on all of the variables except for social well-being and there were no statistically significant differences between the post-test and the follow-up for any of the variables. These findings suggest that in persons with chronic conditions and fatigue, the fatigue management course was successful in improving various aspects of well-being and that these improvements were maintained through the follow-up period.

Operational Procedure for Testing for Statistical Significance in a Paired Data Sample

Step 1. *State the research hypothesis.*
a. *Null Hypothesis: H_0: $\mu_1 = \mu_2$*
b. *Alternative Hypothesis: $\mu_1 \neq \mu_2$*
c. *Directional Hypothesis: H_1: $\mu_1 > \mu_2$*

Step 2. *Select the level of statistical significance.*

α = .05 or .01 level of significance

Step 3. *Decide the test statistic and whether to apply a one-tailed or two-tailed test for statistical significance.*

Step 4. *Look up the critical value for t_{crit} from statistical table.*
a. determine the degrees of freedom: $df = N - 1$
b. level of significance α = .05 or .01

c. one-tailed or two-tailed test
d. t_{crit} derived from table of values. (See Table C–3 in the appendices.)

Step 5. *Calculate the group means and standard deviations for each variable.*

Step 6. *Do an exploratory data analysis by determining if mean differences are greater than standard deviations for each variable.*

Step 7. *Plot a graph (see Independent t-test).*

Step 8. *Calculate t_{obs} using the formula:*

$$t_{obs} = \frac{\Sigma D_1}{\sqrt{[N\Sigma D_1^2 - (\Sigma D_1)^2]/N - 1}}$$

Where
ΣD_1 = sum of differences between each subject's scores on measured variable
ΣD_1^2 = sum of the squared differences on each score
N = total number of subjects

Step 9. Fail to reject the null hypothesis if $t_{obs} < t_{crit}$
Step 10. Reject the null hypothesis if $t_{obs} \geq t_{crit}$
Paired Data Sample

Below is a hypothetical example of correlated *t*-test. Is there a statistically significant difference between performance IQ scores in adults with traumatic brain injury after undergoing an intensive cognitive retraining program?

PERFORMANCE IQ SCORES

SUBJECT	BASELINE (PRE-TEST)	$X_1{}^2$	AFTER TREATMENT (POST-TEST)	$X_2{}^2$
01	97	9409	113	12769
02	106	11236	113	12769
03	106	11236	101	10201
04	95	9025	119	14161
05	102	10404	111	12321
06	111	12321	121	14641
07	115	13225	121	14641
08	104	10816	106	11236
09	90	8100	110	12100
10	96	9216	126	15876
	$\Sigma X_1 = 1022$	$\Sigma X_1{}^2 = 104988$	$\Sigma X_2 = 1141$	$\Sigma X_2{}^2 = 130715$

Step 1. *State the research hypothesis.* There is no statistically significant difference between pre- and post-test IQ performance scores in adults with traumatic brain injury who have undergone an extensive cognitive retraining program. This is a null hypothesis (H_0: $\mu_1 = \mu_2$).

Step 2. Group 1: Select the level of statistical significance. This is usually $\alpha = .05$.

Step 3. *Decide whether to use a one-tailed or two-tailed* test. This problem requires a two-tailed test because the hypothesis is stated in null form and the researcher is examining statistical significance without direction.

Step 4. *Look up t_{crit}.* (See Table C–3 in the appendices.)
a. $df = N - 1 = 9$
b. $\alpha = .05$
c. two-tailed test
d. $t_{crit} = 2.2622$

Step 5. *Calculate the group means and standard deviations for the baseline and retest conditions.*

GROUP 1	GROUP 2
$\overline{X_1} = \Sigma/N = 1022 / 10 = 102.2$ $s_1 = 7.74$	$\overline{X_2} = \Sigma/N = 1141 / 10 = 114.1$ $s_2 = 7.65$

Standard deviation computation formula

$$s = \sqrt{\left[N\Sigma X^2 - (\Sigma X)^2\right] / \left[N(N-1)\right]}$$

$$s_1 = \sqrt{\left[(10)(104988) - (1022)^2\right] / \left[(10)(10-1)\right]}$$

$$s_1 = \sqrt{[1049880 - 1044484] / 90}$$
$$s_1 = \sqrt{5396 / 90}$$
$$s_1 = 7.74$$

$$s_2 = \sqrt{\left[(10)(130715) - (1141)^2\right] / \left[10(10-1)\right]}$$
$$s_2 = \sqrt{\left[(1307150 - 1301881)\right] / 90}$$
$$s_2 = \sqrt{5269 / 90}$$
$$s_2 = \sqrt{58.54}$$
$$s_2 = 7.65$$

Step 6. *Exploratory data analysis.*

$$\overline{X_1} - \overline{X_2} = 102.2 - 114.1 = 11.9$$
$$s_1 = 7.74$$
$$s_2 = 7.65$$

The mean difference between pre- and post-test scores is greater than the standard deviations for pre-test and post-test scores. The difference between the standard deviations is relatively small, indicating a homogeneity of variance for the two groups of scores.

Step 7. *Exploratory graph.* This is displayed in Figure 8–1.

From the exploratory data analysis, there appears to be a significant difference between the pre-test and post-test scores.

SUBJECT	BASELINE TEST	RETEST	D_1	D_2
01	97	113	-16	256
02	106	113	-07	49
03	106	101	$+05$	25
04	95	119	-24	576
05	102	111	-09	81
06	111	122	-11	171
07	115	121	-06	36
08	104	106	-02	4
09	90	110	-20	400
10	96	126	-30	900
	1022	**142**	$\Sigma D_1 = -120$ $(\Sigma D_1)^2 = 14400$	$\Sigma D^2 = 2448$

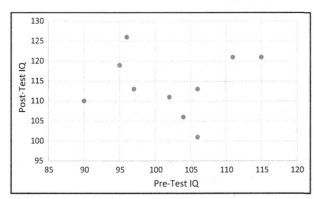

Figure 8–1 Exploratory graph analysis using hypothetical data. The graph shows differences between pre- and post-test performance IQ scores for a group of adults with traumatic brain damage after cognitive retraining. The statistical test being performed is a correlated *t*-test.

Step 8. *Calculate* t_{obs}

$$t_{obs} = \frac{\Sigma D_1}{\sqrt{[N\Sigma D_1^2 - (\Sigma D_1)^2]/N - 1}}$$

$$t_{obs} = \frac{-120}{\sqrt{[(10)(2448) - (14400)]/10 - 1}}$$

$$t_{obs} = \frac{-120}{\sqrt{(24480 - 14400/9}}$$

$$t_{obs} = \frac{-120}{\sqrt{10080/9}}$$

$$t_{obs} - (-120)/\sqrt{1120}$$

$$t_{obs} = (-120)/33.460$$

$$t_{obs} = -3.586$$

Step 9. $t_{obs} = -3.586$. Using Table C–3 in the appendices, we find that $t_{crit} = 2.2622$. The researcher rejects the null hypothesis and concludes that there is a statistically significant difference between the pre- and post-test scores and that cognitive rehabilitation appeared to be effective in raising performance IQ scores in this sample of individuals with traumatic brain injury.[1]

8.3.2 Two Group Pre-Post Intervention Designs [O3]

As its name suggests, the two group pre-post intervention design is different from the one group design because of the additional group. The basic pre-test/baseline, intervention phase, and post-test structure is the same. The addition of a second group, however, acts like a control group. It is possible that this second group doesn't receive any type of intervention during the intervention phase, or it might be that this group receives an alternative intervention. The similarities of the two groups are that each can act as their own controls by virtue of the pre- and post-test respective comparisons, but the difference is that with the addition of the second group, a comparison can also be made between the two groups at the post-test time. There are a number of ways that the statistical analysis/es can be done with this design. One option is for the investigator to take the post-test, pre-test difference scores within each group, then compare the two difference scores using an independent *t*-test. If there was a statistically significant difference, it could be interpreted

---

[1]   Note that the negative sign in -3.5 does not affect the value. Both positive and negative values are interpreted equally when compared with the t_{crit} value for the table.

that the change that occurred in the one group was statistically significantly greater than the change that occurred in the second group. This design provides a more powerful and controlled comparison of the independent variable than just the one group pre-test post-test design.

Lin et al. (2018) used a pre-test post-test design to study the effects of parent participation in occupational therapy development in children with developmental delay. These researchers recruited 30 parent-child dyads who were assigned to one of two groups through a self selection process. The two groups were a control group which involved rehabilitation therapy and the experimental group that received both rehabilitation therapy as well as instruction and tracking of a parent participation program. While, paired *t*-tests showed improvement in both groups on several outcome measures including cognitive ability, verbal ability, gross motor ability, and fine motor ability, the experimental group demonstrated statistically significant improvement in total motor score (gross and fine motor combined), social ability and self-care ability, whereas the control group did not show improvement on these outcomes.

Another option for statistically analyzing the two group pre-test post-test design is to perform a 2 × 2 analysis of variance (ANOVA) where the first factor would be group which is a between-group factor, and the second factor would be time (i.e., pre-test, post-test), a within-group factor. The way this is commonly referred to in the text is that it would be a 2 × 2 ANOVA (group × time) with time being a repeated factor. This type of design would provide three analyses. The first is whether there was a difference between the two groups overall (combining the pre- and post-test scores for each group and then comparing groups). While this may provide interesting information, it doesn't factor in any difference that occurs across time. The second analysis is the comparison between the pre-test and the post-test performance for the two groups combined, but it doesn't parse out the difference between the two groups. Again, this might provide interesting information about what generally happened between the baseline and the post-test, but not if there is a difference between the two groups. The third analysis that comes from this statistical strategy is what is known as the interaction between the two factors of group and time. This interaction analysis, if statistically significant, can be interpreted that the two groups behaved differently from each other across time. For instance, in the group with one level of the independent variable, the participants' performance may have improved across time whereas the participants in the control group showed a performance that remained relatively unchanged across the pre-test and post-test. If this were the case, a good argument could be made that the intervention is what caused the change in performance for the non-control group. Ethically, if the study involved a special population and the intervention was deemed effective and helpful, it would be important to provide the control group

with the same therapeutic condition that the other group received, as soon after the post-test as possible. This way, no participant would be denied the beneficial experience.

Another version of the two-group pre-test post-test design is what is known as a counter balanced repeated measures design. A counter balanced design would have the same two groups only both groups would experience both interventions (or one intervention and the control), however one group would receive the two conditions in one order and the other group would receive the two conditions in the opposite order of the first group. For instance, one group would experience the experimental, then the alternative control condition and the other group would experience the alternative control condition first, then finish with the intervention condition. Doing so would provide for some control of order effects. In this strategy, two separate analyses should be done. First is a one-way ANOVA to test for order effects. If there was no statistically significant difference in the two order of presentation groups, then the investigator can move on to doing the analysis to test the efficacy of the independent variable. This would involve performing either a paired *t*-test or a repeated measures ANOVA between the intervention and the control conditions. The overall advantage of this strategy is that since each participant is their own control, the desired statistical power can be obtained using a smaller sample than if the comparison was between independent groups. A disadvantage, however, is that it could be argued that having the same participant in both groups could reduce the independence between the two conditions. An example of this design was done by Kehoe and Rice (2016) in a study that investigated the influences of materials-based (MB), imaginary (I), and virtual reality (VR) conditions had upon motor performance in a dart throwing activity. The MB condition involved throwing real darts at a real dart board. The imaginary condition involved pretending to throw a dart while imagining doing so, and the VR condition involved a Microsoft Xbox Kinect system loaded with a virtual reality-based dart throwing game. In this counter-balanced design, 34 adults who were novice at dart throwing were randomly assigned to one of three order of presentation groups, namely MB-I-VR, I-VR-MB, or VR-MB-I. Wilcoxon and Paired *t*-tests revealed no difference in the motor performance between the MB and I conditions, but there were differences between the VR with the MB conditions and between the VR and the imaginary conditions. The authors concluded that motor planning processes involved with virtual reality were different from those elicited in the materials-based and imaginary conditions, which were similar to each other.

Another type of design at this level (O3) is the case-control design that uses pre-existing groups. As mentioned earlier, case-control designs are by design retrospective studies. They involve comparing two groups of people, mainly through medical records, or through some other database. One group of people would presumably have been exposed to something or have some experience that was uniquely different from what the other group was exposed to or experienced. Usually, it is desired to have the second group be as close to a control group as possible. However, an inherent challenge is that because all of this happened in the past, there is no way to control the ambient experiences that both groups may have encountered at the time. Regardless, there are rich databases provided by a variety of agencies, not the least of which is the Centers for Disease Control and Prevention which, among others, provides databases on COVID-19, deaths and mortality, alcohol use, cancer, diabetes, and more. Another source of good databases is the United States Census Bureau.

Included at the O3 level is also the prospective type of group comparison as an outcome study. This type of study design was explored when discussing the E3, controlled clinical trial. The difference between the group comparison in the E3 and O3 levels is that the O3 group comparison study design has a feature that keeps it from fulfilling all of the requirements required by the E3 group comparison. The most common reason for this divergence is the lack of random assignment. It may be an intentional decision not to control natural setting variability. Another common reason, as mentioned above, may have its basis in the ethical responsibility to not withhold beneficial treatment to a group, thereby preventing a true control group for the study design. Regardless, the general design would involve the comparison of two or more groups that reflects the manipulation of the independent variable. The simplest form would be a two-group comparison; the statistic of choice would be a *t*-test for independent variables. If the study involved a comparison of more than two groups, then the analysis would likely involve an ANOVA followed up with a post-hoc multiple comparison with a Bonferroni, Tukey, Scheffé, or other multiple comparison statistic. The purpose of the post-hoc multiple comparison is that while the ANOVA will determine if there is an overall statistical significance across all groups, it does not determine the significance of the specific difference between any pair of groups; post-hoc multiple comparisons are designed for this very purpose. For example, if the ANOVA stated there was a significant difference among the three groups, the investigator would depend on the post-hoc multiple comparison to see which specific groups were different from each other. In this example it would compare group 1 with group 2, group 1 with group 3, and group 2 with group 3. There are multiple different types of post-hoc multiple comparison statistics from which to choose. Each has its own unique features and applicability, the scope of which is beyond this textbook.

Instead of calculating an ANOVA with follow up post-hoc multiple comparisons, another strategy may be that the investigator would choose to calculate pre-planned contrast analyses. The advantage of this strategy is that it can be more precise in that the investigator is only interested in comparing group 1 with group 2 and group 1 with

group 3. If this was the plan, then the investigator could adjust the alpha to accommodate two comparisons. If the overall alpha was set at .05, the investigator would set the alpha at .025 (the Bonferroni adjustment). The advantage of this is that this alpha size is larger than what the multiple comparison alpha would be, which likely would be .0167 because by default it compares all possible combinations, in this case three. The use of pre-planned contrasts is not as common as using the traditional ANOVA with follow-up multiple comparisons, however this strategy can provide more precise, and therefore a more powerful analysis if its use satisfies the study's design and sufficiently satisfies testing the hypothesis/es (Marini, 2003).

8.3.3 Two Group Intervention Comparison Designs with Covariate Investigation [O2]

Studies labeled O2 have relatively more rigor than those labeled O3. Studies at the O2 level represent important scientific inquiry into understanding the efficacy of interventions, and how this efficacy may interact with participant factors. For retrospective studies, they are similar in design as to what was described above, but with the addition of a covariate. A covariate is a variable that, as its name suggests, covaries. One such example from the literature is a study by Ownsworth and colleagues (2017) that investigated learning strategies for people with severe traumatic brain injury (TBI), specifically whether error-based versus errorless learning was more beneficial for the participants. In their study, 54 participants with TBI were randomly assigned to an errorless learning group or an error-based group. Both groups involved eight 90-minute occupational therapy sessions involving meal preparation and goal-directed activities. The dependent variable (i.e., outcome) was the number of errors on a cooking task. In their analysis, the researchers employed an ANCOVA with years of education as the covariate. With this covariate in place, the results were that the error-based learning group performed statistically better than the errorless learning group. While it is not known whether the same difference would exist without the covariate in the analysis, with the level of education being statistically controlled through the ANCOVA analysis, the difference emerges.

As mentioned earlier, one of the assumptions associated with traditional parametric inferential statistics (e.g., *t*-tests and ANOVAs) is that the variables studied are independent from the other variables associated with the study. It is possible that through design, or in hindsight, it becomes plausible to suspect that there is a variable that is correlated or covaries with one of the dependent variables. When studying human behavior from an epidemiological perspective, education level, socioeconomic status, and age are variables that often covary with human behavior. This is true for retrospective and prospective research.

In order to understand analysis of covariance or ANCOVA, it is helpful to already have a grasp of analysis of variance as well as regression. This will become apparent once we've explored the concepts of ANCOVA and will see that this statistical procedure is, in a way, an amalgamation of ANOVA and regression analyses. The overall purpose of ANCOVA is to statistically control the effects that one variable has on another variable. Often the variable to be controlled has an unwanted effect upon the results of a regular ANOVA. This concept of controlling extraneous variables has been discussed at length in an earlier chapter, but suffice it to say that a well-controlled research study is designed to measure only the independent variable. Through the research design, extraneous variables are removed from the study. For example, research bias can be mitigated through single or double blind studies. Another example of an unwanted variable may be an order effect in a repeated measures design. A potential way to control order effects is to counterbalance the order of presentation of the experimental conditions so that half of the participants receive condition "A" first, then condition "B," and the other half of the participants receive condition "B" first, then condition "A." These are examples of research design methods for controlling extraneous variable influence upon the dependent variable. With good planning and foresight, well-balanced studies of greater rigor can be designed. Sometimes, however, it is not possible to control for some extraneous variables. Sometimes the variables can be anticipated, and sometimes they are discovered only after the data are collected. It is in these situations that a statistical method for controlling the influence of extraneous variables may be possible. There are some requirements associated with whether variables can be controlled statistically, not the least of which is that they need to be continuous data, there should be no interaction between the variable and the dependent variable, that is, there should be homogeneity of regression slopes, and lastly, the variable needs to covary with the dependent

variable. This last point is important in that the more the variable covaries with the dependent variable, the stronger its influence is upon the dependent variable outcome. Common variables considered to be covariates include, but are not limited to age, intelligence, and education.

The assumptions for the ANCOVA statistic include the following:

- Independent observations (one data point falling where it has no effect on other data points)
- Data are normally distributed (when graphed would appear as a normal curve)
- Homogeneity of variance between groups
  - Levene's test can be used to check for this
- Linearity
- Randomization, or matching (e.g., age, gender, education-matched)
- Homogeneity of regression slopes
  - should be no interaction between the covariate and the dependent variable
- Covariate is measured without error.

In a regular ANOVA, the variance of statistical error is normally attributed to a couple of sources including the "treatment" or the independent variable and just plain "error," the latter of which is a term given to the portion of the variance that can't be accounted for by the independent variable portion of the statistical model. Ideally the independent variable portion of the variance would be 100% which would yield an enormous F-value with an associated minuscule p-value. Alas, we do not live in a perfect world and try as we might, no research methodology is able to remove all extraneous error. If there is an unregulated covariate within the statistical model, it is possible that it inflates the independent variable variance, and henceforth increases the chance of a Type II error. As you recall, a Type II error is when the null hypothesis fails to be rejected when it really should have been. Herein lies the reason for employing an ANCOVA. If there is an important variable that can be identified that covaries with the dependent variable

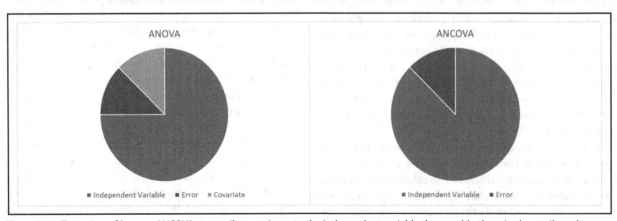

Figure 8–2 Illustration of how an ANCOVA can attribute variance to the independent variable that would otherwise be attributed to error in an ANOVA.

the ANCOVA can statistically remove a portion of the variance that would otherwise be mistakenly attributed to the independent variable. In essence, the ANCOVA gives back the variance that would have been naturally attributed to the independent variable's portion of the variance if the covariate didn't exist. By doing so it allots greater statistical power to the testing of the independent variable which should increase its associated *F*-value and decrease the size of the associated *p*-value, thereby reducing the chance of a Type II error. See Figure 8–2 for an example of the partitioning of the variance comparison in an ANOVA model versus an ANCOVA model. In summary, ANCOVA is a statistical method to remove extraneous variables that covary with the dependent variable that would otherwise increase the chance of a Type II error.

Let's look at some hypothetical data on a class of occupational therapy students. Let's say that the dependent variable is the performance on an occupational therapy exam and the independent variable is the study method. In condition 1 students studied in groups whereas in condition 2 students studied individually. The exam was given and the mean score for group 1 was about 54% and for group 2 it was about 50%. Arguably neither group performs well, but group 1 had a higher mean score, though the ANOVA table indicated a *p*-value of greater than 0.05 (Table 8–1).

Refer to Table 8–1 and pay close attention to the sum of squares. In Table 8–1 the variance attributed to error was 5.036 whereas in Table 8–2, the variance attributed to the error is 0.004. The difference is attributed to the covariate labeled RestQuotient. Moreover, the *F*-value associated with the independent variable is now larger than the *F*-critical value yielding a *p*-value significant at 0.011 compared to the one-ANOVA in Table 8–1.

A fair interpretation is that there is "more to the story" than just study methods. The instructor would be correct in saying that if the RestQuotient score was controlled for, then the method of individual study yielded significantly better exam scores than the method of group study. The significant covariate of RestQuotient appeared to influence the independent variable. If the study methods were employed the evening before the exam, it might be that the students in the group condition had a lower (less desirable) RestQuotient compared to the students who studied individually. Though the instructor can't say for certain from these data, perhaps students in the group spent less time resting than the students who studied independently. While this study didn't capture the amount of time studying or the type of activity beyond studying the day before the exam, it would be a good factor to control in the next iteration of this line of scientific inquiry.

TABLE 8–1

SPSS OUTPUT FOR ONE-WAY ANOVA FOR THE INDEPENDENT VARIABLE EXAMSCORE

DEPENDENT VARIABLE:	EXAMSCORE				
Source	Type III Sum of Squares	df	Mean Square	F	Sig.
StudyMethod	.022	1	.022	.255	.616
Error	5.036	58	.087		
Corrected Total	5.059	59			

TABLE 8–2

SPSS OUTPUT FOR ONE-WAY ANCOVA FOR THE INDEPENDENT VARIABLE EXAMSCORE WITH THE COVARIATE RESTQUOTIENT

DEPENDENT VARIABLE:	EXAMSCORE				
Source	Type III Sum of Squares	df	Mean Square	F	Sig.
RestQuotient	5.033	1	5.033	81713.057	.000
StudyMethod	.000	1	.000	6.992	.011
Error	.004	57	6.159E-05		
Corrected Total	5.059	59			

8.4 META-ANALYSIS OF OUTCOMES STUDIES [O1]

Similar to the other three sides of the pyramid, meta-analyses at the O1 level represent the highest level of evidence available on the outcome side of the pyramid. While a well-designed and implemented outcomes study can provide important information to help guide occupational therapists by informing their clinical reasoning, the value of a single study is somewhat limited, regardless of how well the study was conducted. Meta-analyses, on the other hand, through an established protocol, can provide a stronger level of confidence in the results because the interpretation is based on multiple studies, selected using a prescribed method, all of which investigated a common independent variable. In concept, meta-analyses usually involve incorporating the means and standard deviations from each respective study and pooling the respective sample sizes. In doing so, this provides much greater statistical power because of the increased statistical degrees of freedom. Meta-analysis will be covered in detail in Chapter 10.

8.5 SUMMARY

This chapter explored the levels of research associated with the outcome side of the Research Pyramid. At the lowest level, one-group pre-test post-test designs along with commonly associated inferential statistics were discussed. Retrospective case controlled studies were discussed with and without covariates. Alongside these, outcomes-based group comparison study designs were explored. Meta-analyses based upon outcomes studies were discussed as the highest level of evidence available on the outcome side of the Research Pyramid. The most common aspect that differentiates outcomes-based research from experimental research is that outcomes research often occurs in the field, and as such does not adhere to assumptions (e.g., random selection) associated with the respective levels of experimental studies found on the experimental side of the Research Pyramid. Often these compromises are due to pragmatics associated with involving research participants from special populations; namely, a lack of availability for random recruitment and ethical random assignment to comparison groups. Regardless, outcomes-based research provides valuable information which occupational therapists can use towards forming their clinical reasoning that is based upon scientific evidence.

9

Qualitative Research Models

A qualitative research approach involves the study of the empirical world from the perspectives of the subjects under investigation. As such, it is based on two assumptions. The first assumption is that human behavior is influenced by the physical and psychological context or environment in which it occurs. Consequently, to understand this contextual influence, the researcher must observe the subjects in their natural context... Second, a qualitative approach is based on the assumption that human behavior goes beyond that which can be observed; it lies in the perspectives and meanings held by the individuals in a context.

(Schmid, 1981, p. 105)

OPERATIONAL LEARNING OBJECTIVES

By the end of this chapter, the learner will be able to:

1. Define qualitative research
2. Recognize the differences between quantitative and qualitative research designs
3. Describe the basic types of qualitative research
4. Describe the qualitative research process
5. Identify qualitative data collection methods
6. Identify the techniques of qualitative data analysis and synthesis
7. Identify how methodological rigor is enhanced in qualitative designs
8. Critically analyze an example of qualitative research from the health literature

9.1 Defining Qualitative Research

Occupational therapists, when providing interventions for their clients, must navigate both the physical world of their environments and bodies, but also the psychosocial realm of their lives, where culture, symbolism, and meaning are crucial influences on valued activities. For this reason, qualitative research is particularly important for understanding phenomena that are important for the effective professional reasoning of therapists.

Qualitative research may be defined as a set of inquiry approaches that seek to understand participants in all the complexity of their natural surroundings. It seeks to uncover deeper meanings about the lived experience of the study participants (sometimes called informants). It often attempts to do so without imposing any preset ideas about what is important, valued, or motivating to the participants. At its best, it uses a series of refined techniques to define the research question, select informants, gather information and insights from them, and analyze and synthesize these data into a coherent, well-founded portrayal of their life perspectives. To achieve these aims qualitative researchers have developed approaches with several fundamentally different assumptions from the ones pertaining to most quantitative research. Yet qualitative and quantitative research can often be used effectively in tandem, as described later in this chapter in section 9.13 on mixed methods.

As applied in occupational therapy studies, qualitative research has engaged many questions. The research purpose may be to understand the experience of living with a particular disability or chronic medical condition (Clark, 1993). It may be to understand the lived experience of a client undergoing rehabilitation for that condition (McAlonan, 1996). Informants may include the clients, their family members, or their occupational therapists. A qualitative researcher may seek to understand the meaning of a particular activity for an individual or group of people sharing a characteristic or interest (Taylor & McGruder, 1996).

Among health and rehabilitation professionals, there is a growing interest in exploring the lived experience of clients and their families (Bamm et al., 2015; Ferguson et al., 1992; Llewellyn, 1995; Morse, 1994; Swinth et al., 2015; Westby & Backman, 2010). This interest has been shaped by several factors. The first is the disability rights movement. Consumers of health and related services are actively campaigning against the medical approach to disability and for a positive acceptance of people with disabilities' place in society, and for consumers of health services to be seen not as "patients," but rather as agents of their own destinies (Swain & French, 2008). The second factor is collaboration between researchers in health and social science disciplines (e.g., medical anthropology), contributing to an alternative view of disability from the traditional illness-based one, where the expert treats the depersonalized, impaired patient (Good, 1993). In its place, the handicapping effects of a disability are regarded as socially constructed (World Health Organization, 2007). That is, both social attitudes and the public physical space create impedances to the activities of people with a disability. Socioeconomic conditions also contribute heavily to the incidence and impact of disability (Oliver, 1992; Plantinga et al., 2012). A third factor is the return in occupational therapy to client-centered practice. Collaboration between therapist and client in goal setting and the therapeutic use of self for building a trusting relationship are indicators of this renewed emphasis in the field on the agency of the client for self-determination (American Occupational Therapy Association, 2020; Pollock, 1993). A fourth factor is the re-focusing on occupation-based therapy (American Occupational Therapy Association, 2020; Christiansen et al., 1995) By definition, occupation is a set of activities performed by an individual within a role where the activities have meaning to the person. Qualitative research lends itself particularly well to an exploration of meaning to the individual that is not presumed or assumed by the researcher, but rather uncovered.

Exploring the lived experience of the client requires different research designs from those previously employed in the medical and health sciences. Allied health researchers have turned to sociology (the study of groups, social institutions, and collective behavior) and to anthropology (the study of human cultures) for more appropriate research methodologies (Krefting, 1991). Investigators in these disciplines have been unraveling the complex cultural interactions among individuals since the end of the 19th century (Parsons, 1939).

Qualitative research models differ from those in the quantitative tradition in three fundamental ways. First, qualitative researchers are interested in "participatory and holistic knowing" (Reason, 1988) This contrasts with the distance and objectivity of the researcher, and the isolation of variables sought particularly in experimental research designs. Second, there is an acknowledgement of critical subjectivity in qualitative research. This involves researchers accepting and reflecting upon their own unalterable subjective perspective and thus biases. Qualitative researchers become their own "research instrument"—in direct contrast to the notion of an objective researcher in experimental research designs. Third, qualitative researchers hold the view that there are multiple perspectives and thus multiple realities when it comes to lived experience and the meaning of activities and behaviors to individuals. Not as a neutral observer, but as an engaged participant, can the researcher gain an understanding of the complex phenomena at hand as experienced. Research informants are regarded as "sources of understanding" for these complex realities, rather than as "subjects of study."

9.2 CHARACTERISTICS OF QUALITATIVE RESEARCH

There are four fundamental characteristics of qualitative research:
- Phenomena are investigated and interpreted in their natural settings, considering the socio-cultural-historical context, in a quest for an insider perspective.
- Multiple methods are used to identify, confirm, and offer interpretations of the meanings held by participants about these phenomena.
- The researcher and the study participants (informants) occupy a central place together in the qualitative research process.
- An inductive process is used to develop general principles from the study of specific instances. Ultimately, a theory of human experience under the study circumstances is sought.

9.2.1 Phenomena Are Investigated and Interpreted in Their Natural Settings, Considering the Socio-Cultural-Historical Context, in a Quest for an Insider Perspective

Qualitative research usually takes place in naturalistic, community settings. Qualitative researchers commit to prolonged engagement in the natural setting in order to understand the meanings held by participants about the phenomena under investigation. From this involvement and understanding, qualitative researchers develop insight and theoretical knowledge about the human condition. This knowledge may be in the form of patterns or themes or it may be a fully developed theory about the phenomena studied. Whatever the case, the resulting knowledge is uncovered through and grounded in direct field research experience rather than imposed before data collection through hypotheses or planned analyses among variables (Glaser & Strauss, 1967).

9.2.2 Multiple Methods Are Used to Identify, Confirm, and Offer Interpretations of the Meanings Held by Participants About These Phenomena

Qualitative researchers use an array of methods to collect information about, describe, and interpret events and meanings in individuals' lives. The basic methods used for gathering data are interviewing, observation, and documentary analysis. The strategies most commonly used to analyze data include content analysis or thematic uncovery, grounded theory procedures, critical analysis, and narrative analysis. These strategies are employed in the search for regularities in the meanings that participants hold about the phenomena under investigation. For some researchers, these regularities are viewed as a form of conceptual order; for others, their interest lies in the repetition of patterns across the data.

9.2.3 The Researcher and the Study Participants (Informants) Occupy a Central Place Together in the Qualitative Research Process

In qualitative research, the researcher is acknowledged as an individual located within a historical context and within a research tradition. Researchers bring to the research process particular sets of beliefs about the world that guide their actions. In contrast to experimentally based research designs, qualitative researchers attempt not to impose pre-existing expectations on the phenomena or setting under study. Rather, the researchers' set of beliefs functions as an interpretive framework (Guba, 1990). This interpretive framework guides the research purpose and also shapes the research questions and the methods employed to address these questions. In addition to an interpretive framework, qualitative researchers become familiar with the literature and develop general guiding questions to help bring focus to the purposes of the research.

9.2.4 An Inductive Process Is Used to Develop General Principles from the Study of Specific Instances

In qualitative research, the analysis begins with specific patterns of data and builds toward general principles. This contrasts with the deductive process employed in the quantitative tradition in which hypotheses are constructed prior to data collection and then tested. In qualitative research, preparing the research text is the final stage of the inductive analytic process. The research text is a construction that integrates and interprets data and the researcher's understanding of the topic of study. The completed product is the public text, which may be delivered either as a research report, journal article, book, or conference paper.

9.3 TYPES OF QUALITATIVE RESEARCH

Qualitative research may be categorized in several different ways. Tesch (1990), for example, listed 46 different research approaches under the rubric of qualitative research. Some research methods more closely fit the characteristics described above; others are less closely associated. Several qualitative methods have become common and well accepted in health literature (Luborsky & Lysack, 2017). These include ethnography (section 9.3.1, below), phenomenology (9.3.2), narrative analysis (9.3.3), and some types of participatory action research (9.3.4; see Table 9–1). Other methods, such as discourse analysis, ethnoscience, and critical theory, do not appear as often in the occupational therapy literature. Briefly, discourse analysis and ethnoscience are concerned with the study of the characteristics of language as a communication tool and as culture, respectively. Critical theory involves the taking apart (deconstruction) of a widely adopted set of ideas in society, for example, to determine who benefits and who is disadvantaged by such attitudes and beliefs. (Further detail may be found in DePoy & Gitlin, 2019.)

Historical research and operations research, which may be classified as descriptive research when they exclusively use quantitative methods, may additionally use qualitative research methods, in which case they would be classified as mixed methods research. They will be covered below in section 9.13.

Another approach to classifying qualitative research is by the research purpose. Some approaches are ideal for identifying regularities, patterns, or themes. Others are better suited to generating and refining tentative theoretical propositions. Still others are more useful for intense, intimate study of a phenomenon using personal reflection and personal testimony. There is ongoing debate in the qualitative research literature about this diversity of approaches and associated methodological issues (Denzin & Lincoln, 1994; Higgs, 1997). Each approach has adherents in the core disciplines of psychology, psychiatry, sociology, and anthropology.

9.3.1 Ethnographic Research

About the same time that Gesell (1928) was experimenting with his photographic dome in pursuit of descriptive developmental research, cultural anthropologists developed rigorous methods for collecting data describing the everyday lives of indigenous people and the meanings to them of their activities. Franz Boas, the noted anthropologist, wrote in the foreword to Margaret Mead's classic study *Coming of Age in Samoa* (1928) the following, which articulated one goal of anthropological field research:

> Through a comparative study of these data and through information that tells us of their growth and development, we endeavor to reconstruct, as well as may be, the history of each particular culture. Some anthropologists even hope that the comparative study will reveal some tendencies of

development that recur so often that significant generalizations regarding the processes of cultural growth will be discovered.

(Mead, 1928, p. xiii)

Mead attempted to answer the question "Are the disturbances which vex our adolescents due to the nature of adolescence itself or to the civilization?" (pp. 6–7). She lived in Samoa for six months, and there she analyzed the life and development of 68 girls between the ages of 8 and 20. She was particularly concerned with three villages on the island of Tau.

In her field study, Mead painted a vivid and complete picture of the island life of adolescent girls. She felt that certain characteristics, basically Samoan, enabled adolescent girls to pass through puberty without the upheavals that are an oft-expected aspect of living in a developed, Western society. Chiefly, a Samoan girl may leave her immediate household and go to live with another family at any time, especially if she feels put upon. Other characteristics concern life roles, absence of double standards, familiarity with losses such as death, casual family relationships as opposed to intense ones, and a specific place in society for each member. Further, Mead pointed to a tolerance for sexually diverse behavior and concomitant lack of guilt feelings about such behavior, an absence of extreme poverty, and a less stressful environment as reasons for a more serene adolescence than that found elsewhere in the world.

Mead made a substantial early contribution to the field of ethnography: to reconstruct accurately a particular culture and to search for patterns that can provide theoretical insights into the human condition. Her observations occurred in a natural setting, Samoan villages, and entailed six months of prolonged engagement with her informants. Although her work on Samoa was later severely criticized by Freeman (1983), Freeman's own criticism has since been called into question (Shankman, 2010). What is not in dispute is that Mead and her supervising professor Boas advanced a methodology for understanding an unfamiliar culture or set of experiences that could overcome the preconceived notions of a researcher.

9.3.2 Phenomenology

Edmund Husserl, the Austrian-German philosopher-mathematician, was the principal founder of phenomenology (Husserl, 1901; Husserl, 1913). Throughout his academic career, he sought to develop a science and philosophy of consciousness, which he called "transcendental phenomenology." A very basic idea of Husserl's work is that consciousness is of a fundamentally different nature from the world of objects, but that it can be studied scientifically nonetheless. His work had a profound influence on 20th century philosophy (Stanford Encyclopedia of Philosophy, 2022).

TABLE 9–1

FOUR TYPES OF QUALITATIVE RESEARCH COMMON IN HEALTH CARE LITERATURE

	ETHNOGRAPHY	PHENOMENOLOGY	NARRATIVE ANALYSIS	PARTICIPATORY ACTION RESEARCH
Definition	Examination of a cultural or social group through extended participant observations and interviews, to determine the meanings of behavior and interactions of the group (Creswell, 1998; Vidich & Lyman, 1994). Draws heavily upon the discipline of anthropology in its study of cultures for both its assumptions and its techniques in the research process.	Study of the lived experiences of an individual or group of persons, living under unique or noteworthy conditions. It focuses on consciousness and the meanings applied by the informants to the activities in their daily lives. The approach is derived from the philosophical work of Husserl on human consciousness.	Study aiming to capture the authentic storyline about a client's life. Often is concerned with the client's occupational profile and occupational trajectory. Plot mechanisms of the protagonist, conflict, thwarted expectations, and foreshadowing may be used to organize the data.	Research process in which the researcher forms an equal partnership with informants as *researchers*. Informants play a leading role in defining the research questions, selecting methods of data collection, performing analysis and synthesis of data, and in the composition of the final paper. The focus in on discovering knowledge that will allow the participants to materially change their daily lives for the better (thus the word "action" in the title).

Once consciousness was validated as a legitimate topic of scientific inquiry, studies began on the "lived experience" of various people. Two of the earliest studies to appear in the occupational therapy literature using the term phenomenological were Kibele (1989) and Yerxa and Locker (1990). McCuaig and Frank (1991) used a phenomenological approach to discover, interpret, and portray the lived experience of an adult woman with cerebral palsy (in an indication of the overlap between phenomenology and ethnography, McCuaig and Frank labeled their study an ethnography).

Phenomenological studies can seek insights into the lived experience of clients undergoing health services (McAlonan, 1996, on individuals with a spinal cord injury receiving sexual rehabilitation services), or on former clients reintegrating into their new life roles (Taylor & McGruder, 1996, on the meaning of sea kayaking for individuals with spinal cord injury).

Recent studies using phenomenology as a method include Moen et al. (2022) on the experiences of children and youth with concussion, Levi et al. (2023) on social pain perceptions in individuals with autism, and Smith et al. (2023) on the social experiences of families raising a child with autism.

In virtually every study in occupational therapy using a phenomenological approach, the argument is made, implicitly or explicitly, that understanding the phenomenal world of the client (the lived experience of the client in the pertinent circumstances) is helpful, if not crucial, for the client's therapist. Understanding life from the client's perspective provides the therapist with a context for making better professional, collaborative decisions about the client's care.

9.3.3 Narrative Qualitative Research

A qualitative research approach can also be employed when the goal is to capture an authentic narrative about an informant's life or some aspect of that life. An early example in the occupational therapy literature is Clark (1993), who studied the story-making and story-telling aspects of a client's life as she recovered from a stroke. Techniques of life history ethnography were used, as well as the narrative analysis of Polkinghorne. Clark recounted events from her informant's early childhood that affected her adult occupational trajectory, including during her recovery process. Through their conversations (interviews), the informant realized the crucial importance of coming to feel again that she was the agent in her own life. Clark argued that such research approaches were particularly well-suited for studying questions in occupation science, in addition to having profound implications for the practice of occupational therapy (1993).

9.3.4 Participatory Action Research

This type of qualitative research is different from the first three described in three ways. First, a participatory action research project may not necessarily use a qualitative methodology at all. Second, the researcher forms an equal partnership with the project informants, *as researchers.* The informants identify the questions to be studied, decide upon the methods to be used, and play an integral part in data collection and analysis. They may even have a critical role in the composition of the final paper. Third, as the name indicates, the purpose of gathering data and acquiring insight is to plan and carry out some action that will change the lives of the participants. Taylor et al. (2004) published an early paper in the professional literature describing participatory action research, providing its common characteristics, and giving two case examples of its use. The second case was a project to create an ongoing study with informants who had AIDS and who now, with better pharmaceutical treatments available, had a prognosis of reduced mortality. The ensuing study assisted social agencies construct better programs for individuals in this situation. Large components of the project apparently used qualitative methods of data collection (semi-structured interviews and focus groups; see section 9.5 below).

A recent example of a participatory action research project was Angell et al. (2020). The authors involved 153 individuals with disabilities making the transition from institution to community living. Through focus groups the researchers and informants collectively identified lived experiences, barriers, and ways for therapists to alter their approaches so as to better prepare and assist individuals in such a situation.

All four types of qualitative studies have certain features in common. They seek to portray the actual lived experiences of the informants. They use informant interviews heavily. They perform an iterative analysis as the data are generated, using earlier findings to guide later avenues of questioning. They all create an interpretation of the experienced world of the informants which, if the study was conducted rigorously (see section 9.12 below), can have implications for the wider world of people who are similar. All four types of qualitative study can powerfully inform the practice of occupational therapy.

9.4 Sampling in a Qualitative Study

In contrast to quantitative studies, where the selection of a sample is of profound importance for the type of statistical generalization that may be made, in qualitative studies different strategies are used. In seeking one or more informant insiders to the phenomenon under study (e.g., a culture or an individual's lived experience), the researcher may make use of one of the following sampling techniques:

9.4.1 Nominated Sample

The researcher asks several members of the culture (in an ethnographic study) which individual would be a good (i.e., articulate, authentic, willing) informant for the group. Often this question yields a key informant who knows a great deal about living in that culture, by virtue of longevity in that culture, personality, or connectedness with other members of the culture. It may be the titular leader of that culture (chief of a tribe, president of a group, or the acknowledged, informal leader). The testimony of this key informant cannot automatically be generalized to other members, yet it often provides a deep and comprehensive view of the distinct features of that culture.

9.4.2 Cascading Sample (Snowball Sample)

When informants of the target phenomenon are difficult to identify, and more than one or two are sought for the study, a cascading sample may be useful. Once one informant is found the researcher asks that informant if there are other people who are in the same situation as that person. After enlisting these people as informants, the referral question is asked again. The cascade continues until informants are recommending people who have already been enlisted as informants (the point of sampling saturation). For example, a researcher may know one refugee Cambodian-American family living in the city of the study. They volunteer for the study and recommended several other Cambodian-American families. Each of these families know of other similar families. Soon, virtually the entire local community of refugee Cambodian-Americans has been asked to participate in the study.

9.4.3 Sampling Until Data Saturation Is Reached

When informants are readily available, the researcher may enlist one after another and collect data until no new ideas are being revealed. Then the researcher stops adding informants, under the assumption that the existing set of informants has provided thorough information about their culture or their experiences.

9.4.4 Convenience Sampling

As may be done in quantitative studies, the qualitative researcher may simply post a request for volunteers in a physical community setting or online. Respondents are presented with the purpose of the study and provided the opportunity for informed consent. With such a sampling approach it may be more difficult for the researcher to claim representativeness or transferability, in other words, that the authentic essence of the experience or culture has indeed been captured, and the findings apply more widely beyond just those individuals who were studied.

9.4.5 Research Purpose and Sampling

According to the stated purpose of the research, it may be more strategic for the researcher to study a few individuals extensively (repeated interviews, prolonged observations), or enlist a greater number of individuals for less in-depth data collection. Qualitative studies that have a focused purpose (Shaw et al., 2010, on perceptions of older drivers of safety risks in contemporary vehicles) may lean toward higher numbers of people as informants. Studies that are phenomenological (McCuaig & Frank, 1991) or narrative (Clark, 1993) typically have fewer informants, and their experiences are deeply investigated over longer periods of time.

9.5 QUALITATIVE DATA COLLECTION—INTERVIEWING

The most common data collection method in qualitative research is interviewing. Using interviews as a data collection method rests on the assumption that "the perspective of others is meaningful, knowable, and able to be made explicit" (Patton, 1990). In short, researchers conduct interviews to find out about values, experiences, and meanings that cannot be directly observed. Everyday familiarity with conversational or therapeutic interviews can lead novice researchers to regard interviewing for research purposes as quite straightforward. To effectively use interviewing as a research method, though, requires knowledge of, and practice with, available techniques.

Research interviews take several forms. Interviews can be done face-to-face, over the telephone, or in a group. The format may be structured, semi-structured, or open-ended. Interviewing may be used to collect personal experiences, to understand particular phenomena, or to identify the perspective of a particular group of people. Interviews may be brisk or lengthy. They may be a single one, two per informant, or part of a series.

Oftentimes investigators will employ a combination of interviewing approaches if this suits the purpose of the research and the research questions. For example, an interview may begin with a standardized, structured format, followed by sections made up of semi-structured questions. Alternatively, the interview may begin with an unstructured, open-ended format and conclude with a set of standardized questions. The type of interview that will best suit the research purpose needs particular care and thought.

9.5.1 Structured Interviewing

In this type of interview, the interviewer uses a pre-established set of questions in a uniform manner. Although the questions may be open-ended, the interviewer cannot alter the predetermined format. The aim of this structured approach is to achieve as close as possible a standard format across interviewers (when there is more than one conducting the study) and informants. One disadvantage of this approach is that the interviewer is not able to seek clarification or pursue topics that arise during the interview that could deepen the understanding of the researchers about the phenomenon of interest.

9.5.2 Semi-Structured Interviewing

This type of interviewing utilizes a general interview guide. The issues to be covered in the interview are pre-determined; however, question format and exact content are not pre-specified. Rather, the interview guide can be adapted, as necessary, during the interview. Semi-structured interviewing is an effective use of time while still allowing the interviewer to build rapport and conduct the interview in a flexible way. This approach is particularly appropriate for group interviews (focus groups), where it is important to encourage all participants to contribute to the topic under discussion.

9.5.3 Unstructured (Open-Ended) Interviewing

The purpose of this approach is to interview respondents without imposing any prior categories on the content, vocabulary, or format of the interview. The emphasis is on listening and on understanding each informant's point of view, not on explaining their perspectives within a predetermined interpretive framework (Holstein & Gubrium, 1995).

Unstructured interviews are particularly useful for starting an interview process that will eventually contain multiple encounters for conversation over a period of time. Subsequent interviews can then be used to elaborate on information gathered in the opening, unstructured interview. One disadvantage of unstructured interviewing is the time involved. Another is the resources needed to analyze the quantity and variety of data gathered.

Since Mead (1928), qualitative researchers have refined the techniques of interviewing informants such that the data collector would not be suggesting words or ideas to the informant (Spradley, 1979, 1980). These approaches are used in unstructured (open-ended) or semi-structured interviews. In a study of the culture of the unhoused, starting an unstructured interview with an open, "grand rounds" type of question, such as "Tell me

about living in the open," or "Tell me about not having a fixed home," gives the informant the greatest latitude for addressing what is of importance to that individual. A general opening question also avoids using particular words that might be leading to the informant. Spradley advocates, in its purest form, that the ethnographic interviewer only utter words the informant has used, once the grand rounds question has been posed. Subsequently, the interviewer must strike a balance between letting the informant totally determine the path of the conversation and having the discussion veer off topic. To stay on target often a semi-structured interview approach is used. In either type of interview, it is permitted and in fact encouraged for the interviewer to use probes ("Tell me more about that"), contrasts ("What's an example of a rain that is not gloomy?"), or challenges ("Yesterday you told me living rough was freeing; today you just said it was a burden. Can you explain that?") (Spradley, 1979). Interviewing of one or more informants continues until no further new information or ideas are obtained (the point of data saturation).

9.5.4 Audio or Video Recording of Interviews

In virtually all qualitative data studies the researcher will audio-record or video-record the informants giving their testimony. Using an audio-recorder is an efficient and accurate method to record an interview, although this needs to be done unobtrusively so as not to inhibit an informant's responses. Usually, verbatim transcripts are made from the recordings, including all words uttered as well as non-verbal utterances such as sighs or other non-verbal noises that may indicate resignation, disgust, surprise, or anger. The transcribed recordings allow the researcher to read and listen to the interview multiple times. It also allows for other researchers to engage directly with the interview material. This process will be amplified in the section below on data analysis.

There may be a very few instances where audio-recording is not suitable. Using an audio-recorder in public may invade the privacy of the participant by drawing attention to the informant. Circumstances may mitigate against adequate sound recording, particularly in open and crowded public places such as a coffee shop. Audio-recording may be inappropriate when the aim is to keep interviews as informal as possible.

Experience suggests that informants frequently share valuable information just after the recording process is turned off. No matter how relaxed informants become with an audio-recorder, there are still occasions when information is withheld for privacy reasons or because of personal embarrassment. It is, therefore, important for the researcher to document extensively in field notes (see section 9.7 below).

9.5.5 Group Interviewing

Interviewing people in groups has gained popularity in allied health research. Group interviews are commonly called focus groups. Focus groups may be structured, semi-structured, or unstructured. Group interviews are a cost-effective and efficient way to gather data. Interviewers need to be experienced in managing group processes, however. For example, aspects of group interaction, such as the tendency of one or more members to dominate the group or of the group members to slide into "group think," may impede the process of gathering comprehensive information from the informants (Frey & Fontana, 1991).

9.5.6 Attentive Listening

Interviewing requires a commitment to, and practice in, eliciting and understanding another's point of view. Developing skills as an attentive listener is as important as becoming a skilled questioner. To avoid hearing informant testimony in predetermined categories requires careful practice of listening and posing non-leading and non-judgmental questions. A novice qualitative interviewer must practice unstructured or semi-structured interviewing under the supervision of an experienced qualitative researcher. Ideally such training interviews would be conducted with a person simulating the informant who has some experience with what led to the inclusion of the informant. Then the experienced researcher can look on, interject feedback as indicated, and summarize the novice's strengths and weaknesses after the practice has concluded.

9.6 QUALITATIVE DATA COLLECTION—FIELD OBSERVATION

Observation is essential for understanding human occupation. As Adler and Adler (1994) noted, "as long as people have been interested in studying the social and natural world around them, observation has served as the bedrock source of human knowledge" (p. 377). The main purpose of field observation in an ethnography is to describe accurately the social structure, social processes, and behaviors engaged in by a group of people; the meanings these experiences hold for the informants; and the settings and spaces in which these processes take place. The investigator observes the interactions among members of a group and records their responses to various situations. The researcher seeks to understand their formal codes for communications and the unwritten rules that guide their behaviors (Mead, 1928; Thrasher, 2013). In a field study, the investigator may become a participant observer, that is, to the extent possible performing the occupational roles and enacting the forms of activities of the people studied, in order to gain deeper insight into their meanings. Hence the requirement in many anthropological studies for the researcher to spend at least a year with people in the target culture, so as to experience one entire cycle of life through the seasons.

One major advantage of field observation is that data obtained from this technique are collected in authentic, community settings, not under artificial laboratory or clinical conditions. Another advantage is that the investigator observes and performs behavior directly rather than by eliciting verbal responses alone, such as through surveys. A third advantage is that the observer, who is not an indigenous member of the culture, will interpret patterns and behaviors differently from the way that these are acknowledged by those within the culture. Indeed, the "outsider" assists in bringing to the forefront patterns that, being embedded in "insider" behavior, are sometimes not readily described or consciously recognized by members of the group.

The duration and scope of observation, just as with interviewing, needs to be carefully considered and designed. It may better suit addressing the research topic by planning an in-depth observation of a few occasions. For another research question it may be warranted to spend time observing a greater number of situations for a shorter period of time.

9.7 FIELD NOTES—BEFORE, DURING, AND AFTER INFORMANT ENCOUNTERS

Field notes are a basic tool for the qualitative researcher. As Patton noted, "There are many options in the mechanics of taking field notes... *What is not optional is the taking of field notes*" (Patton, 1990, p. 239, italics in original). Note taking can also be used to expand the recorded account, for example, with enriching descriptions of visual "pictures" of participants' facial expressions, gestures, and other non-verbal behaviors. Taking notes also expands the opportunities to collect data. For example, taking notes can provide a documented account of participants' reactions and interactions.

The first step in planning field notes is to decide on a format. Field notes can be composed in a notebook or entered into a laptop computer, tablet, or smart phone. The second step is to organize the different types of field notes according to their purpose. The purposes of field notes include maintaining a transcript file, a personal log, and an analytical log (Minichiello et al., 2008).

The transcript file contains descriptive data about the observation or interview setting. This includes where the observation took place, who was present, and what social interactions and activities took place. This file may also contain a diagram of the setting. The transcript file may contain pointers to direct informant quotations that seem important.

The personal log is the repository for the researcher's thoughts on the field research. This log includes personal impressions, reactions to the study experience, and personal reflections during the study. Writing this log needs to be done during, or as soon as possible after each encounter in the field (observation or interview). It is not possible at the end of a study to go back and capture the feelings, reactions, and reflections that occurred during informant encounters. Keeping the personal log in the form of a journal may be helpful. Using headings and subheadings will help to organize the material and make it easier to review the contents and connect ideas to the primary source material (field observations and interview transcripts) in the analysis stage. The headings will vary according to research focus.

The analytical log contains the researcher's insights and reflections on data collection and analysis in the context of the theoretical framework of the study. Minichiello et al. (2008) suggested that this is where the researcher asks and answers questions such as: What is it that I know so far? What do I not know? What do I need to know? How do I collect this information? This log also provides a record or audit trail of the analysis and theoretical propositions as these develop throughout the study.

A rigorous qualitative researcher expends effort during a study in documenting their "intersubjective reflexivity." That is, the researcher recognizes their own values, biases, and filters toward reality. There is no claim that the researcher is objective toward informants. Instead, the researcher documents through field notes what is anticipated before informants are met for interviews. What expectations or anxieties does the researcher have?

During interviews, the researcher takes notes to amplify what will become the verbatim transcript of the process. In addition to writing cues for questions to return to, or new topics to open a discussion around, the researcher records any impression during the interview that may be of later help in interpreting what the informant meant. The researcher should document the evolving relationship with the informant(s).

Immediately after interviews the researcher is advised to record their impressions of the informant, the physical context, the informant's testimony, and the researcher's own reactions to what was said during the interview. Comments on the "intersubjective reflexivity" as an ongoing theme are appropriate. The researcher may find value in sketching the physical setting where the interviews or observations took place. It is also important at this point for the researcher to document future questions for the informant that arose from the just-completed interaction.

9.8 Other Data Sources— Personal Journals, News Sources, Archives

In order to comprehensively collect data about the culture under study, the researcher may seek out other documentary source material. This material may have been created by the informant (diary or journal) or by other participants in or observers of the culture (news articles, medical or legal records, online or paper archives). These materials may either confirm what has been observed or recorded during interviews, or may serve to enrich the portrayal of the experience or the culture, or may even reveal seeming contradictions. All such outcomes may assist the researcher in being more thorough when it comes time for analysis.

The cumulative total of data gathered from different sources allows the researcher to perform triangulation. Findings verified by two or more sources of data are said to be triangulated. Such findings should carry more weight in the final outcome of the study.

9.9 Qualitative Data Analysis

There is a diverse variety of methods for analyzing qualitative data (for example, see Flick, 2013; Miles et al., 2014; Stevens, 2022). Stevens (2022) contains chapters on grounded theory, narrative analysis, and thematic analysis, among others. At the start of the data analysis in a qualitative study, researchers sometimes spend time going through the documented information over and over. This technique is to build familiarity with the data as a whole and in particulars. Often direct quotations will later be drawn from the informant's words to illustrate certain findings of the study. The final outcome for the analysis, in both content and format, is open. The researcher aims to end with a thick, authentic description, interpretation, and portrayal of the experience, life, or culture, drawn directly from all data sources.

Qualitative data analysis methods are based on the following general principles.

9.9.1 Iterative Data Analysis

A distinctive feature of qualitative research is that the data analysis process is iterative. That is, rather than having planned in advance to run a certain set of statistical tests on the complete data set, as in quantitative research, the qualitative researcher expects the data analysis process to evolve as it is being undertaken. First, analysis is conducted concurrently with data collection. As analysis occurs, the researcher develops further questions that guide ongoing data collection. The researcher may formulate propositions that are checked in reference to the existing data. This proposing and verifying illustrates the movement between inductive and deductive processes typical of qualitative analysis.

9.9.2 Open Coding

Next begins the process of identifying key ideas throughout the transcripts, field notes, and other data sources, called "coding the data," or "open coding," the latter term coined by Straus and Corbin (1998). The identifying codes or labels may take the form of "strips" (Agar, 1996), semantic networks (Good, 1993), or themes, dimensions, essences, clusters, theories, typologies, stages, or hierarchies (Hasselkus, 1993). Agar's strips consist of coded information (informant quotes, for example) that illustrate one pattern at one level of the data. Good's semantic network (1993) consists of a web of terms, with lines drawn between pairs of terms to indicate the existence and strength of relationship between the two. Themes are coding labels that have coalesced into a coherent illustrative pattern.

9.9.3 Code-Recode

Often passages of data are coded by more than one researcher, called *peer checking*. Codes at first are expansive, flexible, and may overlap. Codes may be recoded, combined, or transformed.

9.9.4 Pattern Detection

At some point in the analysis a firm set of codes coalesces out of the fluidity. Comparison is the main intellectual tool employed by the researcher in performing this step. Comparison is used to "discern conceptual similarities, to refine the discriminative power of categories, and to discover patterns" (Tesch, 1990, p. 96). Glaser and Strauss (1967) developed the term *constant comparative analysis* to describe the process whereby the researcher compares and contrasts elements of data in a search for recurring regularities. These regularities are further compared and contrasted to develop concepts. These concepts are then compared and contrasted to form internally consistent and mutually exclusive categories.

Frequently in studies published in the occupational therapy literature this is the point of establishing themes and sub-themes. For a single published study of article length, typically 3–6 themes are used. One or more of them might have sub-themes associated, to further elaborate the hierarchy of ideas about the informant experience. In some studies, the researcher infers and formulates one or two over-arching themes.

9.9.5 Data Analysis Software Applications

Qualitative data are, most frequently, text derived from interview transcripts, questionnaire responses, field notes, and documents such as case records. The researcher may also use photographs and video (Harper, 1988). The volume of text data gathered can create a data management challenge. Miles and Huberman (2014) provided a useful summary of storage and retrieval requirements (Table 9–2).

TABLE 9–2
WHAT TO STORE, RETRIEVE FROM, AND RETAIN
• Raw material: field notes, tapes, site documents
• Partially processed data: write-ups, transcriptions. Initial version and subsequent corrected, "cleaned," "commented-on" versions
• Coded data: write-ups with specific codes attached
• The coding scheme or thesaurus, in its successive iterations
• Memos or other analytic material: the researcher's reflections on the conceptual meaning of the data
• Search and retrieval records: information showing which coded chunks or data segments the researcher looked for during analysis, and the retrieved material; records of links made among segments
• Data displays: matrices or networks used to display retrieved information, along with the associated analytic text; revised versions of these
• Analysis episodes: documenting of what was done, step by step, to assemble the displays and write the analytic text
• Report text: successive drafts of what is written on the design, methods, and findings of the study
• General chronological log or documentation of data collection and analytic work
• Index of all the above material
Source: Adapted from Miles and Huberman (1994, p. 48). © 1994 Sage.

Qualitative researchers need to develop a data management system that suits their own style or that of the research team and the purpose of the research. Traditional methods for organizing data include using notebooks, file folders, card systems, filing cabinets, and the like. Newer methods include word-processing programs, databases, spreadsheets, and other computer-based programs. Storage and retrieval of data can be done quickly and efficiently by computer. Recent developments in computer software mean that researchers can also get help with data analysis. Several computer-based text analysis programs, known ti http://atlasti.com/). Reviews of available programs, their functions, advantages, and shortcomings are available at the CAQDAS Networking Project (http://caqdas.soc.surrey.ac.uk/) and Qual Page www.qualitativeresearch. uga.edu/QualPage/). For many studies they may not be necessary. Thinking long and hard on the part of the researcher, though, is not optional:

> You can color code or cut up transcripts, transfer things onto three by five cards, whatever. You mainly need to spend enough time with the data that you detect patterns and themes emerge. You can tag and sort using any devices you wish or no devices but pens and scissors. You can roll in the data like a canine. There is nothing magic about software programs that manage data. They don't do the analysis. You do. Software can count frequencies of certain word strings or find all instances in which a word is used. But the analysis happens in the researcher's cerebral hemispheres.
>
> (McGruder, 1999)

9.9.6 Member Checking—Getting Feedback from Informants about the Findings

Researchers who bring tentative findings back to their informants for their feedback are performing *member checking*. Usually, it is performed during the last or next to last interview with an informant. It may be one of the strongest techniques for accurately solidifying the findings in a qualitative study. When there are time constraints, however, it is unfortunately often omitted by qualitative researchers.

9.9.7 A Posteriori and A Priori Analysis

With or without member checking, the researcher settles upon a set of themes, a semantic network, or some means of concisely conveying the findings made about the experiences, life, or culture studied. Developing these themes from scratch would be called performing an *a posteriori*

analysis. That is, the analytic structure is built up from nothing during the course of the study. Themes are illustrated by direct quotations from the informants in the study, and preferably are confirmed by the informants themselves (member checking).

An alternative is when a researcher collects data in order to test the thematic structure developed in an earlier study. In this case the researcher "tests" the data to determine how well they fit with the earlier structure. This analytic approach may be used with or without member checking. This comparative, testing approach is called *a priori* analysis. The conclusion may be that there was a good fit, a partial fit, or very little fit with the interpretive structure of the earlier study or studies.

9.9.8 Grounded Theory as an Approach to Data Analysis

Glaser and Strauss (1967) and Strauss and Corbin (1998) articulated a technique for building up concepts from the data, by constantly comparing new data with prior patterns uncovered, until the researcher reaches a theory. By using their *constant comparative* method, one arrives at a *grounded theory*. Their approach may be used in many types of qualitative studies, and therefore has not been given its own category as a type of qualitative research in this textbook.

9.9.9 Ultimate Aim of Data Analysis and Synthesis

The ultimate goal of the analysis and synthesis of data in an ethnography, a phenomenological study, or a life narrative is to portray the complexity of life with accuracy, coherence, and consistency. This "thick description" (Geertz, 1973) has the ring of authenticity. There can be contradictions. They are an inevitable result of human subjectivity and the existence of multiple representations of reality. There should be variability in the data and in the findings, but both variability and contradictions should make sense within the patterns that were uncovered in the wider context of the informant world.

9.10 EXAMPLES OF THE APPLICATION OF ETHNOGRAPHY TO OCCUPATIONAL THERAPY

Health care related qualitative research studies using an ethnographic approach include:

- Daily occupations of Orthodox Jewish couples (Frank et al., 1997).

- Ethno-geriatric studies of African-American and Asian-American elders (McBride & Lewis, 2004).
- Cultural competency of health care professionals (Noble et al., 2009).
- Community-based therapy for individuals with traumatic brain injury, their caregivers, and their therapists (Doig et al., 2009).
- Women leaving violent relationships in Sierra Leone (Njelesani et al., 2021).
- Autistic adults and their caregiver families (Bagatell et al., 2023).
- Everyday occupations among Rohingya refugees in a camp (Alve et al., 2023).

Note that none of these studies attempted to portray an entire culture, but rather, the collective experiences of a group of people who faced similar occupational/health challenges.

9.11 Examples of the Application of Phenomenology to Occupational Therapy

- Financial management dependence post brain injury: Survivor experiences (Koller et al., 2016).
- Liminal space in psychosis: Effect on social participation (Fox & Bailliard, 2021).
- Volunteering as occupation in recovery from mental illness (Pérez-Corrales et al., 2022).
- Caregiver perceptions of weight management programs for individuals with spinal cord injury (Pedersen et al., 2023).
- Roles of caregivers of autistic adults (Bagatell et al., 2023).

The insights generated by the above studies can not only increase empathy in therapists, but also bring about an increased understanding of these life challenges, giving therapists greater scope of view and expertise for collaborating effectively for improved interventions and outcomes. In this way, qualitative studies also contribute to evidence-based practice: the improvement of practice decisions on the basis of carefully analyzed empirical data.

9.12 Rigor in Qualitative Research

In qualitative research designs, the aim is to make sense of the meanings that people apply to phenomena in personal and social worlds. Traditionally, the rigor of experimental designs and other quantitative methods for collecting and analyzing data are judged by means of the constructs of objectivity, reliability, and validity (internal and external). Decades ago, however, investigators began to question the appropriateness of using the traditional meanings of objectivity, reliability, and validity as ways to address rigor and trustworthiness in qualitative research (Kielhofner, 1982). An early comprehensive formulation of an alternative approach to judging the rigor of a qualitative study was Guba (1981). Guba's "model of trustworthiness" was introduced into the occupational therapy literature by Krefting (1991).

Guba described four elements of rigor for qualitative studies that were meant to supplant the classical notions of objectivity, reliability, and internal and external validity. These elements are confirmability, dependability, credibility, and transferability.

9.12.1 Confirmability

Rather than seeking to be objective toward the participants and the outcome of a study, in Guba's model the desirable alternative is confirmability (Krefting, 1991). In order to establish the rapport necessary between researcher and informant for the latter to be comfortable revealing deeper experiences and meanings, objectivity in the researcher would be undesirable. The researcher in a qualitative study is unavoidably enmeshed with informants. Nonetheless, neutrality toward data recording, analysis, and synthesis is desirable. Objectivity is thus replaced in Guba's model with confirmability. Is the data collection design and implementation auditable in a step-by-step manner? Would another researcher, given the audit, reach the same conclusions? If so, then the original researcher demonstrated neutrality and not bias toward the data processing in the study.

9.12.2 Dependability

Dependability corresponds to the notion of quantitative reliability. Instead of a quantitative consistency in the numerical data, though, dependability in qualitative research means establishing trackable variability. The term "trackable" means that methods and interim decisions are thickly described, so that in theory a complete audit of the process could be done. In dependable qualitative research, such an audit would show that the data collection, analysis, and synthesis are thoroughly documented, are seen to be fair, and are, in principle, replicable in a future study. Techniques for achieving dependability also include peer checking and code-recode (mentioned above) and triangulation (elaborated upon below).

9.12.3 Credibility

Because qualitative studies are not expected to employ (and usually cannot use) methods of randomization and control, the traditional notion of internal validity should not apply. Guba's model replaces this notion with credibility. Since the ultimate goal of most qualitative research is the portrayal of human experience, one of the main criteria for credibility is the extent to which the findings of a study are recognizable by people (other than the informants) who themselves live in the situation portrayed. Findings should be sufficiently sophisticated so as to have captured the multiple realities of the informants. Another marker of credibility is prolonged engagement of the researcher with the informants. Kielhofner (1982) noted the value of intense participation, as it increased "intimate familiarity and discovery of hidden fact" (Krefting, 1991, p. 217). Immersion in the experience and in the data enables the researcher to more readily discover patterns, themes, and values, as experienced by the informants (Krefting, 1991).

Credibility can be undermined if informants alter their testimony so as to say what they think the researcher wants to hear. Besides developing a closer relationship of trust with the informant, the researcher can use interview techniques to lessen the "social desirability" contaminant. Probes and contrasts (Spradley, 1979), mentioned above, can serve this purpose. Testing alternative explanations of a phenomenon with informants can increase the credibility of a study. So can "non-cases," such as, in the prior example of a study of unhoused individuals, "Tell me about having a day that is not good" (if the informant has just described a "good day"), or "What's an example of when you are not frustrated" (when the informant has just described circumstances of becoming frustrated). Pursuing outlier cases with the informant can also deepen understanding of the experience under study ("Do you know someone who does not feel that way about the police?").

Qualitative researchers who are able to spend an extended time with informants are more likely to observe less frequent situations, or those that arise only seasonally. Researchers seeking data from the informant in different settings or times of the day also strengthens credibility (Krefting, 1991). Qualitative researchers, on the other hand, will also be wary of becoming over-involved. The technique used to monitor the level of involvement is reflexive analysis or reflexivity (Krefting, 1991). Keeping a field journal helps researchers track their own reactions, insights, and wishes, and make adjustments to their approach if an over-involvement is detected (Krefting, 1991). As noted below, triangulation is another powerful technique for avoiding mis-portrayal of informant experiences and their meanings.

Member checking, that is, having informants provide feedback on the interim and final findings, is another way to strengthen the credibility of a study. Krefting (1991) wisely cautions the researcher to first consider the possible effect on the informants to be shown the tentative research findings. Depending on the focus of the research, seeing the findings could be upsetting to the informants.

Triangulation has come to mean the use of multiple methods, sources, analysts, or theoretical perspectives to verify the information gained in different arenas (Triangulation, 2014). The aim of triangulation is "to guard against the accusation that a study's findings are simply an artifact of a single method, a single source, or a single investigator's bias" (Patton, 1990, p. 470).

Triangulation of sources involves comparing the consistency of information derived from varying sources, for example, comparing the data gathered from interviews and observations, from public and private documents, or from different informants making the same claim independently. Triangulation across data analysts is becoming more common. This triangulation could take the form of the extent of agreement between the field notes of one observer and the observations made by another, for example. Last, some investigators have suggested triangulation of theoretical perspectives. This means applying more than one theoretical perspective to the research findings to reveal any differences and similarities (Patton, 1990).

As mentioned at the beginning of this chapter, the researcher is an integral part of the qualitative research process. Concern for the credibility of the researcher is therefore an integral part of the verification process. Researcher credibility is dependent on training, experience, and acknowledgment of the researcher role in the research process. Researcher credibility requires a clear and concise explanation of the researcher role and contribution to the study findings. It is the researcher's responsibility to explain the extent of possible researcher effect on the study and whether changes in perceptions or responses occurred during the study or to what extent predispositions, background experiences of the researcher, or biases influenced the study findings. A description of the researcher's interpretive framework allows the reader to understand with which paradigm the researcher framed the research question and collected and analyzed the data. Frank and open explanation in reporting research enhances credibility (Linkov et al., 2009).

9.12.4 Transferability

External validity in quantitative studies is understood as the extent to which the findings from the selected sample of participants can be generalized to the population from which the sample was chosen. Rarely in qualitative research is there an attempt to randomly select a sample from a population, as noted above in section 9.4, in order to generalize back to that population in some quantitative way (e.g., with confidence intervals). Instead, Guba's model explores applicability through transferability, which, Guba claims, is the responsibility of the reader of the study, not the researcher (Krefting, 1991). The author of the study is responsible for providing enough background information about the informants, the researcher, and the contexts of their interactions so that readers can make up their own minds about the transferability of the findings to some other group of people. In some qualitative studies, such as in a narrative analysis or a phenomenology of a single individual, there is no intention of transferring the results to someone else. Rather, the transferability comes into play on a different level. First, the data analysis itself represents a transfer "from an instantiation to an interpretation" (source of quote unknown; see Christensen, 2008, p. 113, where the phrase "instantiation to interpretation, or the intentional explanation" is used in discussing phenomenology). That is, from the singular particulars of the informants, patterns are detected, meanings are documented, and unifying themes of experience are determined through interpretation. To the extent that this process provides valuable insight to readers, then it is said to have transferability. Second, the findings of the study may result in the articulation of a theory. To the extent that this theory has applicability to other people, places, and times, then the study of its origin is deemed to have transferability.

Each of these four elements of rigor in qualitative studies can be strengthened by one or more of the techniques mentioned above. They are summarized in Table 9–3.

While a study may not use all of these techniques, it is usually the case that the more that are used, the better the rigor of the study. In acknowledgement of these

TABLE 9–3

TECHNIQUES FOR QUALITATIVE RIGOR

Nominated sample
Prolonged engagement
Sampling to data saturation
Reflexive analysis
Triangulation of data, analysts, theoretical perspectives
Peer checking
Code-recode
Audit trackability
Member checking

techniques, the classification of a qualitative research study in the Research Pyramid system is Q4 for a study of one individual (addressing transferability unknowns), Q3 for a study of more than one informant and a few of the techniques for increasing rigor, and Q2 for a study employing many or most of these rigor-enhancing techniques. Then level Q1, similar to a meta-analysis in levels E1, O1, and D1, is assigned to studies that perform a systematic synthesis of qualitative studies, called a meta-synthesis. Both meta-analysis and meta-synthesis are covered in Chapter 10.

Before leaving this chapter, we will explore the combination of quantitative and qualitative approaches to a study, called mixed methods.

9.13 MIXED METHODS RESEARCH

Triangulation of methods may involve collecting both quantitative and qualitative data for comparison and potential reconciliation. This helps to expand and elaborate the quality of information gained by one method alone. Despite contrasting paradigms of research, quantitative and qualitative approaches have been increasingly used together in studies.

Until about 2000, the positivist experimental tradition of quantitative research was predominant in medicine, rehabilitation, and related health professions. As this textbook makes clear, both quantitative and qualitative approaches contribute to scientific inquiry in occupational therapy. Perhaps it is the fact that therapists are equally concerned with both the physical world of the client (including their body's biological system) and the subjective world of agency in the client (where occupational meaning is derived). It is a challenge for researchers in occupational therapy to incorporate qualitative and quantitative approaches into their studies. An example of integrating both qualitative and quantitative research was carried out by Uhlig et al. (2010), exploring the effectiveness of Tai Chi with patients diagnosed with rheumatoid arthritis. Quantitative analysis was used to measure muscle function in the lower extremities and qualitative measures were applied in discovering subjective lived experiences in the study. Uhlig et al. concluded that "the combination of qualitative and quantitative research methods shows that Tai Chi has beneficial effects on health not related to disease activity and standardised health status assessment, and may contribute to an understanding of how Tai Chi exerts its effects" (2010, p. 43). More recently, Chilton et al. (2022) applied both qualitative and quantitative methods in a study of the knowledge and attitudes of occupational therapy practitioners about the sexual health of older adults.

9.13.1 Historical Research

Definition

Historical research is a systematic method for reconstructing events that happened in the past to describe and understand them. As applied to occupational therapy, historical research pertains to (a) the chronology of events in occupational therapy, (b) the interrelationship between these events, and (c) the critical factors influencing them. For example, one might want to describe the events and identify the individuals that led to the formation of the discipline of occupational therapy in 1917. In studying historical data in occupational therapy, the investigator examines the individuals who were significant in shaping events and creating change, and the institutions or organizations that were part of the historical process. The scientific approach to collecting historical data is similar to all methods of research in that the investigator proposes a research problem, states guiding questions, collects data, interprets the results, and arrives at conclusions and implications. The main differences between historical research and other types of research models are in the format of guiding questions and in the use of related literature. In historical research the guiding questions serve as the rationale for collecting data and the literature review and examination of artifacts provide the data, while the literature review generates guiding questions in other qualitative methods.

Purposes

Fraenkel and Wallen (2012) suggested five purposes for historical research:

1. "To make people aware of what has happened in the past so they may learn from past failures and successes" (p. 411): For example, cone stacking has been used rather than craft activities to increase fine motor coordination. The craft activity is client centered and increases motivation, whereas the cone stacking is a non-meaningful repetitive activity.

2. "To learn how things were done in the past to see if they might be applicable to the present day problems and concerns" (p. 411): The model used in adult day centers from the 1950s and 1960s was successful in treating individuals with psychosocial illnesses. Adult day care centers now use this model in caring for individuals with Alzheimer's disease.

3. "To assist in prediction" (p. 412): Special education has alternated between placing students with special needs into self-contained classrooms and into the general education program. Examination of mainstreaming in the 1980s demonstrated that these students would not succeed in the general education program without support from special educators, occupational therapists, and other allied health personnel.

4. "To test hypotheses concerning relationships or trends" (p. 412): Over the last 80 years, an examination of trends of employment settings has shown a change for occupational therapists from hospital-based settings to schools, home health care, and other community-based settings.

5. "To understand present educational practices and policies more fully" (p. 412): To understand Medicare reimbursement, occupational therapists study previous legislation and litigation leading to the present policies.

Historical Research Related to Occupational Therapy

- Bockoven, J. S. (1971). Occupational therapy—A historical perspective. Legacy of moral treatment–1800s to 1910. *American Journal of Occupational Therapy, 25*, 223–225.

- Cockburn, L. (2005). Canadian occupational therapists' contributions to prisoners of war in World War II. *Canadian Journal of Occupational Therapy, 72*, 183–188.

- Frank, G. (1992). Opening feminist histories of occupational therapy. *American Journal of Occupational Therapy, 46*, 989–999.

- Friedland, J., & Silva, J. (2008). Evolving identities: Thomas Bessell Kidner and occupational therapy in the United States. *American Journal of Occupational Therapy, 62*, 349–360.

- Gutman, S. A. (1995). Influence of the US military and occupational therapy reconstruction aides in World War I on the development of occupational therapy. *American Journal of Occupational Therapy, 49*, 256–262.

- Hamlin, R. B. (1992). Embracing our past, informing our future: A feminist revision of health care. *American Journal of Occupational Therapy, 46*, 1028–1035.

- Horghagen, S., Josephsson, S., & Alsaker, S. (2007). The use of craft activities as an occupational therapy treatment modality in Norway during 1952–1960. *Occupational Therapy International, 14*, 42–56.

- Newton, S. (2007). The growth of the profession of occupational therapy. *US Army Medical Department Journal*, 51–58.

- Peloquin, S. M. (1991). Occupational therapy service: Individual and collective understandings of the founders, Part 2. *American Journal of Occupational Therapy, 45*, 733–744.

- Reitz, S. M. (1992). A historical review of occupational therapy's role in preventive health and wellness. *American Journal of Occupational Therapy, 46*, 50–55.

- Stecco, C., & Aldegheri, R. (2008). Historical review of carpal tunnel syndrome. *La Chirurgia degli Organi di Movimento. 92*, 7–10.

- Woodside, H. H. (1971). Occupational therapy – A historical perspective. The development of occupational therapy 1910–1929. *American Journal of Occupational Therapy, 25*, 226–230.

Hypothetical Historical Questions to Explore in Occupational Therapy

- How did occupational therapists treat individuals with polio during the 1950s?
- What treatment techniques were used by occupational therapists in large mental hospitals during the 1930s?
- What were some of the experiences and education of noted individuals in occupational therapy?
- How is occupational therapy treated in the literature by individuals who write about their disability experiences?
- How have different philosophical viewpoints in occupational therapy influenced intervention in the schools?
- What is the history of the use of arts and crafts in occupational therapy?
- What are the major theories that have influenced clinical treatment trends through time?

Format of Historical Research

The outline of historical research is as follows:

Part I: The statement of problem and significance of the study (e.g., how the study impacts on occupational therapy)

Part II: Guiding questions and methods for collecting data

Part III: The results, including the collection of data from primary and secondary sources

Part IV: A discussion of the results based on previous data from other studies

Part V: Conclusions, implications of results, and recommendations for further study

Part I: The Statement of Problem and Significance of the Study. What are potential areas for historical research in occupational therapy? How does one determine its significance? These are issues of concern for the historical researcher or historiographer planning a study. Jacques Barzun (1974), in a discussion of psychohistory, stated that the primary purpose of the new history is explanation, and the ulterior motive is action. He wrote, "The type of explanation sought is the scientific; that is, showing a connection ("durable link") between the facts and a definable cause. Classification, then analysis, then prediction is the sequence that leads naturally to action" (p. 60). Barzun suggested that the historiographer's main motive is to obtain evidence in support of a cause. In effect, the historical researcher is a tool for change. This approach to medicine and health care can lead to research supporting causes that advocate change in the delivery of health care, public health education, and the training and preparation of health professionals. The vulnerability of this approach is that the researcher could subjectively determine what evidence to cite. The historiographer should start with a relevant problem and objectively collect data. Table 9–4 outlines the relationship between the researcher's motive and the problem being investigated using the historical research model.

Part II: Guiding Questions and Methods for Collecting Data. After narrowing the area of investigation to a researchable question, the researcher states any assumptions underlying the study. These assumptions are the researcher's preliminary opinions, attitudes, and knowledge in the area. For example, if a researcher is interested in what factors led to the development of the rehabilitation movement in the 20th century, tentative assumptions could be proposed. These are:

- The rehabilitation movement developed in response to the health needs of the individual who is chronically disabled.
- The rehabilitation movement was facilitated by governmental legislation related to social security.

TABLE 9–4	
RELATIONSHIPS BETWEEN RESEARCHER'S MOTIVE AND INVESTIGATED PROBLEM	
MOTIVE OF RESEARCHER	**STATEMENT OF PROBLEM**
Establishing the occupational therapist as an independent practitioner	How did the independent health practitioner evolve historically?
Integrating the individual with cognitive disabilities into the community	What factors led to the institutionalization of individuals with intellectual disability from 1900 to 1950?
Incorporating wellness in health education of public schools	What is the history of health education in public schools?
Assuring the right of access to primary health for every individual	Historically what are the determining factors regarding access to health care?
Gaining parity in health insurance coverage for psychosocial disabilities	Why have insurance companies typically restricted reimbursement for psychosocial disabilities?

- The industrialized countries were first to educate specialized rehabilitation workers.
- World War I and World War II generated the need for developing a technology for restoring function in soldiers who were severely wounded.
- The first leaders in the rehabilitation movement were social reformers.

Continuing with the above examples, the researcher generates the following questions:

- What was the historical chronology of the rehabilitation movement?
- How did social welfare programs influence rehabilitation legislation?
- How did advances in medical treatment influence rehabilitation of individuals with chronic disabilities?
- When did the allied health professions emerge and affect the rehabilitation movement?
- What scientific technology facilitated advances in rehabilitation medicine?
- Who were the leaders and supporters of the rehabilitation movement?

These guiding questions provide the content areas for the literature search and collection of data. The plan for collecting the data should be carefully formulated. The research plan is the outline of primary and secondary sources to be used in the data collection procedure. These sources include the following:

- Published books, periodicals, newspapers, and pamphlets
- Unpublished conference proceedings and minutes of meetings
- Official records and vital statistics
- Governmental documents, archives, and publications
- Personal letters, diaries, and memoirs
- Collateral interviews of eyewitnesses
- Audio recordings and films

Part III: Data Collection. The essential task of the historical researcher is to collect data and evaluate it for reliability and validity. By obtaining various sources of information, the researcher can crosscheck the data, thereby substantiating conclusions. This procedure is called *triangulation*. Primary sources that represent "first hand" data, such as eyewitnesses and contemporary documents, are the best evidence for the historical researcher. In comparison, secondary sources are the interpretations and critiques of historical evidence based on primary data. Primary sources are the raw data for historical research, while secondary sources serve as supportive evidence. In researching a problem the investigator should seek evidence that is direct, objective, and verifiable. It should be clear that one unit of datum is not conclusive. The "personal equation," which is the observer's effect on what is being observed and measured, must be controlled by the investigator's substantiating evidence from more than one primary source in eyewitness accounts.

Secondary sources such as encyclopedias, textbooks, and critical essays are useful in initially obtaining an overview of a historical problem. These sources represent the generally accepted versions of historical events that have been "retold" in a reductive manner. The critical historiographer need not accept any evidence until primary data can substantiate the facts.

Part IV: Discussion of Results, and Part V: Conclusions and Recommendations. The raw data of a historical study must be critically analyzed by the investigator for its validity before any conclusions or generalizations can be made. The historical researcher must examine every document and piece of evidence with a skeptical eye, seeking substantiating proof for the authorship and the accuracy of its contents. *External criticism* of a document is a testimony of its authenticity. The Hippocratic writings are an example of unknown authorship and unknown copyright date. It is important for the historical researcher to substantiate the author of every document, the date it was written, and the place of origination or presentation, as evidence for external validity. Indirect means for collecting evidence are frequently used by historians. These methods include archeology and paleography (e.g., study of ancient manuscripts and examination of art objects). Ancient medical instruments used in surgery were discovered through archeological evidence. Questions that might be asked when examining external validity are (Fraenkel et al., 2012):

- Did the purported author actually write the document or report the event?
- Do we know the exact date that the document was written?
- Do we know where the document was written or where the observation took place?
- Are we sure that the writing of the document and the observation were not influenced by external events or individuals?
- Are we sure the document is genuine?

The next step of the historical researcher is to establish the validity or truth contained in a document. This process is called *internal criticism*. The purpose of this process is to establish as near as possible the actuality of an event. Fraenkel and Wallen (2012) suggested the following types of questions:

- Was the author an eyewitness to the event?
- Did the author participate in the event?
- What expertise did the author have to discuss or report the event?
- Was the author biased or subjective in the observation, or did the author have a vested interest in the event's interpretation?

Historical surveys of medical progress are frequently filled with interpretative statements that go beyond the evidence and selective omissions that fail to give a true perspective of events or individuals who had an impact on treatment. It is left to the historical researcher in occupational therapy to carefully evaluate the biases of the authors when interpreting evidence. Generalizations and synthesizing statements should be carefully documented. In examining the causes of events, the historiographer takes a multidimensional point of view when examining the influences of contemporary practices of treatment, discoveries, patterns of dysfunction, governmental and community intervention, war, and natural disasters. One variable rarely changes the course of history.

A good example of historical research is a scholarly manuscript by Saul Benison (1972), "The History of Polio Research in the United States: Appraisal and Lessons." In this article, Benison documented the chronological events that led to a safe and effective vaccine for preventing polio. He analyzed the problem from three perspectives: (a) time of events, (b) settings where research took place, and (c) individuals and scientists who had an impact on the problem and facilitated progress in the development of a vaccine. These three factors are detailed in Table 9–5.

In documenting the chronology of events and the individuals who made important contributions to the development of a successful polio vaccine, Benison used the following primary sources:

- Contemporary accounts of the early polio epidemics from 1894 to 1910
- Autobiographical notes
- History of the Rockefeller Institute
- Foreign journals
- Scholarly articles by Flexner (2002) and associates

- Conference proceedings
- Research articles
- *Bulletin of the History of Medicine*
- National Foundation Archives
- History of Warm Springs
- Private communication
- Minutes of committees
- Files from the National Foundation
- Biographical essays
- Final reports of research grants
- Congressional hearings

In total, Benison used 117 citations to document his article. He concluded that the development of a successful polio vaccine was a cooperative effort by researchers in major universities funded by two private organizations—The Rockefeller Foundation and the National Foundation—with external support from the United States Public Health Service. Benison's lesson in the article was that modern medical progress is a cooperative effort where researchers from diverse settings are supported by the federal government, private foundations, and voluntary health agencies.

The historical research article by Benison is an example of rigorous documentation providing strong external validity. Benison's article should serve as a model for research in occupational therapy. (See Box 9–1 for another example of historical research.)

TABLE 9–5

HISTORY OF POLIO RESEARCH IN THE UNITED STATES

TIME	EVENT	SETTING	CONTRIBUTORS
1884	Polio epidemics identified in the US		
1907	Initial research in polio	Rockefeller Institute	Flexner
1910–1913	Poliovirus implicated	Rockefeller Institute	Flexner and associates
1920–1930	Transmission of polio	Rockefeller Institute	Olitsky et al.
1938	Warm Springs Foundation	Georgia	Roosevelt et al.
1938	Electron microscope	Germany	Borries
1946	Immunization of monkeys	Johns Hopkins	Morgan
1948–1951	Identification of poliovirus	U. California Johns Hopkins U. of Pittsburgh	Kessel Bodian Salk
1949	Cultivation of poliovirus	Harvard	Enders et al.
1952	Salk vaccine (dead intramuscular vaccine)	U. Pittsburgh	Salk
1954	Mass vaccinations	U. Michigan	Francis
1958	Sabin Vaccine (oral live vaccine)	U. Cincinnati	Sabin

Source: Adapted from Benison (1972, pp. 308–343). © 1972 W. Norton.

Box 9-1. Example of Historical Research

1. Bibliographical Notation

Sachs, D., & Sussman, N. (1995). Historical research: The first decade of occupational therapy in Israel: 1946–1956. *Occupational Therapy International, 2,* 241–256.

2. Abstract

The present study examined the first decade of the development of occupational therapy in Israel: 1946–1956. The structural-functional approach to the study of professions, which provided the theoretical framework for this study, identifies three formal organizations in the professions: the practice, the educational system, and the association. The purpose of this article was to follow the development of occupational therapy and to examine the interrelations of the profession's three formal organizations in the reviewed period. The methodology of the study was based on qualitative historical methods. Data collection included oral histories, and published and unpublished written material. Data organization and analysis were within the framework of the structural-functional approach. Data analysis indicated that "expansion" was a major theme affecting the development of occupational therapy, the reason for which lies within the historical background of the period under investigation. In addition, data indicated that the practice was the strongest and most active organization in occupational therapy and that expansion in practice was beyond the capacity of both the educational system and the professional association. The interrelations of the three formal organizations, and the rapid expansion of occupational therapy practice, had a lasting effect on the development of occupational therapy in Israel (p. 241).

3. Justification and Need for Study

Because "historical research sheds light on present behaviors and practices" (p. 242), this study was completed to "understand current theories and practices more accurately, and to plan intelligently for the future" (p. 242).

4. Literature Review

Forty-two references were cited in the study. Articles came from a wide variety of sources, including files at the Occupational Therapy School at the Hebrew University from 1947 to 1954; archives of Hadassah 1941–1949; *Israeli Journal of Occupational Therapy; Health Services in Israel: A Ten Year Survey 1948–1958;* and *Trade Unions in Israel.*

5. Research Hypothesis or Guiding Questions

The guiding questions explicitly stated were (a) "How did the practice [in occupational therapy] develop and how did it adapt itself to the growing needs of the healthcare services?" (b) "How did the educational system cope with practice needs?" and (c) "How did the association [Israeli Occupational Therapy Association] meet the needs of the profession?"

6. Methods

Interviews were held with nine female occupational therapists who had been practicing between 1946 and 1956 and who were considered prominent leaders in the development of occupational therapy in Israel. Primary documents including memoirs and archived materials were accessed by the investigators. These materials were analyzed using the structural-functional approach (Parsons, 1939). The credibility of the data was obtained by validating oral testimonies with contemporary documents.

7. Results

The historical development was organized into three periods, each covering the practice, the education system, and the professional association: (a) Preliminary Period, 1941–1945; (b) The Formative Years, 1946–1948; and (c) Expansion: 1949–1956.

(continued)

BOX 9-1. EXAMPLE OF HISTORICAL RESEARCH (CONTINUED)

8. Conclusions

"Analysis of the data indicates that the practice was the strongest and most active organization [as compared with education and professional association] in the function of occupational therapy. Expansion in the practice was beyond the capacity of the education and the association—By employing historical research methods and a conceptual framework to the study of professions, this study exposed the origin of some of the problems faced by occupational therapy in Israel" (pp. 254–255).

9. Limitations of the Study

The study only interviewed nine individuals when collecting the bulk of the data. Also, some contemporary documents were not available and presumed to have been lost due to war conditions.

10. Major References Cited in the Study

Archives of Hadassah (1941–1949). *Occupational therapy correspondence services* (RQ, 1 HMO, Box 51). Hadassah.

Files at the occupational therapy school, 1st class. (1947–1949). Hebrew University.

Files at the occupational therapy school, 2nd class. (1949–1951). Hebrew University.

Files at the occupational therapy school, 3rd class. (1952–1954). Hebrew University.

Grushka, T. (1959). *Health services in Israel: A ten year survey 1948–1958*. Ministry of Health.

Grushka, T, (1968). *Health services in Israel*. Ministry of Health.

Sussman, N. (1989). *The history of occupational therapy in Israel: The first decade—1946–1956*. Unpublished master's thesis, New York University.

Potential areas for historical research in occupational therapy include:

- Biographies of founders of the discipline of occupational therapy
- Development of innovative assistive technology
- Development of social attitudes toward psychosocial illness
- Chronological analysis of the treatment of a disability
- History of the occupational therapy discipline
- History of a hospital, health facility, organization, or institution
- History of reimbursement practices
- History of movements in occupational therapy (e.g., rehabilitation and normalization)

9.13.2 Operations Research

Ackoff and Rivett (1963) described the three essential characteristics of operations research: "(1) systems orientation, (2) the use of interdisciplinary teams, and (3) the adaptation of scientific method" (p. 10). Operations research was originally developed in Great Britain during World War II mainly for the purpose of using radar effectively to combat German air attacks (Crowther &

Whiddington, 1948). Subsequently, during the 1950s, large corporations employed operations research teams to analyze production methods as a way of increasing efficiency. Norbert Wiener's (1948) contributions in cybernetics and in the application of the feedback principle expanded systems theory so as to have biological, sociological, and psychological dimensions. For example, using the technology of cybernetics, the methodology of operations research, and systems theory, researchers have examined the processes used to implement evidence-based care in a primary care practice (Huebsch et al., 2015), physiology of respiration (Pribram, 1958), equipment design and human engineering (Shrader, 2006), the city as a system (Blumberg, 1971), physician clinical rotation (Reid et al., 1991), higher education (Cheng, 1993), family planning (Huezo, 1997), obstetric care (Sibley & Armbruster, 1997), and rehabilitation (Doarn et al., 2010). The feedback in these systems represents input, output, and the resultant changes in the total system of production from feedback deriving from the output.

The concept of operations research and systems theory have more recently also been applied to problems in health care (Dickinson et al., 2010; Jacob & Shapira, 2010; Uomoto & Williams, 2009). For example, hospital management provides an excellent ground for operations research.

For hospital administrators, the problems of expanding costs and depersonalized care for health consumers have become increasingly aggravated during recent decades. Although society seeks improved, expanded health care for larger portions of the population, hospitals have to find more efficient methods to service more clients and to provide them with sophisticated diagnostic methods for detecting and treating illnesses with the most advanced technology. Specifically, these problems include (a) architectural design, (b) medical equipment, (c) adequate hospital staffing including the availability of consultants, and traveling nurses, (d) cost sharing for expensive machinery, (e) maintaining staff morale and preventing burnout, and (f) health policy evolution and the arrival of new options of paying for care, such as managed care. Operations research as applied to the fields of allied health and rehabilitation uses observational, interview, and survey data along with systems analysis to identify critical issues and indicate problem solutions. Health care studies that may be considered operations research include the following:

- Recurrence of chronic disease among vulnerable populations (Woods et al., 1997)
- Depersonalization of clients in long-term care (Kliebsch et al., 1998)
- Inadequate funding for long-term care (Xakellis Jr et al., 1998)
- Characteristics of TBI assessed in the workplace (Bootes & Chapparo, 2002)
- Integrated care for returning veterans (Uomoto & Williams, 2009)
- Learning difficulties in children with ADHD (Bennett et al., 2009)
- Roles of non-medical health care workers (Mitchell, 2009)
- Computer-based cognitive remediation for schizophrenia (Dickinson et al., 2010)
- Lack of rehabilitation services in forensic psychiatry (Muñoz et al., 2016)

In all the foregoing problems, the underlying assumption is that a system, a unified interconnected whole, exists. The operations researcher analyzes the components of the system and their interrelationships. From the identification of these relationships and how they function in practice under the influence of input, output, and feedback, comes an understanding of the essential dynamics of that system. Box 9–2 provides an example of an operational research study.

BOX 9-2. EXAMPLE OF OPERATIONS RESEARCH

1. Bibliographical Notation

Bennett, A. E., Power, T. J., Eiraldi, R. B., Leff, S. S., & Blum, N. J. (2009). Identifying learning problems in children evaluated for ADHD: The Academic Performance Questionnaire. *Pediatrics, 124*, e633–e639. doi: 10.1542/peds.2009–0143

2. Abstract

OBJECTIVE: The objective of this study was to assess the usefulness of the Academic Performance Questionnaire (APQ) to identify low reading and math achievement in children who are being evaluated for attention-deficit/hyperactivity disorder (ADHD).

METHODS: Charts of 997 patients who were seen in a multidisciplinary ADHD evaluation program were reviewed. Pupils who were in first through sixth grade and had completed APQ and Wechsler Individual Achievement Test II (WIAT–II) Basic Reading and Numerical Operations subtests were enrolled in this study. The 271 eligible pupils were randomly assigned to a score-development group (*n* = 215) and a validation group (*n* = 56). By using data from the score-development sample, APQ questions that predicted low academic achievement were identified and the scores for these questions were entered into a logistic regression to identify the APQ questions that independently predicted low achievement.

RESULTS: Only two APQ questions, one about reading and one about math, independently predicted low achievement. By using these two questions, the area under the receiver operating characteristic curve was 0.834, and the optimal combination of sensitivity and specificity occurred when the total score for the two items was > 4. This cutoff had a sensitivity of 0.86 and a specificity of 0.63 in the score-development group and a sensitivity of 1.0 and a specificity of 0.53 in the validation sample.

CONCLUSIONS: The APQ may be a useful screening tool to identify children being evaluated for ADHD who need additional testing for learning problems. Although the predictive value of a negative screen on the APQ is good, the predictive value of a positive test is relatively low.

(continued)

Box 9-2. Example of Operations Research (continued)

Keywords: attention-deficit/hyperactivity disorder; learning disorder; screening; developmental-behavioral pediatrics; school-aged children

3. Justification and Need for Study

The authors state that learning disorders co-occur with ADHD in 20 to 30% of children and are typically identified by a psychoeducational assessment. Primary care physicians who evaluate children for ADHD often find it difficult to identify which children they should refer for additional assessment of academic skills. The purposes of this study were to (a) examine the test-retest reliability of the APQ and (b) evaluate the validity of the APQ with regard to predicting low achievement in reading and/or math.

4. Literature Review

The authors cited 17 references. The primary sources came from the journals, *Pediatrics*, *Journal of Pediatric Psychology*, *Journal of Learning Disabilities*, *School Psychology Review*, and the *Journal of Developmental Behavior Pediatrics*.

5. Research Hypothesis or Guiding Question

Is the APQ helpful in identifying those students with ADHD who will have difficulty in reading and math achievement?

6. Methods

The charts of 997 students who were seen in a multidisciplinary ADHD evaluation program were reviewed. Students who were in first through sixth grade and had completed APQ and WIAT–II Basic Reading and Numerical Operations subtests were enrolled in this study. The 271 eligible students were randomly assigned to a score-development group ($n = 215$) and a validation group ($n = 56$). By using data from the score-development sample, APQ questions that predicted low academic achievement were identified and the scores for these questions were entered into a logistic regression to identify the APQ questions that independently predicted low achievement.

7. Results

Results of this study demonstrate that using only two questions from the APQ, one about math and one about reading, as a screen produces a test with acceptable test-retest reliability and sensitivity.

8. Conclusion

The APQ may be a useful initial screening tool for assessing learning problems among children who present with symptoms of ADHD or other school problems. Before the APQ can be implemented as a primary care screening tool, additional research is needed to confirm its predictive validity in a primary care setting assessing children with a diverse range of demographic characteristics.

9. Limitations of the Study

This study was a retrospective chart analysis of children with ADHD who attended a multi-disciplinary center. The results of this study should be considered in the context of the following limitation. The children in this study did not have a full psychoeducational assessment. For clinical efficiency, only the two subtests of the WIAT–II that best correlate with overall reading and math scores were selected. A more complete academic assessment may have changed the classification of some children who scored near the cutoff. In addition, we did not assess other important skills, such as writing, spelling, and phonics. Thus, the ability of the APQ questions to detect children with low achievement in these areas could not be assessed.

(continued)

Box 9-2. Example of Operations Research (continued)

10. Major References Cited in the Study

Glascoe, F. P. (2001). Can teachers' global ratings identify children with academic problems? *Journal of Developmental and Behavioral Pediatrics, 22*, 163–168.

Gresham, F. M., & MacMillan, D. L. (1997). Teachers as "tests": Differential validity of teacher judgments in identifying students at-risk for learning difficulties. *School Psychology Review, 26*, 47–60.

Leslie, L. K., Weckerly, J., Plemmons, D., Landsverk, J., & Eastman, S. (2004). Implementing the American Academy of Pediatrics attention-deficit/hyperactivity disorder diagnostic guidelines in primary care settings. *Pediatrics, 114*, 129–140.

Polaha, J., Cooper, S., Meadows, T., & Kratochvil, C. J. (2005). The assessment of attention-deficit/hyperactivity disorder in rural primary care: The portability of the American Academy of Pediatrics guidelines to the "real world." *Pediatrics, 115*, e120–126.

9.14 Summary

In summary, qualitative research offers a diversity of methods well suited to the interests of researchers in occupational therapy. It contains many techniques that can be used by the researcher to strengthen the rigor of individual studies. The increasing popularity of qualitative methods is evident in the growing number of qualitative studies reported in the occupational therapy literature and the appearance of health journals devoted specifically to qualitative research studies.

10

Evidence Synthesis
Meta-Analysis, Meta-Synthesis, and Evidence Reviews

When a review is performed following predefined steps (i.e., systematically) and its results are quantitatively analyzed, it is called meta-analysis. Publication of meta-analyses has increased exponentially in pubmed.gov; using the key word "meta-analysis," 1,473 titles were yielded in 2007 and 176,704 on January 2020. Well-designed and reported meta-analyses provide valuable information for clinicians, researchers, and policymakers

(Hernandez et al., 2020).

OPERATIONAL LEARNING OBJECTIVES

By the end of this chapter, the learner will:

1. Understand the importance of accumulating evidence from multiple research studies
2. Appreciate the differences among a literature review, a systematic review, a scoping review, an evidence review, a meta-analysis, and a meta-synthesis
3. Describe the steps in conducting a meta-analysis
4. Describe ways to strengthen a meta-analysis
5. Describe approaches for conducting a meta-synthesis
6. Use a risk of bias table and an evidence table, and know the current criteria for judging the overall strength of evidence for a given topic
7. Understand the issues and challenges with knowledge translation

DOI: 10.4324/9781003523154-10

10.1 NEED FOR A SYNTHESIS OF STUDIES

Thus far in this textbook the methodologies and means of analysis for *individual* studies have been presented (whether descriptive, experimental, outcome, or qualitative studies). Neither scientists nor health care practitioners should place too much reliance, though, on a single study. Before making important decisions, it is better to gather findings from multiple studies, carefully critique them, and then synthesize them into a set of conclusions in a replicable and defensible way. Several ways of doing just that appear frequently in the health care literature. This chapter will cover the most common, important approaches to evidence synthesis in health care fields.

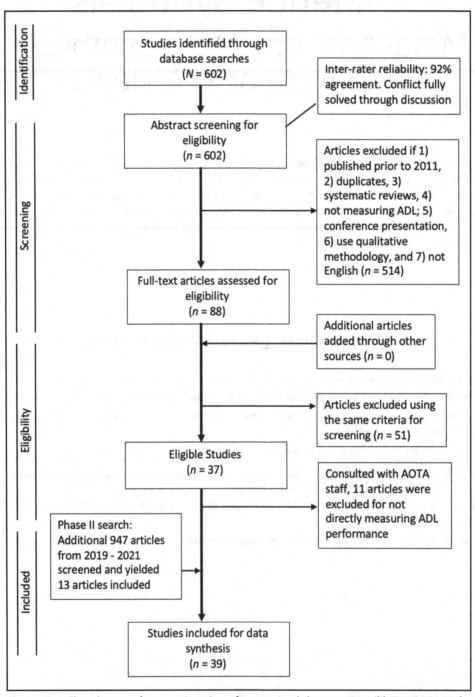

Figure 10–1 Flow diagram of systematic review of occupational therapy-compatible interventions for improving activities of daily living performance and participation of adults with multiple sclerosis.

10.2 SYSTEMATIC REVIEW VERSUS LITERATURE REVIEW

When a scholar or practitioner collects several sources of information, found by convenience, reads them, analyzes them, and writes a summary, that would be considered a literature review. There is no attempt to be comprehensive and discover all relevant sources on the given topic. There is no documentation of how these sources were found, or why these sources were kept while others were discarded. Although the author of the summary may articulate some useful insights, the review itself has weak or unknown reliability (replicability), and unknown validity (comprehensiveness, representativeness, and accuracy).

A systematic review, on the other hand, intentionally strengthens the replicability, the representativeness and comprehensiveness, and the accuracy of the conclusions by taking certain methodological steps. First, the keywords, databases, and years of inclusion used in searching the literature are presented. Inclusion criteria (how a study qualified for the review) and exclusion criteria (what would result in a study being deleted) are explicitly given. The number of potential studies retained at each step in the process (the "hits"), and the number excluded (with reasons why) are presented for each stage of the review (see Figure 10–1). The final number of reviewed sources is clearly stated. (See Liberati et al., 2009, for the format for portraying these steps in a PRISMA diagram, commonly required for health journal review articles.) Each source used in the review will have a full citation in the reference list at the end of the study (APA, 2020). In this way another researcher could replicate the study (repeat it exactly), and presumably come to the same conclusions as the original author(s).

10.3 SYSTEMATIC REVIEW VERSUS SCOPING REVIEW

When the purpose of a review is to perform an overview of the existing literature on a topic (rather than an exhaustive review of individual variables, as is typical with a systematic review), often a scoping review is conducted (Munn et al., 2018). Considerations for replicability and accuracy are still present, but comprehensiveness is not as high a priority. A scoping review may also seek to identify where there are gaps in the literature (Munn et al., 2018), for example, whether people with a certain diagnosis within a specific range of ages have ever been studied, or whether only people with a mild form of a disease have ever been researched. These gaps point naturally to possible future studies. A scoping review format can also be used to clarify concepts used over time in the literature (Munn et al., 2018).

A recent example of an occupational therapy scoping review is Lynch et al. (2023). They systematically reviewed the literature on school-based therapists using a multi-tiered approach to intervention in schools. Of the 40 studies they found, published between 1990 and 2020, 22 described single tier interventions (e.g., for children with a known diagnosis, or for children identified as at risk), and 18 discussed multi-tiered approaches (Lynch et al., 2023). In these latter studies the school therapists used a consultative approach with teachers, rather than providing intervention at the level of the entire school (for handwriting or student self-regulation), which Lynch et al. (2023) pointed out was a gap in the literature on school-based practice.

Another recent scoping review on occupational therapy published in a medical journal is Rocamora-Montenegro et al. (2021). They reviewed studies on the use of occupational therapy for clients with severe mental illness. From the 35 studies they included in the review, they identified that the most frequently used intervention approaches were those they labeled as psychosocial (using groups to address symptoms, occupational balance, and social and work integration for individuals with schizophrenia). Next most frequent were those labeled psychoeducational (to improve disease management, social abilities, and leisure skills). Other approaches in the literature were cognitive- and exercise-based (Rocamora-Montenegro et al., 2021). They noted the relative methodological weakness in many of the studies.

10.4 META-ANALYSIS FOR QUANTITATIVE STUDIES

When the purpose of a review of quantitative studies is to attempt a mathematical combination of their results, usually to indicate quantitatively the superiority of one intervention over another, or of an intervention versus a placebo or usual care, then a meta-analysis may be used. In the Research Pyramid model of evidence, it is labeled an E1 (if experimental studies are analyzed; 1A in AOTA terminology) or O1 (if outcome studies are analyzed; 2A in AOTA terms), or E1/O1 if both types of studies (AOTA Levels 1B, 2B, and 3B) are included. The term "meta-analysis" is said to have been coined by Glass (1976), an educational researcher. Unlike any of the prior listed review types, in a meta-analysis there is an actual mathematical calculation combining the results of multiple studies. In order for this mathematical formulation to be accurate, the studies must be similar in design and focus. For example, it would not be preferable to combine the findings of two studies mathematically if one study had a dependent variable of self-esteem, and another study used the dependent variable of quality of life, since these are two different constructs. In the occupational therapy literature, the study result of interest, usually, is the effect size of the intervention (Cohen's *d*, if the design is testing a single variable, or η^2, pronounced "eta-squared," if two or more constructs were investigated simultaneously in the study). Each study in the meta-analysis must provide enough information in order for these effects sizes to be calculated, if they were not reported directly. Note that in other disciplines effects based on correlation coefficients (economics) or odds ratios/relative risk (medicine) may be used in the meta-analysis (Hansen et al., 2022).

In the following subsections (10.4.1 to 10.4.8), the specific steps in conducting a meta-analysis will be presented. (The first four also apply to conducting or critiquing a meta-synthesis for qualitative data; see section 10.5 below.) These steps are adapted from Hansen et al. (2022), and enhanced by the experiences of the current text authors in conducting and supervising review studies. These eight subsections can also be used to critique a published meta-analytic study, that is, to determine to what extent the study followed each of the procedural steps, and presented this explicitly in the published text.

10.4.1 Formulation of the Research Question

This first step is a crucial one. The constructs (topics) of interest must be carefully specified (Hansen et al., 2022). In an intervention meta-analysis, for example, the results will be garbled if studies are collected where different types of intervention protocol were used (the independent variable). Even when there is good uniformity among the studies on a single intervention approach, the outcome (dependent) variables, if they vary among studies, may cloud the implications of the analysis. Care to select studies for their compatible independent and dependent variables is all the more important for the following reason: the statistical program calculating the meta-analytic combined effect of the studies processes the numbers as numbers. That is, any set of studies with effect sizes could be the input for a statistical software package, and an overall effect size will be calculable. The meaning and implications of the output, however, must be subject to careful interpretation. For example, a meta-analysis could be conducted where the intervention of interest is "all programs for cognitive deficits." The meta-analysis might produce an output finding that there is, overall, a small effect size from such programs. This finding might mask the fact that some programs (e.g., those that are client-centered and occupation-based) are more effective than others. The output might also mask that the effect is greater when the outcome variable is measured through functional cognition, rather than through neurophysiological skills such as speed of stimulus processing. Defining and screening the variables of interest is a crucial step at the outset of any meta-analysis (Hansen et al., 2022), and for any review study, for that matter.

Likewise, the population of interest is crucial. In the prior example, if the meta-analysis included people with different origins of cognitive deficit (CVA, TBI, dementia), the overall result could obscure which programs are most effective for which diagnoses. Unfortunately, when the literature on a given topic is thin, there may be a need to widen the diagnostic categories included, in order to have enough studies to perform the analysis. A more substantial field of literature allows for a more focused design of the study, which then permits more precise conclusions.

10.4.2 Construction of the Search Strategy

As with any systematic review, the search strategy for locating articles must be carefully designed and explicitly documented (Hansen et al., 2022). Are the keywords, search parameters, and databases accessed described in enough detail that another researcher could replicate the search? One caveat for replication in contemporary internet-based searches is that some search engines use a type of artificial intelligence algorithms to customize the findings shown to the user. Traditional databases such as PubMed, CINAHL, PsychInfo, and ERIC, do not (as yet) customize the search results. These and similar scholarly databases should be most heavily relied upon for the initial searching.

Other search techniques that will boost the comprehensiveness of the study include the following. First, any article on the topic that is itself a meta-analysis should be screened carefully. It is best practice for a meta-analysis that when an existing meta-analysis is found, it not be included in the new meta-analysis as if it were a single, independent study like the others found. Doing that could result in some studies being counted twice in the analysis (once on their own, once as part of the existing, published meta-analysis). The reference list of that existing meta-analysis can be mined for articles that are not found by a search engine. Any references found inside the existing meta-analysis can be added to the list of studies for the new meta-analysis with a note as to where they were found.

Second, the reference lists of all articles that are deemed suitable for the study can be another rich source of relevant literature. Again, that these articles were found in this way needs to be documented, as well as how many were found this way. A third technique is to examine the list of included studies for researcher names which appear in multiple studies. These names represent scholars who are productive in researching this topic. Their names can become input for the search engines, and their other publications, which the original search did not locate, may be found in this way. Relevant ones again are added to the list of studies to be used.

A final technique for a comprehensive search strategy is to examine the list of hits for journal names that appear often. These are most likely journals that frequently publish studies on the topic of interest. Most journals have a website where it is possible to search the contents of the journal for the given window of years (e.g., 2000–2020). Other relevant articles may be found in this way that were not located via the keyword search. As before, it is important for the sake of replication that the author of the new meta-analysis documents how such additional articles were found and how many were found in this way, so as to complete the PRISMA diagram (Liberati et al., 2009).

10.4.3 Inclusion/Exclusion of Studies

Defining the search strategy carefully is in essence setting the stage for the inclusion criteria for the search. Diagnosis (or diagnoses) of interest, used in the keywords of the search, for example, will yield many articles where people with that diagnosis were studied. For a given study, however, were people of other diagnoses included? Thus, an inclusion criterion for the meta-analysis might be that 50% or more of the participants in a study needed to have the diagnosis of interest. One could also justify setting this criterion at 100%, depending on how rigorous the meta-analysis needed to be, and on what the intention for generalizing the results is. Age ranges for the participants might also be specified in the inclusion criteria. A study, for example, to be included needs to have 90% of its participants within the ages of 21–65 years old. Another inclusion specifier might be the severity of the condition. For a meta-analysis on interventions for people with MS, for instance, there could be specific interest in individuals with a moderate form of the condition. This criterion might be specified as, "participants needed to have a score between 2.0 and 6.5 on the Expanded Disability Status Scale."

There will inevitably be studies that appear as relevant on the first list of "hits" that turn out not to be eligible for the meta-analysis. Exclusion criteria for eliminating these studies from consideration need to be explicitly given. For example, the author of a meta-analysis seeking worldwide generalizability may choose to exclude studies where the participants were receiving concurrent pharmaceutical treatment for the deficits of interest that is not accessible in many countries. Sometimes the need to exclude such a study can be determined from the title of the article. Sometimes it only becomes apparent when the abstract is reviewed. In many cases, it is only during the review of the full text of the article that the trigger for an exclusion criterion is found. For this reason, it is important for the author of any review to read the entire text of each article under consideration.

Other reasons for excluding studies can be that the study was actually only a description of a protocol (i.e., a plan for an intended study, one that has not yet been conducted). The author of a meta-analysis may also choose to exclude studies that are a pilot study, a feasibility study, or a conference abstract of a presentation. Of course, the

thicker the empirical literature on a given topic, the more selective the review author can be. Studies where the topic for the meta-analysis was not the main purpose of the study, but was only addressed secondarily, may be deleted if this is an exclusion criterion.

10.4.4 Rating of Studies

Just as with individual studies, it is important in a meta-analysis to appraise the rigor of the individual studies included. Note the size of the sample in each study. Note how intensively and for how long the intervention in each study was provided. Note whether the people providing the intervention were specifically trained to do so. The authors of the meta-analysis may wish to rate each included study on a "risk of bias" scale, such as described below in section 10.6.1. Ranking the included studies on the level of possible bias in their designs and implementation may help with the interpretation of results, as described in the next section.

10.4.5 Analysis of Studies

Once the final list of studies to be included in the meta-analysis is formulated, it is time to begin data extraction and analysis. Meta-analysis software formats vary, but most will allow for the input of the main variable (the effect size per study, or per construct within a study) and one or more covariates. The covariate data points can be used in a post-analysis, to explore hypotheses as to why the results turned out the way they did. That is, why did some studies indicate that the traditional intervention worked better than a new intervention, while other studies showed the reverse? Perhaps the difference was due to differing sample demographics.

Effect Size

The main data point for each study in a meta-analysis will be the effect size of the intervention of interest. If Cohen's d is being used for effect size, then the data point might be +0.2, which would indicate that, for this study, the intervention improved the performance of a group of individuals by an average of one fifth of a standard deviation. Cohen considered this size of effect size to represent a small effect. Moderate beneficial effects are represented by a d = +0.5, and large effects by a +0.8 or larger. If the studied intervention creates a negative effect size (e.g., –0.2), that would indicate that the intervention caused a group average performance to decline by one fifth of a standard deviation—a small detrimental effect.

Correlation: Effect Size to Sample Size

Meta-analytic researchers often perform this check on the data early in the analysis. If there is a large, inverse correlation between sample size of the studies and the effect sizes, then studies with smaller samples tended to generate greater effect sizes. Such an outcome here could indicate that the data are subject to high sampling error. That is, the results of the studies overestimate the actual effect of the intervention, due to the inaccuracy of small samples. If there is little to no correlation between sample size of studies and effect size of studies, then the researcher can be more confident that the set of studies being used is not biased or subject to high sampling error.

Homogeneity/Heterogeneity Statistic Cochrane's Q, I²

Another check of the data in a meta-analysis is calculating Cochrane's Q statistic. Cochrane's Q is used to determine whether the studies in a meta-analysis show expected variations around a common mean value, or whether instead they cluster around two or more mean values (in which case, they show heterogeneity). Technically, Q is the sum of squared differences between individual study effects and the pooled effect across studies. The sum of squared differences may be weighted (by giving more importance to some studies than to others), in which case Q is the weighted sum of squared differences between individual effects and the pooled effect across studies. The larger the value of Q, the more likely the collective studies show heterogeneity in their results.

An alternative indicator of homogeneity of studies *is* I^2, which is defined as the proportion of the study variability attributable to heterogeneity in the studies. It ranges in value from 0 to +1.0 (like a squared correlation coefficient) and because it is unitless, the values of I^2 can be compared across multiple meta-analyses. A higher value for I^2 (i.e., closer to +1.0) would mean that in that particular meta-analysis, the studies were more heterogeneous, that is, more likely to represent findings from truly different populations or from truly different constructs. The advantage of using I^2 over Q is that I^2 is independent of the number of studies in the meta-analysis, thus more easily compared between meta-analyses.

Confidence Intervals

A sample mean, as a point estimate of the population parameter, is often reported more meaningfully as a confidence interval (that we can be 95% confident that the population mean lies within a 95% confidence interval). Also with effect sizes, an individual study's effect size is a point estimate of the effect size that intervention would have in the population. More meaningful is to calculate an effect size confidence interval (ES CI), based on the size of the sample in the study and also on the variability within that sample. Then a researcher can say that there is 95% confidence that the true effect size of the intervention in the population lies within the ES CI. A larger ES CI (indicating more uncertainty) would be due to a smaller sample in the study, or the sample having greater variability of scores. Larger samples with less variability would give rise to shorter (more precise) ES CI's. A more precise (shorter) ES CI is more likely to fall entirely on one side of the vertical "null hypothesis" line between the

intervention being better or the intervention being worse than an alternative. How this plays out visually will be shown in the section below.

Forest Plots

For each study in a meta-analysis, the effect size confidence interval is placed in a forest plot (see Figure 10–2). The central vertical line indicates the null hypothesis being true (that there is no difference between one intervention and another, or between an intervention and placebo, in the population of interest). On one side of the central vertical line is the area where the experimental intervention is better for the population (creates a stronger beneficial effect). On the other side of the central line is where the control intervention (traditional therapy or a placebo therapy) would yield a stronger beneficial outcome in the population.

Each study in the meta-analysis is represented in the forest plot by a horizontal line segment. The shorter the line segment, the narrower the 95% CI estimate of ES for that study would be. Studies whose ES CI lies entirely on one side of the vertical line or the other provide evidence for that side's intervention to be clearly (statistically significantly) superior. An ES CI that crosses the vertical line is like a CI of the population mean that crosses zero (contains both negative and positive values, such as CI = –3.5 to +2.8). In this case in a meta-analysis, that would mean that the researcher cannot reject the null hypothesis that there is no real difference

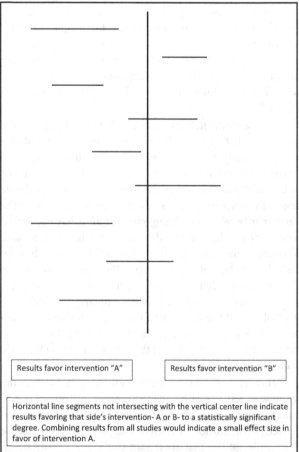

Figure 10–2 Meta-analysis plot of effect size confidence intervals.

between the interventions. The researcher is left with the conclusion that not enough evidence of a difference was assembled for the researcher to be 95% confident that one intervention is truly better than the other in the population.

The forest plot displays one line segment per study in the meta-analysis, thus providing a quick visual overview of how all the studies included in the analysis turned out. In the meta-analyses published by the Cochrane organization, a diamond shape will be inserted at the bottom of the forest plot. The diamond's top and bottom points indicate the location of the overall ES of the intervention, calculating the ES CI of all the studies together. The diamond may fall on one side of the null hypothesis line or the other, or it may fall on or very close to the vertical line (see www.cochrane.org/about-us/difference-we-make for an example). The more clearly it falls on one side or the other (i.e., the farther away the diamond is from the vertical line) the stronger the overall evidence is, pointing to that intervention as superior. Of course, if the ES CI's of most studies fall on one side of the vertical line, then the diamond is most likely to fall on that side, too. The exception would occur if it were many small sample studies falling on one side of the line, and a few very large sample studies falling on the other side, as the larger sample studies carry more weight in the meta-analysis calculation.

10.4.6 Sensitivity Checks

Even after the calculation of the overall ES location in a meta-analysis, a researcher may question how influenced this result was by a single study. Thus, some meta-analyses add a step to the analysis. After finding the location of the overall ES with all studies included in the calculation, the researcher has the software recalculate the position, excluding one study at a time, until all have been excluded exactly once from the calculation. How much the overall location moves while doing these repeated calculations is an indication of the sensitivity of the finding to the presence or absence of a single study. If the location does not move very much during the sensitivity analysis, that means that no one study is overly influencing the final result.

10.4.7 Post-Analysis of Covariates or Interactions

Once the forest plot has been generated, and the overall ES calculated, there remains the question: why did some studies show one intervention was superior, while other studies found in favor of the other intervention (or no intervention). That is, why were some of the line segments (the ES CI's) on one side of the vertical line, while others were on the other side? The null hypothesis explanation would be that there isn't any reason for it, that all that variation is due to random error. What if the variation, though, is not due to random error?

For example, a hypothetical meta-analysis compares the effect of intervention A versus intervention B. Some

individual studies' ES CI's fall to the left of the vertical line (i.e., outcome of A > B). Others fall to the right of the line (outcome of B > A). The forest plot by itself cannot explain why the studies varied in this way. A post-analysis, however, might reveal that the vast majority of the studies where A > B were conducted with women participants, and those where B > A were with men. Clearly, intervention A works better for women while intervention B works better for men. This situation is the exact description of an interaction between sex and intervention type. Unless demographic or other variables are investigated as part of the meta-analysis, this insight could be overlooked. If there are enough studies included in a meta-analysis (e.g., 20 or more) it may be possible to investigate the role of multiple covariates (age, severity of disease, the way the intervention was implemented, the way the outcome variable was measured). One or more of these covariates might turn out to have had a discernible effect on the study outcome. Even without a higher order statistical post-analysis, such an examination of other variables can give rise to hypotheses, which may one day lead to further research and deeper knowledge.

10.4.8 Implications of the Findings

Even a meta-analysis on a large number of studies will not answer all questions about the effectiveness of an intervention. Before applying the findings, careful consideration must be given to the generalizability of the meta-analytic findings. What range of participants were included in the studies (by age, severity of diagnosis, time since onset, other concurrent occupational issues or ethnic or geographical diversity in the participants)? How and where was the intervention provided (specially trained therapists, in which setting, under which conditions)? How exactly was the outcome variable measured?

Each scholar citing a meta-analysis and each practitioner considering how to implement the findings of the meta-analysis must take care not to over-generalize. A well-conducted meta-analysis may be the highest level of quantitative evidence available, but no one study (even a meta-analysis) is fully comprehensive. Its strength relies on the depth of literature on the topic and on the clarity of the concepts on this topic in the literature.

10.4.9 Meta-Analyses of the Effectiveness of Occupational Therapy

Two of the earliest meta-analyses to appear in the occupational therapy literature in the United States were authored by Baker and Tickle-Degnen (2001) and Murphy and Tickle-Degnen (2001), on the effects of occupational therapy for clients with multiple sclerosis and Parkinson's disease, respectively. From 23 studies available at the time, Baker and Tickle-Degnen (2001) found that occupational therapy was effective both for client factors (strength, ROM, mood) and for ADL (effect size $r = +0.52$ to $+0.57$, which roughly converts to a $d = +1.22$ to $+1.39$). It was noted by the authors that the studies had not addressed therapy to help clients with life role challenges, nor did they display high levels of methodological rigor (Baker & Tickle-Degnen, 2001).

Murphy and Tickle-Degnen (2001) investigated the results from 16 included studies and found small to moderate positive effects of occupational therapy for both client factors and functional activities for clients with Parkinson's disease (overall $r = +0.26$, which converts to $d = +0.54$). They also called for greater rigor in future studies.

About 20 years later, while occupational therapy meta-analyses were still being published in occupational therapy journals (Ikiugu et al., 2017, on mental health interventions; Lau et al., 2022, on self-management for survivors of stroke living in the community; Lockwood & Porter, 2022, on the effectiveness of occupational therapy on preventing hospital readmissions; Song, 2015, on community care occupational therapy for people with dementia), studies on the effectiveness of occupational therapy were appearing in journals outside the field. Bennett et al. (2019), meta-analyzing studies on home therapy for people with dementia and their care-givers, was published in the *British Medical Journal Open*. Tofani et al. (2020) meta-analyzed studies on the effects of occupational therapy on quality of life for clients with Parkinson's disease. Their work was published in *Movement Disorders Clinical Practice*. Chen et al. (2022) conducted a meta-analysis of studies concerning the use of virtual reality training for improving ADL and cognitive function in persons post-stroke, and their study was published in the *Archives of Physical Medicine & Rehabilitation*. He et al. (2023) combined studies on occupational therapy and quality of life for clients with breast cancer in a meta-analysis, published in *Medicine (Baltimore)*. Finally, McCarthy et al. (2023) published their meta-analysis in *BMC Geriatrics*, on the effects of multidisciplinary rehabilitation for older adults with COVID-19. The trend of meta-analytic studies of occupational therapy interventions both within and outside the field points to a growing, recognized body of literature on the overall effectiveness of the profession on clients of varying diagnoses.

10.5 META-SYNTHESIS

The body of qualitative literature on health topics in general and occupational therapy in particular has grown rapidly over the past 30 years. Many topics now offer opportunities for systematic review and meta-synthesis of the findings of studies conducted on these topics. Quantitative studies can be systematically reviewed and meta-analyzed using the techniques described above. Similar rigorous approaches for synthesizing qualitative studies have been developed for at least 35 years (Noblit &

Hare, 1988). These techniques began to be discussed in the occupational therapy literature about 15 years ago (Gewurtz et al., 2008). Below is a summary of the main techniques, and a discussion of how they have been applied in literature relevant to the field of occupational therapy.

As methodologies for conducting a meta-synthesis evolve, it is worth noting that there is a divergent use of terminology. Dole et al. (2021) called their synthesis of practice guidelines of multiple professions on carpal tunnel syndrome treatment a meta-synthesis. Carrera et al. (2023) called their study of parent experiences schooling their children with autism spectrum disorder a meta-analysis, although it fits the definition of a meta-synthesis as used in this textbook. Finally, Dépelteau et al. (2021) described their review of studies on individuals living with fibromyalgia as a thematic synthesis.

The first four steps in the meta-synthesis process are virtually identical to those in a meta-analysis. See sections 10.4.1 to 10.4.4 above.

10.5.1 Rating Study Rigor

In a meta-synthesis, it is also important to consider the methodological rigor of the studies included. For such qualitative research studies, different elements of rigor will be evaluated, compared to those in quantitative studies. These elements of rigor were described in section 9.12 in the preceding chapter of this book. ENTREQ is a formulation of qualitative study rigor evaluation designed to be used in meta-syntheses (Tong et al., 2012).

10.5.2 Synthesis Approaches (Summarizing, Aggregating, Synthesizing)

Early reviews of qualitative literature involved summarizing the findings from several studies without attempting to rigorously synthesize those findings. Another approach is to aggregate findings across studies using the manual of the Johanna Briggs Institute (Aromataris & Munn, 2020). In the late 1980s resources began to appear to help scholars actually synthesize the findings across qualitative studies (Jensen & Allen, 1996; Noblit & Hare, 1988). These were codified into an oft-used book by Sandelowski and Barroso (2006). Nurse scholars Jensen and Allen specified three steps in the process of meta-synthesis: (a) evaluating each study's methodology, (b) aligning codes and themes for translation, and (c) interpreting the meta-reality portrayed by the studies, including their variability (Jensen & Allen, 1996).

Thomas and Harden, social scientists concerned with human health, described the process similarly (2008). They advocated using thematic analysis for a meta-synthesis in a similar way to the original thematic analysis in individual studies: (a) line-by-line coding, (b) development of descriptive themes, close to the original study data, and (c) generation of analytic themes, where the synthesis and interpretation occurs (2008). An early appraisal of meta-synthetic techniques in the occupational therapy literature was Gewurtz et al. (2008). Despite the challenges of devising a meta-interpretation, they advocated for meta-synthesis as a means to "advance knowledge about occupation and occupation-based practice," and "develop deeper insights and understandings" (Gewurtz et al., 2008, p. 301). These "insights and understandings" can include the identification of factors related to an outcome, as in McGrath et al. (2019), a meta-synthesis on the experience of sexuality after a stroke. A meta-synthesis can also support claims of causality, as in Boshoff et al. (2021). They identified ways in which the parents of children with autism spectrum disorder experienced poor service for their children in health care facilities. By implication, the difficulties could be attributed to lack of knowledge on the part of health care professionals. Their recommendation for more education for those professionals entailed the claim that if health professionals better understood these parents, client–therapist communication would improve, and the parents and the child would receive better service (Boshoff et al., 2021).

10.5.3 Generalizability and Implications for Practice

The question of how to apply the findings of a meta-synthesis to practice does not have a simple answer, just as is the case with the outcome of a meta-analysis. Careful consideration must be given by a practitioner to the representativeness of the studies that went into the meta-synthesis. Finfgeld-Connett, a nurse scholar, concluded that generalizability of meta-syntheses is enhanced when the authors used "systematic sampling, second-tier triangulation, maintenance of well-documented audit trails and the development of multi-dimensional theory" (Finfgeld-Connett, 2010, p. 246). Systematic sampling strengthens the extent to which the meta-synthesis captured the true variability in the experiences of the people studied in the contributing research. Second-tier triangulation refers to the intentional incorporation of findings derived from different sources of data (observation in naturalistic settings, participant interview, documentary evidence). Developing a multidimensional theory consists of generating the analytic themes of Thomas and Harden (2008). All three of these steps strengthen the comprehensiveness, representativeness, and authenticity of the interpretation of reality created in the meta-synthesis. A meta-study with these qualities in place will be worthy of consideration for transfer to professional practice. How the practitioner actually applies them in practice will be influenced by the relevance of the findings and the ease of implementation of the insights. One of the strengths of qualitative research (both the original studies and a meta-synthesis) is that it provides a clear window into the lived experience of clients. Having a clear view of what clients often experience in these circumstances offers to the practitioner a powerful tool for building a therapeutic relationship. Such qualitative findings can also widen a therapist's perspective on client occupations and priorities, which can aid in collaboratively setting goals and choosing intervention approaches (Tomlin & Swinth, 2015).

10.5.4 Recent Meta-Syntheses Relevant to the Practice of Occupational Therapy

Meta-syntheses are published in increasing number in the health literature in general, and in occupational therapy journals in particular. A PubMed search in late 2023 for meta-syntheses from the last five years relevant to occupational therapy yielded 22 results. Those published in occupational therapy journals covered studies of people with the unusual or complex and not well understood diagnoses of autism spectrum disorder (Carrera et al., 2023) and fibromyalgia (Depelteau et al., 2021), or the experiences of clients undergoing or using complex interventions (self-initiated management approaches to cognitive impairments for people with dementia or brain injury (Nygård et al., 2022), or heretofore unstudied aspects of recovery, such as "reablement" in the elderly after a health setback (Bergström et al., 2023). One study synthesized the findings of studies on the experiences of allied health students performing a less typical international fieldwork placement (Levitt et al., 2021). In journals outside the field were found meta-syntheses on the experience of ethnic minority youth with disabilities (Lindsay et al., 2023), sexuality in adults after a stroke (McGrath et al., 2019), and the health care system experience of parents who had a child with autism spectrum disorder (Boshoff et al., 2021). In these studies, the topics were ones that were not well understood or often addressed by therapists. For the sake of more effective interventions, it was deemed important to present a comprehensive, synthesized portrayal of the issues in the lived experience of clients and their caregivers. As with primary qualitative research, this lived aspect of intervention is where meta-syntheses can make a distinct contribution to the field. The deeper understandings that these syntheses make possible are readily applicable in professional practice, because they can help prevent misunderstandings between client and practitioner that impede the flow of therapy.

10.6 SEARCHING FOR EVIDENCE TO INFORM OR SUPPORT PROFESSIONAL PRACTICE

In the era of evidence-based practice, every health care practitioner needs to be a skilled consumer of evidence reviews. Most practitioners should also become

TABLE 10–1

RISK OF BIAS FOR NON-CONTROL (PRE-POST INTERVENTION) RESEARCH STUDIES

RISK OF BIAS FOR NON-CONTROL (PRE-POST INTERVENTION) RESEARCH STUDIES

Citation	Study objectives clear; consistent with variables selected for design	Eligibility and selection criteria clear	Participants representative of population of clients accessible to researchers	All eligible participants invited for participation	Sample size appropriate (power calculation done)	Intervention clearly described (frequency, length, intensity and by whom provided) and fidelity of delivery documented
Hoogewerf (2017)	+	+	+ representative by sex, age, type, severity of diagnosis	-	+	+

Evaluation: + = yes, - = no, NR= Not reported (counts as a -)
Scoring: Count yes scores for each study and divide by 11, yielding the
Risk of bias rating: Low (L)-75-100%, Moderate (M) 25-75%, or High (H) 0-25%
Source: Modified from the original tool: www.nhlbi.nih.gov/health-topics/study-quality-assessment-tools which contains detailed instructions for carrying out the risk of bias appraisal, item-by-item.

competent at designing and conducting their own evidence reviews. So that these reviews can be implemented rigorously, this section provides an outline of the process, with further explanation of where challenges may occur.

An evidence review to address a question from professional practice may differ from a scholarly systematic review. Often a meta-analysis may have ten or fewer studies taken into consideration, whereas a practitioner's review results in 50 to 75 studies being included. For example, a practitioner may phrase an evidence question as, "What is the published, empirical evidence supporting any major type of intervention for cognitive impairments?" This question is stated very broadly, in order to capture the evidence available on this broad topic, and the number of included studies is accordingly greater. A related scholarly systematic review may be much more specific, for example, "What is the empirical evidence for the effectiveness of outpatient interventions addressing impairments in executive functioning among home-dwelling individuals recovering from a traumatic brain injury?" The practitioner may be interested in casting a broad net into the literature. The researcher is often concerned about articulating a focused question in order to reduce variability in the findings and thus increase statistical power, or uses the precise form of a question due to the awareness that there is a knowledge gap on this exact topic.

Considerations of rigor for the scholar's systematic review have been detailed in previous sections of this chapter. Specific aspects of implementing a review and appraisal process by practitioners or students will be described below.

10.6.1 Defining the Search Topic of an Evidence Review

First, the importance of carefully selecting the search topic has been given in section 10.4.1 above. Practitioners may use a "PICO" or "PACO" template to help focus their question. PICO stands for patient, intervention, comparison, outcome, and is used when the practitioner seeks evidence about intervention effectiveness. An example would be

Patient—For adults with intention tremors

Intervention—do weighted wrist cuffs

Comparison—compared to weighted utensils or other adaptive devices

Outcome—reduce the amount of food spilled, increase food consumed, or increase efficiency of eating (amount consumed per minute)?

For a PACO question, the "intervention" is replaced by "assessment," and would be used when the practitioner is seeking the best means of assessing a certain type of client (diagnostically/demographically) on a designated performance construct. For example,

Patient—For adults at risk for lymphedema after breast cancer surgery

Assessment—does Indocyanine Green (ICG) lymphography

Outcome measures pre-defined, operationalized, valid and reliable, and assessed consistently (inter-rater reliability established)	Assessors blinded to participant exposure to intervention	Loss to follow up after baseline 20% or less	Statistical methods used to examine changes in outcome measures from before to after intervention	Outcome measures were collected before and multiple times after intervention	Overall risk of bias assessment (low, moderate, or high risk)
+	-	-	+	+	M

Comparison—compared to other traditional methods of early detection of lymphedema

Outcome—result in earlier detection of lymphedema or fewer false positive findings?

In practitioner or student evidence reviews, the exact parameters of the PICO or PACO question may need to be revised once the initial literature search has been conducted. A revision may be necessary if the search resulted in too few articles (thus, widen the search) or too many articles (thus, narrow the search) being identified.

10.6.2 Outlining the Search Strategy

For a student evidence project, often a formal proposal will be required. This proposal will be reviewed and approved by the faculty supervisor of the project. The search strategy section of the proposal will include a comprehensive list of all the search terms to be used while gathering evidence. Likewise, with the help of a library liaison staff, a list of databases to be searched will be given. A knowledgeable project supervisor may guide students into considering more search terms than the students initially developed themselves.

If there are explicit criteria that the proposers wish to follow (such as including literature published from a certain year forward, articles in other languages than English if fluent readers are available, or an explicit inclusion of qualitative research studies), then these should be explicitly listed as part of the search strategy.

A faculty supervisor may also wish for students to commit to screening the reference lists from relevant articles for more possible sources, and examining meta-analyses and meta-syntheses on the topic to determine if those authors used any articles that have not been found by other means. A decision may also need to be made whether to include dissertations, theses, conference presentation abstracts, or other grey literature. These types of sources may need to be included if there are very few peer-reviewed, published articles on the topic.

Inclusion and exclusion criteria for articles can thus be succinctly stated. These criteria will be essential when the reviewer must make a decision about whether to include an article or not, as explained in section 10.6.3 below.

10.6.3 Master Citation List

Once the search strategy has been fully implemented, the evidence gatherer should compose a list of citations of all studies being considered for the review. The original total number of hits should be documented, and the number of articles excluded based on a review of their titles indicated. This information will be needed in constructing the PRISMA flow chart (Liberati et al., 2009) at the end of the search process, to indicate how many articles were used in the review, and the reason why excluded articles were deleted from the review.

The master citation list will include articles that are deemed "yes" (definitely qualifying), and "maybe" (in need

TABLE 10-2

EVIDENCE TABLE: ADL INTERVENTIONS FOR PERSONS WITH MS

AUTHOR YEAR COUNTRY	LEVEL OF EVIDENCE / STUDY DESIGN / RISK OF BIAS (QUALITY ASSESSMENT)	PARTICIPANTS (# PARTICIPANTS, MEAN AGE, GENDER PERCENTAGES) / INCLUSION CRITERIA / STUDY SETTING	INTERVENTION AND CONTROL	OUTCOME MEASURES OF INTEREST	RESULTS (INCLUDE SIGNIFICANCE OF THE FINDINGS)
MINDFULNESS ON SLEEP					
Cavalera et al. 2018 Italy	**Level:** AOTA- 1B Pyramid- E2 Randomized, two-group, repeated measures **Risk of Bias:** moderate	**Participants:** N (enrolled, completed, follow-up) = (139, 112, 96); 139 included in intention to treat Intervention= 54 (36 Female) Mean age: 42.26 yrs Control= 67 (42 Female) Mean age 43.19 yrs **Inclusion:** neurologist diagnosed RRMS or SPMS; no change in treatment prior 3 mos; no relapse or steroid use 4 wks prior; 18+yo; owned computer, tablet, or smartphone	Duration: 8 wks **Intervention:** Kabat-Zinn mindfulness modified for online format (added music meditation and discussion of symptom acceptance) led by expert Mindfulness Based Stress Reduction trainer. Videoconference with home exercises **Control:** psycho-education course on stress management, relaxation, sleep hygiene, fatigue, social relationship.	Medical Outcomes Study Sleep Pretest, Posttest (2 mos), and 6 mos follow-up	**Significant results:** Intervention group had statistically significantly fewer sleep problems (p < .001, eta^2 = 0.130) at 2 mos compared to Control group. **Non-Significant results:** At 6 mos no statistically significant difference seen.
Hoogerwerf et al. 2017 Netherlands	**Level:** AOTA- 3B Pyramid- O3 One group pre-post; with 10-wk waiting period as Control **Risk of Bias:** moderate	**Participants:** N (enrolled, completed) = (59, 20) Female 83% Mean age 48 yo EDSS range, 1-7.5 **Inclusion:** diagnosis of RRMS or SPMS; 18-60 yo; with severe fatigue; fluent in Dutch	**Intervention:** Mindfulness-Based Cognitive Training group protocol in 8 weekly meetings of 2.5 hrs over 10 wks, led by 2 certified trainers **Control:** N/A	Symptom Checklist-90, sleep subscale Pretest, posttest & 3 mos follow-up	**Significant results:** None **Non-significant results:** Symptom Checklist-90 no change
AEROBIC EXERCISE FOR SLEEP					
Siengsukon et al. 2016 USA	**Level:** AOTA- 2B (< 30 participants) Pyramid- E2 Pilot, Randomized, two-group, pretest/ posttest- block randomized by disease type/sex **Risk of Bias:** low	**Participants:** N (enrolled, completed) = (28, 24) Intervention= (14, 12) (11 Female) Mean age 48.9 yrs Control= (14, 12) (8 Female) Mean age 50.9 yrs **Inclusion:** 18+ yo; RRMS or SPMS; independent ambulatory with/without assistive device; ≥ 24 MMSE	Duration: 12 wks, 3 times/wk **Intervention:** mod intensity aerobic **Control:** walking & stretching	PSQI Epworth Sleepiness Scale for daytime sleepiness Pretest, Posttest	**Significant results:** Intervention group had statistically significant reduction in daytime sleepiness (p = .016, ES = +0.63) **Non-Significant results:** Control group had better outcome than the Intervention group for PSQI (p = .033, ES = -0.51)

Note: EDSS- Expanded Disability Status Scale; ES – effect size; hr(s)- hour(s); MMSE – Mini-Mental State Examination; mo – month(s); mo(s) – month(s); PSQI – Pittsburgh Sleep Quality Index; RRMS- Relapsing-Remitting Multiple Sclerosis; SPMS – Secondary Progressive Multiple Sclerosis); wk(s) – week(s); yo – years old; yrs- years of further review). A reading of the article abstract may enable the reviewer to resolve cases of "maybe." Sometimes a careful reading of the full text of the article will be necessary. At some point, all the maybe articles will be resolved into being a yes or a no. Then all the yes articles constitute the final list of studies included in the review.

10.6.4 Risk of Bias Table

For each included article, an appraisal of the methodological rigor of that study should be conducted. Often this step entails using a template checklist such as the PEDro score, or a Risk of Bias table (as used in the AOTA-sponsored evidence reviews). Filling out this template for all studies will provide the reviewer with a quick overview of the trustworthiness of the set of included articles. The rigor score may also influence certain conclusions about the state of the evidence. See Table 10–1 for an example of a rigor rating template.

10.6.5 Evidence Table

Next the heart of the review is constructed: the evidence table. Information is carefully extracted from each included article and entered into the columns of the evidence table (see Table 10–2 for an example). Somewhat different column headings are used for articles with a qualitative methodology, compared to those for quantitative articles. Different column headings may be used for descriptive studies and single case experimental design studies. Different templates exist for meta-analytic

studies, and a different set of columns may be used for a meta-synthetic study. For all types of studies, though, the first column contains the first author's last name, the year and journal of publication, and the country in which the study was conducted. The second column contains the study objectives, which the article authors may have constructed as a research question, a hypothesis, or a statement of investigation purpose. The third column contains a brief description of the study design and indicators of the study's level of evidence (e.g., from the AOTA hierarchy of evidence or the Research Pyramid level of evidence). The fourth column is for a description of the research participants, their numbers, and the inclusion and exclusion criteria used in their selection (crucial for estimating generalizability later). The next columns are for intervention descriptions (including the "dosage" of the intervention given), outcome measures used, results, and study limitations. Results that were reported as statistically significant must be explicitly recorded as such in the evidence table. Comparisons where there was found to be no statistically significant difference should also be reported.

The master citation table may have contained all included articles listed alphabetically by first author's last name. This order is not necessarily the best, however, for the listing of articles in the evidence table. It may be helpful to sort the articles into sub-categories, depending on which versions of the interventions of interest that article employed. It may also be illustrative to sort the articles (if all used essentially the same intervention) by which exact outcome measures they used, since there are many

TABLE 10–3
STRENGTH OF EVIDENCE TABLE
STRONG
Two or more Level 1A/1B studies (AOTA); E1/E2 studies (research pyramid)
Available evidence indicates consistent results from well-designed, well-conducted studies.
MODERATE
At least one Level 1A or 1B high-quality study (E1/E2) or multiple moderate-quality studies, Level 2A/B or Level 3A/B, (E3/O2/O3/O4)
Available evidence is sufficient to determine the effects on health outcomes, but confidence in the estimate is limited by such factors as number, size, or quality of individual studies, or inconsistency of findings across studies.
LOW
Small number of low-level studies, flaws in the studies, etc.
Available evidence is insufficient to assess effects on health outcomes, due to limited number or size of studies, important flaws in study design or methods, inconsistency of findings across studies, or lack of information on important health outcomes.

Note. The strength of the evidence is based on the guidelines of the US Preventive Services Task Force (www.spreventiveservicestask force.org/Page/Name/grade-definitions).

ways to measure such constructs as pain, quality of life, or ADL function, for example, and different means of measurement may lead to different outcomes.

Abbreviations may be freely used inside the evidence table in order to save space. Every abbreviation used should be documented and expanded out in an abbreviation note at the end of the evidence table. While the risk of bias table and the master citation list rarely appear in a published review article, it is common for the evidence table to be published in its entirety. For an example of a section of a completed evidence table, see Table 10–3.

10.6.6 Strength of Evidence Findings

Once the evidence table is complete, it is time to compose the evidence findings. Practitioners are seeking to know how strong a recommendation in favor of the selected intervention or assessment the reviewer can make. This describes the question of the strength of the evidence. For PICO questions, while there is no universal table to determine when the evidence found should be labeled "strong," or "weak," or "none," or even "clearly contraindicated," it is helpful for readers of the literature to know that some consistent system of labeling strength of evidence was used. The system used in AOTA-sponsored intervention evidence reviews, for example, is as follows:

Strong evidence—two or more studies at evidence level 1A or 1B, with low or moderate risk of bias, indicating that an intervention is reliably effective, without there being any contradictory evidence.

Moderate evidence—at least one 1A or 1B study with low or moderate risk of bias indicating that the intervention is effective.

Note: Multiple studies at lower levels (several 2A or 2B, or 3A or 3B studies for moderate evidence, for example) may substitute for higher level studies in fulfilling these criteria. Such lower-level studies must be carefully evaluated for rigor.

Low evidence—small number of lower level studies, or only studies with weakness in rigor, are present in the literature.

Of course if the evidence indicated that the intervention in question actually does harm to (from side effects) or brings about a decline in functional performance of clients, then that intervention would accordingly be contraindicated.

For reviews with a PACO question, the challenge to fairly present findings is more complicated. Even if only two instruments are being compared for their accuracy, reliability, and feasibility, there are many parameters on which they may have differed in published studies. These include their intended population, their face validity, content validity, concurrent validity, predictive validity, construct validity, ecological validity, their test-retest reliability, intra- and inter-rater reliability, as well as the feasibility of their administration (time, space, and training needed), and the test cost (for the kit itself, for the scoresheets, and perhaps even for the online scoring of the scoresheets). This list constitutes a great many aspects upon which to compare the instruments. The answer to the question as to which test would be better to use may depend on the anticipated type of clientele (ages, diagnoses), on the constructs the therapist would find most valuable to be measuring, or indeed, in the end, on the cost of using that assessment.

10.6.7 Practice Guidelines

From such strength of findings, practice guidelines can be composed. The categories of recommendation used by AOTA in their evidence work are listed below.

A: There is strong evidence that occupational therapy practitioners should routinely provide the intervention to eligible clients. Strong evidence was found that the intervention improves important outcomes and that benefits substantially outweigh any harm.

B: There is moderate evidence that occupational therapy practitioners should routinely provide the intervention to eligible clients. There is high certainty that the net benefit is moderate, or there is moderate certainty that the net benefit is moderate to substantial.

D: It is recommended that occupational therapy practitioners not provide the intervention to eligible clients. At least fair evidence was found that the intervention is ineffective or that the harm outweighs the benefits.

(AOTA, 2022)

Practitioners should keep in mind that the latest recommendations are only temporary until a new evidence review leads to new findings, which may result in a change of recommendation.

10.6.8 Challenges in the Synthesis and Application of Evidence

Systematically gathering evidence from the literature to answer a practice question involves a long and exacting process. Attention to avoiding the following pitfalls can both speed up and strengthen a project of evidence review.

1. Compose the PICO or PACO question using up-to-date terminology (e.g., from the latest OTPF). Taking care in this step will increase the chances of finding the most relevant recent information on the topic.

2. When searching the literature published over a longer period of time, be sensitive to the evolution of terminology on the topic of interest. Use older terms, too, if older studies are intended to be found.

3. Screen the list of potential studies carefully to detect duplicates. Occasionally, despite publishing protocols to the contrary, a study is published twice, in two different journals. More common is that two publications appear, one reporting on results that are pertinent to the evidence review, and another reporting on those results and on other, newer results. If both studies were kept in the review, that would give an inappropriate "double vote" to the corresponding findings. One article or the other should be deleted from the master citation list.

4. Publications now appear in journals that are protocols (proposals) for a future empirical study. They should be deleted from the inclusion list because they do not yet have any results.

5. Carefully ascertain which citations are conference presentation abstracts or posters. Such scholarly work does undergo a type of peer-review process (for conference selection), but typically this process is far less rigorous than the scrutiny provided by a peer-reviewed journal.

6. The evidence reviewer should be very clear on how broad the membership in the pertinent family of interventions will be. Including all studies using "cognitive behavioral therapy" may result in articles testing quite different interventions.

7. Reviewers should read articles looking for evidence that the intervention was indeed delivered to the participants as intended. Does the article report rates of absenteeism from sessions, attrition rates, or the percentage of times participants declined to complete the session, due to fatigue, pain, or any other reason?

8. If a study only pursued the intervention of interest in the PICO question as its secondary purpose, carefully consider how much weight the study should carry in the final conclusions.

9. For some constructs there can be a large number of outcome measures that are used in studies. Pain, quality of life, and ADL function, for example, each have numerous instruments available for their measurement. All such related instruments may not measure exactly the same construct. If possible, sort studies into sub-groups that used a uniform instrument for the outcome measure. Often this step is not possible.

10. Take extra care drawing conclusions from studies that only used client self-report measures. Such measures are particularly susceptible to the "socially desired" response bias, and to the placebo effect.

11. Pay attention in drawing conclusions to the countries in which the studies were conducted. Rigorous research is conducted in many countries around the world, that is, the concern is not with the internal validity of such studies. Rather, it is prudent to be reasonably concerned that the social, cultural, economic, and geographic conditions prevailing in other countries may not automatically allow the results to be generalized to the country of the reviewer. This phenomenon is a well-recognized issue when a reviewer in a resource-scarce country consumes studies conducted in places with vastly greater access to resources. Reviewers in resource-rich countries, though, may not as readily appreciate this issue of generalizability.

10.6.9 Knowledge Translation

From the beginning of the evidence-based practice era it has been recognized that implementing practice recommendations is often easier said than done. A host of organizational, individual, and communication factors may complicate the process of ending one intervention approach long used, and adopting a new one. There can be many steps in the successful implementation of new instruments or interventions, not the least of which is ascertaining the time and costs involved. There are known factors which facilitate knowledge translation, and there are factors known to inhibit it.

Sometimes, even strong evidence, left to itself, does not self-implement. A careful, intentional, carefully planned process must be undertaken to ensure the translation (the transition) is successful. Some knowledge by practitioners and health care managers and administrators of implementation science (the study of knowledge translation) can be very useful. There now exist journals entirely devoted to implementation science, and there are excellent articles appearing in occupational therapy journals (e.g., Juckett et al., 2021), which can help practitioners through the process.

10.7 Summary

This chapter has examined how to combine the findings of several similar research studies together, in order to formulate better recommendations for therapy practice. This combining can be done in the form of a systematic review of published studies. Another form of this combining is a meta-analysis, conducted on quantitative studies, where the results of each study contribute to a mathematical conclusion about the outcomes of the studies. A third way of combining is meta-synthesis, which is a set of procedures to bring together or synthesize the results of several qualitative studies. Each of these combining methods contains approved steps to strengthen the validity of their overall findings. In therapy disciplines there is a currently accepted method of assessing the risk of bias of published studies, extracting key segments of information from them about their design and results, and making a claim about the strength of evidence they convey together as a set of studies. These steps form the essence of evidence-informed/evidence-based practice. Finally, procedures and challenges in the application of this new knowledge to practice, called knowledge translation, were addressed.

11

Evaluation, Assessment, and Testing

Evaluation is an essential part of the occupational therapy process, quality improvement, and enhancing the accuracy of research. When done well, it can help identify problems, inform decision making and build professional knowledge.

The Health Foundation (2015)

The evaluation process is focused on finding out what the client wants and needs to do; determining what the client can do and has done; and identifying supports and barriers to health, well-being, and participation. Evaluation occurs during the initial and all subsequent interactions with a client. The type and focus of the evaluation differ depending on the practice setting; however, all evaluations should assess the complex and multifaceted needs of each client.

American Occupational Therapy Association (2014)

OPERATIONAL LEARNING OBJECTIVES

By the end of the chapter, the learner will be able to:

1. Define key concepts in testing
2. Identify the major purposes of testing
3. Know where to look for bibliographies of tests in books, test catalogues, and online
4. Know how to select a test for a specific function and target population
5. Know how to evaluate the reliability and validity of tests
6. Know how to incorporate tests into a capstone project or research study
7. Determine the skills necessary in:
   a. administering tests
   b. scoring tests
   c. interpreting the results of tests
8. Develop an objective attitude in selecting a test instrument and evaluating its effectiveness
9. Identify the potential sources of error in testing

This chapter addresses using standardized assessments as dependent variable measures in research studies. We discuss some of the important issues regarding testing and evaluation in occupational therapy research as stated in the questions below:

What are the key concepts that underlie testing and evaluation in research studies?

How do you select the most appropriate test or evaluation for a research study or capstone project?

Why is testing and evaluation an intrinsic part of occupational therapy research?

What are some exemplary evaluations and tests used in occupational therapy and occupational therapy research?

What are the important factors such as reliability and validity in the accuracy of a test or evaluation as it relates to research?

What are examples in occupational therapy research or capstone projects of applying a specific test or evaluation procedure?

11.1 Key Concepts in Testing

- Measurement and testing are one of three sources of information in the evaluation of clients (interview, observation, and testing), and are the focus topic of this chapter.

- Measurement and testing tools in general are designed for three purposes in therapy: to describe the current level of a person's ability or functioning, such as daily living skills or muscle strength, or to conduct a needs assessment of a group (diagnostic); to measure changes in function, such as improvement in social skills (evaluative); and to predict future functioning, such as the ability to drive an automobile safely (predictive).

- Test data may be collected through self-report (survey or checklist), proxy-report (parent or teacher report on a child), or a functional performance test (the core measurement contribution of occupational therapists to the medical or educational team (Rogers & Holm, 2022).

- A measurement scale is a system of assigning scores consistently to a trait or characteristic. Its precision determines whether it is a nominal, ordinal, interval, or ratio scale of numbers (see Chapter 3).

- A test or an evaluation instrument ideally is an objective and standardized measure of a sample of behavior.

- The value of a test depends on its stated purpose, the extent to which its consistency and precision (reliability and validity) have been established empirically, and the feasibility for the practitioner attempting to use the test.

- The degree of accuracy of a test is based on its ability to be consistent (reliability) and to test what it claims to measure (validity).

- Measurement error of a test is derived from factors such as weakened reliability or validity of the instrument when used by this practitioner on this client in the given setting, bias or inattention of the test administrator, fatigue, anxiety, inattention, or lack of motivation on the part of the client, and adverse testing conditions such as a noisy environment.

- Data from heterogeneous populations tend to be normally distributed, while data from homogeneous populations tend to be skewed. For example, in a normal heterogeneous population we expect the average or median height of a male to be 5 feet 9 inches. In a homogeneous population such as basketball players in the NBA, the average height of a player is around 6 feet 7 inches and is positively skewed (approaching a ceiling effect).

- A norm-referenced test (NRT) is a standardized sampling of behavior that uses data such as mean averages from a heterogeneous group of individuals in interpreting results.

- A criterion-referenced test (CRT) is a standardized sampling of behavior that bases the measurement of performance on accepted standards of competency such as in driving skills and behavior.

- An important quality of a diagnostic test is its ability to distinguish between clients who have a deficit or problem and those who do not.

- An important quality of an evaluative test is its ability to accurately detect changes in an individual's behavior (e.g., improvement from pre- and post-intervention in independence in performing ADL and IADL).

- An important quality of a predictive test is its ability to accurately measure a behavior that is indicative of a client's ability to perform in the discharge setting.

See Table 11–1.

11.2 Reliability

Reliability in general is defined as consistency in performance such as in a job where an individual performs dependably and accurately without variance or unpredictability. The reliability of a measuring instrument is in the consistency of its readings. For example, in measuring joint range of motion with a standard goniometer, we expect that trained testers will have similar results. The reliability of an instrument can be affected by ambiguity such as poorly worded instructions for completing a task to the person being tested. It can also be compromised by test environments that are noisy, visually distracting, or too hot or too cold. In a research study it is extremely

Table 11-1

Key Concepts in Tests and Measurements

- **Assessment** refers to the entire process of obtaining, interpreting, and documenting an individual's functional status (American Occupational Therapy Association, Uniform Terminology Task Force, and the Commission on Practice, 1993; Powell, 2008). Assessment involves gathering data from client records, the client, family members, administration of one or more assessment tools or procedures, and integrating the information so that appropriate therapy can be planned (Powell, 2008)
- **Evaluation** refers to "gathering data on performance, such as activities of daily living (ADL) or observation, or using a specific tool or tools in one or more areas" (Powell, 2008, p. 390).
- **Measurement** is "a process of assigning quantitative values to objects or events according to certain rules" (Sattler, 2008, p. 92).
- A **measurement scale** is a system of assigning scores to a trait or characteristic.
- A **test** is essentially an objective and standardized measure of a sample of behavior (Anastasi & Urbina, 1997).
- A **major purpose** of a test is to predict future performance based on a current sample of behaviors.
- An **important quality** of an evaluative test is to accurately detect change in an individual's behavior (e.g., improvement).
- The **value** of a test depends on its purposes, ability to predict outcome, and the degree of consistency and precision in defining a variable.
- The **degree of accuracy** of a test is based on its ability to be consistent (reliability) and to test what it claims to measure (validity).
- The **sources of error in measurement** are derived, for example, from the unreliability of the instrument, bias of the test administrator, behavior from the client, and adverse test environment.
- **Distributions of data** from heterogeneous populations tend to be normally distributed, while data from homogeneous populations tend to be skewed.
- A **norm-referenced test** is a standardized sampling of behavior that uses data from a heterogeneous group of individuals in interpreting results.
- A **criterion-referenced test** is a standardized sampling of behavior that bases performance on accepted standards of competency.

Note. Adapted from *Psychological testing* (7th ed.) by A. Anastasi and S. Urbina, 1997, and *Assessment of children* (3rd ed. Revised) by J. M. Sattler, 1992.

Source: Adapted from Anastasi and Urbina (1997) and Sattler (1992).

important for the researcher to provide the established empirical reliability of the test. The reliability of a test is usually stated as a correlation coefficient, such as $r = .90$, or as an extent of agreement (Intraclass Correlation Coefficient or ICC). The higher the coefficient the higher the reliability of a test. A perfect value would be $r = 1.00$, but this perfection is never expected to be seen, given inevitable measurement error.

11.2.1 Test-Retest Reliability

Test-retest reliability is usually measured by administering the test twice to a group of individuals and calculating the extent of agreement between each individual's scores. Note that using a simple correlation coefficient to indicate agreement could lead to an erroneous conclusion. The two sets of scores could be highly correlated (coefficient of 0.80 or above) yet one set of scores is shifted upward compared to the other set (i.e., the agreement is lacking). For this reason, most calculations of

reliability now use a statistic based on ANOVA, which directly measures the extent of agreement. The most commonly used one is called the Intraclass Correlation Coefficient.

11.2.2 Internal Consistency Reliability

For split-half reliability, the test is divided into two equal parts (often, even versus odd-numbered items) and the scores on these two parts are examined for agreement. High disagreement would indicate that the test unevenly measures the individual's ability, or that different sections of the test measure distinct abilities.

11.2.3 Intra- and Inter-Rater Reliability

In both therapy and research study settings it is highly desirable that the taker of measurements does so consistently from day-to-day. It is also important to show that a group of testers all generate the measurement data in a consistent way. Test developers will establish these types of reliability of the test through empirical studies, where the same group of clients is tested repeatedly by the same individual (for intra-rater reliability) or by a group of testers (for inter-rater reliability). Desired levels of agreement are ICC values of .8 to .9.

11.3 VALIDITY

Validity reflects the authenticity and accuracy of a test. Does the test measure what it purports to measure and nothing else? A test may measure a concept consistently or reliably, but it may not, in fact, measure what the researcher identifies as the target of the test. Tests purporting to measure variables such as cognitive ability, stress management, sensory integration, and attitudes toward individuals with disabilities may also be measuring other variables. The degree to which a test is valid is the amount of empirical evidence that corroborates that the test is actually measuring what it claims to measure.

For example, tests that purport to directly measure an observable trait, such as joint range of motion, have a higher probability of measuring that trait and only that trait. In contrast, tests that claim to measure a trait indirectly, such as self-esteem, will have a greater challenge establishing their validity. With such indirect measurements other factors can too easily interfere. For example, personality, attitude, values, perceptions, interests, and motivations can interact in complex ways, affecting self-esteem at a given moment. Researchers seeking to validate a test are always limited by their ability to precisely corroborate the findings. Traditionally, validity is established on the following bases.

11.3.1 Face Validity

Face validity is the most basic and sometimes crude measure of a test's validity. It is based on informal and superficial inspection of test items. Clients who have had the test administered to them, as well as trial testers and other experts, are shown the test and asked, "On the face of it, does it seem (or feel) to be measuring what it claims to measure?" A large majority answering in the affirmative establishes the test's face validity.

11.3.2 Content Validity

Content validity is the degree to which the test appears to measure all aspects of a concept, according to experts in the field. Each item is analyzed for accurately and appropriately measuring the concept of interest, such as clinical depression. In this example, experts would evaluate whether the test touched on all aspects of depression, and did not include items that were actually measuring

educational background, leisure skills, or independence in IADL. A high percentage of agreement among experts as to the comprehensiveness and precision of the content of the test is sought, usually 80–90%.

11.3.3 Concurrent Validity

Concurrent validity is the strength of correlation with another standardized instrument that has previously been established as having good reliability and validity (called, "having good psychometrics"). A new test may be developed because it is less time-consuming and less expensive than another established, validated instrument. Concurrent validity is determined by administering both tests to the same group of individuals, and then calculating the correlation coefficient between the two sets of test scores. A correlation coefficient of .7 or above is desirable.

11.3.4 Predictive Validity

Predictive validity is the degree to which a test can predict a client's performance accurately over a period of time (longitudinally). For example, a test devised to predict success in a graduate program for occupational therapy students, or a test to indicate whether a client will experience a safe and successful discharge home from a rehabilitation program after a stroke are cases where predictive validity will be important. In the examples, follow-up data from longitudinal studies would determine the correlation between the initial test predictor score and subsequent success in the program or at home. A predictive coefficient of .7 to .8 would be desirable for most purposes. A clinical example of predictive validity can be found in Brown and Finlayson (2013). They discovered that a performance-based assessment, the Performance Assessment of Self-Care Skills (PASS) predicted the odds of an aging client receiving home care within the follow-up period better than self-report measures of ADL.

11.3.5 Discriminative (Diagnostic) Validity

Discriminative validity is the extent to which a test can differentiate between individuals who have an occupational performance problem and those who do not. A cut score on the test is established after trialing the test on many individuals. Those scoring above the cut score are said to have the problem; those scoring below the cut score are said to not have the problem. For example, Rodakowski et al. (2014) found that performance of daily activities could discriminate between older adults with normal cognition and those with a mild impairment.

Discriminative validity is numerically established by examining the false positive (falsely indicating someone has the problem) and false negative (missing someone who has the problem) rates generated by the test across many individuals. A well-designed discriminative test will have rates of 10–20% or less for each of these "false" outcomes. Note that once a test is finalized, attempting to reduce the false positive rate by changing the cut score will inevitably increase the false negative rate. To reduce both false rates simultaneously, a better test would need to be developed.

11.3.6 Construct Validity

Construct validity is considered to be the highest form of empirical evidence that is most sought after by researchers. Construct validity assumes a solid theoretical rationale underlying the test. In establishing construct validity for a test, the researcher uses statistical analysis of empirical data to substantiate the position that the test is in fact measuring all of the defined variable and only the defined variable. High concurrent validity coefficients with similar tests, and low coefficients with other tests that measure different constructs, would contribute to a test's construct validity. Naturally, all other types of validity would be called upon to bolster the claim for construct validity. For example, an investigator devising a test to measure self-image would first adopt or construct a theory that underlies the concept. The theory would include developmental factors, relationships with other variables, and behavioral observations supporting the definition of the construct. Then empirical data would be assembled from the administration of the test in conjunction with other tests, and coefficients would be calculated. Finally, the test developer would assemble all the information together to support the claim of construct validity for the new test. In cases where the construct is thought to have a physical or physiological underpinning, it may be possible to check for the presence of the construct. In the case of dementia, for example, a cognitive test developer could eventually have the test results checked for accuracy through MRI or even brain autopsies, but the high cost prevents this step from being taken very often.

11.3.7 Ecological Validity

Given a test that demonstrates adequate levels of reliability and validity of all types, there remains the question of whether results from such a test actually have meaning in the community life of a client. The question is analogous to asking of a research study of high internal validity, whether it has external validity (generalizability). This test relevance to real life has been called ecological validity. To establish it for a test, the developers show a correspondence between test outcomes and actual performance in the community settings where clients lead their lives. An example is described in Hamera and Brown (2000), where a performance measure for persons with schizophrenia, the Test of Grocery Shopping Skills,

was shown to measure the ability to shop for food in the community for these clients.

11.4 Item Analysis

When devising a test, test developers are interested in the effectiveness of individual test items for differentiating between higher and lower scoring individuals. The developer is also interested in eliminating those items that are ambiguous and have a low discriminative level. Item analysis is a method of gauging the difficulty value and ambiguity of each item. In item analysis, the percentage of successes and failures are calculated for each item. For example, if items 1, 2, and 3 are completed successfully by 80%, 60%, and 40% of the participants, respectively, we can infer that item 3 is either more difficult or more ambiguous than item 1 or 2. Another method is analyzing items to determine which items were passed by high overall scorers and failed by low overall scorers. This analysis will enable the researcher to separate out those items that have discriminative value. Items that are passed by all examinees have little discriminative value but may indicate the level at which all members of the group are functioning. This may be particularly important in criterion-referenced tests where the test administrator is most concerned with issues related to competency.

TABLE 11–2
STEPS IN THE EVALUATION PROCESS
1. Identify the function to be measured.
2. Identify a published instrument to measure condition, or develop a new standardized procedure for evaluation of function.
3. Identify the skill level necessary to use a test instrument.
4. Identify the possible factors in the environment, tester, subject, or test instrument that can potentially distort the test results.
5. Identify the target population for which the test is intended and for which norms have been established.
6. Strictly follow the directions and procedures for administering and scoring the test, or modifying the test procedure to enable the client with disabilities to perform at a maximum level.
7. Interpret the results based on a. norm-referenced data based on the general population, or b. criterion-referenced data for client performance or competence.

11.5 Outline of Overall Evaluative Process of Testing

The steps in the overall evaluative process of testing are listed in Table 11–2 and are elaborated upon in the following section.

The first step in the process of testing is to determine what will be measured and to operationally define the variable. The researcher must be precise and state clearly what is to be discovered. For example, a researcher is interested in evaluating visual perception. Visual perception consists of a number of different skills, such as discrimination, spatial orientation, form-constancy, memory, figure ground, closure, and visual-motor integration. Although it is possible to evaluate visual perception as a whole, effective intervention necessitates an understanding of the individual's ability in each of the various components.

Once the researcher has identified the function to be measured, an instrument to measure that function is selected. Often a published instrument is available. Sometimes published instruments may be better because of the known psychometric properties; however, it may be that there is no instrument, and the researcher has to develop one. This is frequently true when a researcher wishes to use a standardized interview, survey, or observation scale to gather research data.

11.5.1 Qualifications for Administering a Test

If the researcher chooses to use a published instrument, then it will be necessary to determine what qualifications

Level A

There are no special qualifications to purchase these products.

Level B

Tests may be purchased by individuals with:

A master's degree in psychology, education, speech language pathology, occupational therapy, social work, counseling, or in a field closely related to the intended use of the assessment, and formal training in the ethical administration, scoring, and interpretation of clinical assessments.

OR

Certification by or full active membership in a professional organization (such as ASHA, AOTA, AERA, ACA, AMA, CEC, AEA, AAA, EAA, NAEYC, NBCC, CVRP) that requires training and experience in the relevant area of assessment.

OR

A degree or license to practice in the health care or allied health care field.

OR

Formal, supervised mental health, speech/language, occupational therapy, social work, counseling, and/or educational training specific to assessing children, or in infant and child development, and formal training in the ethical administration, scoring, and interpretation of clinical assessments.

OR

Work for an accredited institution

Level C

Tests with a C qualification require a high level of expertise in test interpretation, and can be purchased by individuals with:

A doctorate degree in psychology, education, or a closely related field with formal training in the ethical administration, scoring, and interpretation of clinical assessments related to the intended use of the assessment.

OR

Licensure or certification to practice in your state in a field related to the purchase.

OR

Certification by or full active membership in a professional organization (such as APA, NASP, NAN, INS) that requires training and experience in the relevant area of assessment.

Anonymous. (2023a)

are needed to administer the test. Qualification levels are set by the APA Standards for Educational and Psychological Testing (AERA et al., 2014), and most test publishers adhere to this policy. Levels A, B, and C qualifications are required by Pearson Test Publishers.

11.5.2 Test Contaminants

The next step in the process involves identifying the possible factors in the environment, tester, participant, or test instrument that can potentially distort the test results. These factors are outlined in Figure 11–1. The researcher will want to eliminate as many of these contaminating factors as possible and take steps to mitigate the remainder of the distorting factors.

11.5.3 Target Population

Once the researcher has identified the variable to be measured, the tests to be used, and the potential sources of error that need to be addressed, the researcher must identify the target population for which the test is intended and for which norms have been (or will be) established.

11.5.4 Standardized Protocol for Administration

Whether the researcher is administering a published standardized test or one that was self-developed, the instrument must be administered in an objective, standardized

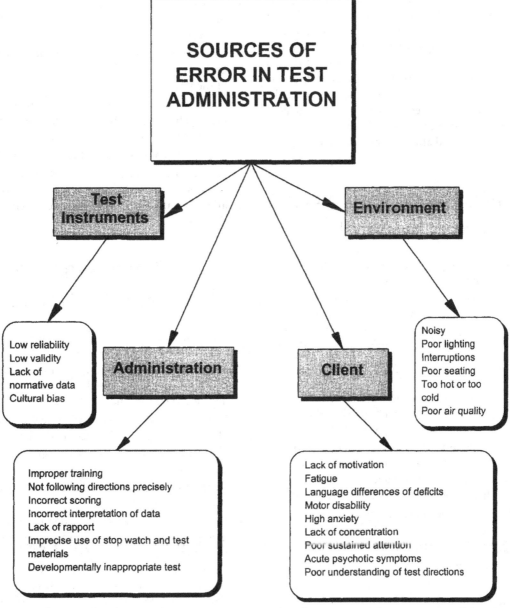

Figure 11–1 Potential sources of error in test administration. Errors come from four main areas: the instrument itself, the administration of the test, the client or subject, and the environment.

way every time. An alteration in the test directions or in how much cuing is given the test taker or client can confound the results, making them less reliable. When the directions or procedures must be modified for the comfort or understanding of the participant, this must be documented in the final test report. Keep in mind that the alteration or modification of the administering of a test will render comparing the score to the norms invalid.

11.5.5 Interpreting Results of the Test

The final step is to interpret the results based on either the typical performance as determined by the norms from a general population (norm-referenced tests) or by a standard that is set prior to the administration of the test (criterion-referenced tests). For example, a researcher wants to evaluate the effects of a cognitive rehabilitation program with individuals who have incurred a traumatic brain injury. The researcher has a choice of measurements: for example (a) a standardized test that measures cognitive ability such as the SCATABI (Scales of Cognitive Ability for Traumatic Brain Injury) or the BTHI (Brief Test of Head Injury) and compare the results with the expected level based on the norms for the general population, or (b) a custom-designed self-evaluation administered before and after the intervention.

11.6 CHARACTERISTICS OF A GOOD TEST IN RESEARCH

The consistency and precision in evaluating a participant's performance or improvement in a research study depend on the quality of the test instrument used for this purpose. The desired test characteristics are listed below.

- For which population is the test designed (e.g., children with learning difficulties, individuals with schizophrenia, persons with muscular dystrophy)?
- What are the specific purposes of the test (e.g., diagnosing an occupational problem, planning intervention goals, determining prognosis, establishing baseline data, or documenting progress)?
- What are the areas of function identified in the test (e.g., social development, leisure interests, perceptual-motor abilities, handwriting, ADL skills, ability to live independently, or cognitive level)?
- What are the methods used to evaluate a client? Primary sources for evaluating a client include:
  - *medical records:* demographics, previous treatment, and outcomes
  - *educational records:* educational attainment, achievement scores

  - *observation of performance:* therapists and teacher observations
  - *interviews:* formal or unstructured individual interviews
  - *objective tests:* objectively scored paper-and-pencil tests, performance scales, and verbal tests
  - *survey questionnaires:* group tests, forced choice or open-ended questions
  - *self-reports:* evaluation of intervention effectiveness through client's perspective
  - *reports from peers, teacher/therapist, or family:* informal reports or observations
  - *biomechanical or physiological measurement of human factors:* devices or machines used to measure the traits.

- Is there a standardized procedure or manual of instructions for administering the test and interpreting results? Are there tables of normative data?
- Are there special skills or certifications that are necessary to administer, score, and interpret results of the test?
- Is the scale of measurement used in collecting data identifiable (i.e., continuous, such as interval or ratio, or discrete, such as nominal or ordinal)?
- Are sources of error controlled or mitigated?
- Are research data reported (such as those derived from previous studies, including reliability, validity, and normative scores), called the psychometrics of the test?

11.7 ASSUMPTIONS IN PROFESSIONAL EVALUATION

The major assumptions in evaluation that guide a therapist in assessment are outlined below.

- Evaluation is an essential factor in the occupational therapy process. It is used to determine the client's abilities, interests, and potentials.
- Evaluation is used to establish baseline data so as to allow comparison with outcome results.
- Evaluation is based on reliable and valid instrumentation. The degree of accuracy in measurement depends on the degree of reliability (consistency) and validity (precision).
- Error is always present to a degree in evaluation, owing to anomalies in the examiner's presentation of test materials, degree of client anxiety or fatigue, client's motivation, less-than-perfect reliability of the test, and a less-than-ideal testing environment. Test scores obtained are a sample of the client's

performance and represent an approximation in a given time frame of actual abilities.

- The reliability of the test score is increased by mitigating potential error factors that could distort the test results.

- Evaluation can provide data for documentation and can be the basis for establishing intervention efficacy and quality assurance. Careful evaluation is an essential method for objectively determining client progress.

11.8 MAJOR PURPOSES OF TESTING IN RESEARCH

The major purposes of testing are as follows:

- Establish baseline data (experimental and quasi-experimental research: pre-test)

- Evaluate outcome or effectiveness of interventions (experimental research and quasi-experimental research: post-test)

- Assess the degree of relationship between two variables (correlational research)

- Evaluate the quality of health care or educational progress for certification or accreditation (evaluative research)

- Assess developmental landmarks (developmental research)

- Assess individual values, interests, or attitudes (descriptive survey research)

- Evaluate differences between groups (experimental and quasi-experimental research research)

- Evaluate functional performance (inclusion criteria for selecting participants from the target population)

11.9 CONCEPTUAL MODEL FOR SELECTING A TEST INSTRUMENT FOR RESEARCH

Whether to select a test from a published source or to construct a new test to measure a defined variable is a frequent dilemma. The measuring instrument is an essential part of a research study and represents the operational definition of a variable. Figure 11–2 shows this process.

The conceptual definition of a variable should lead the investigator to a specific test that is the most appropriate for operationally defining a variable. In research, it is crucial that the investigator select a measuring instrument that has a high reliability and is a valid measurement of outcome. Measuring improvement in such areas as physical capacities, cognitive functions, independent living skills, vocational skills, or perceptual-motor abilities depends directly on the adequacy and sensitivity of the instrument to measure change. A measuring device that does not have the capacity to record subtle changes in an individual's functioning or behavior is of less value to the researcher studying intervention efficacy.

When deciding on the instrument to use for the outcome measure, the researcher must ask the following questions:

- *What is the target population?* Examples include:
  - typical children, adolescents, adults, elderly

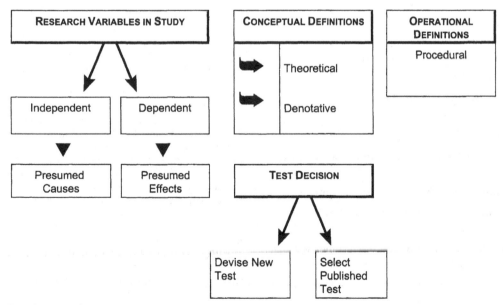

Figure 11–2 Critical steps in determining an appropriate test instrument.

- individuals with an intellectual deficit
- people with a psychiatric diagnosis
- people with physical challenges (specify diagnosis)
- whether there are specific demographic or diagnostic variables to consider.

- *What are the specific areas of function to be measured?* Examples include:
  - manual dexterity
  - cognitive abilities
  - independent living
  - work experiences
  - work tolerance
  - social skills
  - self-care
  - communication
  - mobility and transportation.

- *Where will the client be assessed?* Some places include:
  - home
  - sheltered workshop
  - clinical environment
  - school
  - office
  - hospital.

- *What are the methods for evaluating function and how will the individual be assessed?* Some methods include:
  - observation of performance
  - paper-and-pencil tasks
  - interview
  - self-report and self-evaluation
  - direct measure of function through a standardized test instrument
  - evaluation by teacher, therapist, or parent
  - work samples
  - parent, therapist, or teacher report
  - computerized test.

- *Is the test reliable and valid?*
  - Are there standardized directions for administration of the test?
  - Are norms available for comparison purposes?
  - How many participants were used in collecting the normed values?
  - How was reliability of the test established (e.g., test-retest, split half, equivalent forms)?
  - How was the validity of the test established (e.g., concurrent, construct, predictive)?

- *Are the test results easily interpreted?*

- *What is the scale of measurement (i.e., ordinal, nominal, interval, or ratio, affecting which statistical analysis may be appropriately used)?*
- *How will the individual be tested?*
  - In a single session? (summative evaluation) or over several sessions? (formative evaluation)
  - In a large group, small group, or individually?

11.10 BIBLIOGRAPHIC SOURCES

Another consideration for testing involves asking the following question: Where can I find the most appropriate test instrument? Examples of test instruments related to occupational therapy can be found in a number of sources, including:

Asher, I. E. (Ed.) (2014). *Occupational therapy assessment tools: An annotated index* (4th ed.). American Occupational Therapy Association.

Bortnick, K. (2014). *Occupational therapy assessments for older adults: 100 instruments for measuring occupational performance.* SLACK.

Carlson, J. F., Geisinger, K. F., & Jonson, J. (Eds.). (2021). *The twenty-first mental measurements yearbook.* University of Nebraska Press.

Enderby, P., John, A. & Petheram, B. (2013). *Therapy outcome measures for rehabilitation professionals: Speech and language therapy, physiotherapy, occupational therapy* (2nd ed.). Wiley.

Fischer, J., & Corcoran, K. (2007). *Measures for clinical practice: A sourcebook.* Vol. 1: *Couples, family and children* (4th ed.). Free Press.

Gardner, B. T., Dale, A. M., Buckner-Petty, S., Rachford, R., Strickland, J., Kaskutas, V., & Evanoff, B. (2016). Functional measures developed for clinical populations identified impairment among active workers with upper extremity disorders. *Journal of Occupational Rehabilitation, 26*(1), 84–94. https://dx.org.doi: 10.1007/s10926-015-9591-4

Hemphill-Pearson, B. J. & Urish, C. K. (Eds.). (2020). *Assessments in occupational therapy mental health: An integrative approach* (4th ed.). SLACK.

Hinojosa, J., & Kramer, P. (Eds.). (2014). *Evaluation in occupational therapy: Obtaining and interpreting data.* American Occupational Therapy Association.

Klinkman, M. S. (2009). Assessing functional outcomes in clinical practice. *American Journal of Managed Care, 15*(11 Suppl), S335–S342.

Lezak, M. D., Howieson, D. B., Bigler, E. D., & Tranel, D. (2012). *Neuropsychological Assessment* (5th ed.). Oxford University Press.

Mulligan, S. E. (2003). *Occupational therapy evaluation for children: A pocket guide* (2nd ed.). Williams-Wilkins.

Power, P. (2013). *A guide to vocational assessment* (5th ed.). Pro-Ed.

Rashid, M., Harish, S. P., Mathew, J., Kalidas, A., & Raja, K. (2022). Comprehensive rehabilitation outcome measurement scale (CROMS): Development and preliminary validation of an interdisciplinary measure for rehabilitation outcomes. *Health Quality of Life Outcomes, 20*(1), 160. https://dx.org.doi:10.1186/s12955-022-02048-z

Rubin, S. E., Chan, F., & Thomas, D. L. (2003). Assessing changes in life skills and quality of life resulting from rehabilitation services. *Journal of Rehabilitation, 69*(3), 4–9.

Sattler, J. M. (2020). *Assessment of children: Cognitive foundations and Applications* (6th ed.). Author.

Vroman, K., & Stewart, E. (2013). *Occupational therapy evaluation for adults: A pocket guide.* Lippincott Williams & Wilkins.

11.11 Test Instruments

Testing instruments and procedures can be found for almost every functional area that health professionals might want to assess. Figure 11–3 diagrams the major categories of tests used in occupational therapy, while the following paragraphs and sections describe the major tests. We have tried to select tests that are commonly used or are important for specific reasons (e.g., they have normative data for populations of individuals with special needs; they are used more frequently by occupational therapists; they have high validity and reliability). We recognize that not all tests are listed. For a more complete list, the reader should refer to one of the books on assessment and testing listed in the previous section or to a publisher's catalog (listed in section 11.14). As a caution, new tests are developed yearly, and established tests are revised frequently. Thus, even the most up-to-date book may not have a current description of a test. In case of doubt, it is wise to contact the publisher directly.

11.11.1 Psychosocial Tests

Assessment of psychosocial functioning occurs in several different ways. Observation of a client may occur in a hospital or residential setting. Professionals and paraprofessionals may complete checklists or rating scales as part of the evaluation. Self-report scales used for assessment of self-concept, role identity, stress management, and leisure activities are valuable in the assessment of a client's perceptions. Some of the more widely used psychosocial scales are described in Table 11–3 (cognitive and general assessments) and Table 11–4 (independent living skills). Additional tests are described in the following paragraphs. Other examples can be found in the publishers' catalogs.

Behavior Rating Scales

Behavior rating scales are used by therapists, teachers, and caregivers to obtain information about a client's behavior. Usually, the rating scales are paper-pencil instruments filled out by the client's parents or family. Occasionally, rating scales may be completed by a member of the peer group (e.g., another student in the classroom) or as a self-report measure.

Although rating scales are widely used, there are some disadvantages and cautions to be considered when using them. Because the rating scale is a subjective measurement, response bias is possible. For example, the responder may rate the individual either too harshly or too positively (e.g., the Halo effect) than is realistic, or the respondent may

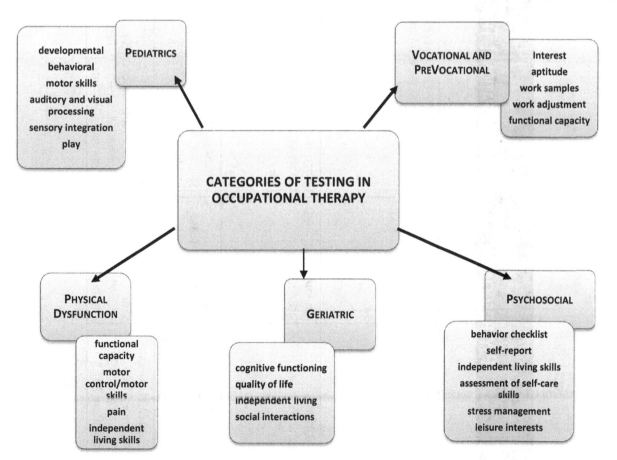

Figure 11–3 Categories of tests used in occupational therapy assessment.

TABLE 11-3

PSYCHOSOCIAL ASSESSMENT IN OCCUPATIONAL THERAPY: COGNITIVE AND GENERAL ASSESSMENT

TEST	TARGET POPULATION	PURPOSE	VARIABLES ASSESSED	PUBLISHER
Allen Cognitive Level Screen (ACLS; Allen, 1985; Allen et al., 2007)	Clients with psychiatric or cognitive impairment	Screening tool to classify people into one of six cognitive levels based on Allen's theory	Six cognitive levels: • automatic actions • postural actions • manual actions • goal-directed actions • exploratory actions • planned actions	Available from: S & S Arts 75 Mill St. Colchester, CT 06415
B. H. Battery (Hemphill-Pearson, 1999)	Children and adolescents	Structured instrument to assess the psychological area of human function	Cognitive and psychosocial factors, including problem-solving and abstraction, frustration tolerance, organization and internal structure, and self-awareness	In B. J. Hemphill-Pearson (1999), *assessments in occupational therapy mental health: An integrative approach* (pp. 139–152)
Burns Cognitive Performance Test	Adults with Alzheimer disease	Assesses cognitive function in daily activities. Based on the Allen Cognitive Disability Theory	Uses performance on six activities of daily living to predict function in context and assess safety needs	In Burns, Mortimer, & Merchak (1994), *Journal of Geriatric Psychiatry Neurology,* 7(1), 46–54.
Canadian Occupational Performance Measure (COPM; Law et al., 1991; Latest edition, 2019)	Individuals age 7 through adults; individuals with disabilities	Designed to detect changes in client's perception of occupational performance. Based on the Model of Occupational Performance	Three subareas are measured (self-care, productivity, and leisure) with total scores obtained for performance and satisfaction.	Canadian Association of Occupational Therapists

TABLE 11–4

PSYCHOSOCIAL ASSESSMENT OF INDEPENDENT LIVING SKILLS

TEST	TARGET POPULATION	PURPOSE	VARIABLES ASSESSED	PUBLISHER
Bay Area Functional Performance Evaluation (BaFPE, 2nd ed.; Williams & Bloomer, 1987; Klyczek & Stanton, 2008)	Adults with psychosocial dysfunction	Two components: Task Oriented Assessment (TOA) which assesses goal-directed abilities, as well as cognitive, performance, and affective areas of function. Social Interaction Scale (SIS) assesses social behaviors observed in 5 different settings.	Twelve functional parameters (e.g., memory, organization, attention, abstraction, task completion, affective and behavioral impression) and seven categories of verbal and non-verbal social interaction.	Available from Allegro Medical
Canadian Occupational Performance Measure (COPM, 4th ed.; Law et al., 1991; Law et al., 2004)	Clients with disabilities; can be used with children as young as age 7	Outcome measured designed to detect changes in client's perception of occupational performance	Self-care, productivity, leisure, performance and satisfaction; based on the Canadian Model of Occupational Performance	Canadian Association of Occupational Therapists
Comprehensive Occupational Therapy Evaluation (COTE; Brayman, & Kirby, 1976; Brayman, 2008)	Adults with acute psychosocial dysfunction who are hospitalized	Provides standard, objective means of rating behaviors of hospitalized patients on a frequent basis	General behavior, interpersonal behavior, task behaviors	In B. J. Hemphill-Pearson (2008), *Assessments in occupational therapy mental health: An integrative approach* (2nd ed.; pp. 113–124; 406–412)

(continued)

TABLE 11–4 (CONTINUED)

PSYCHOSOCIAL ASSESSMENT OF INDEPENDENT LIVING SKILLS

TEST	TARGET POPULATION	PURPOSE	VARIABLES ASSESSED	PUBLISHER
Independent Living Skills Evaluation (ILSE; Johnson et al., 1981; 2008).	Adults (age 18 and above) with chronic psychosocial dysfunction who are living in independent living arrangements or living independently	Assess levels of living skills in areas necessary for independent community living	Ten major categories of independent living in home, community, and personal areas	Community Living Experiences, Inc., The Independent Living Project San Jose, CA 95112
Kohlman Evaluation of Living Skills (KELS, 4th ed. (2016); McGourty, 1988; Pickens et al., 2007)	Clients with acute psychiatric disorders, elderly patients in acute care hospitals; adolescent through elderly; must be used cautiously with individuals hospitalized for more than 1 month	Quick assessment to provide information about a person's ability in everyday functioning in daily living skills, independent living, and work/leisure	Seventeen living skills in areas of self-care, safety/health, money management, transportation/telephone, work/leisure	American Occupational Therapy Association
Milwaukee Evaluation of Daily Living Skills (MEDLS; Leonardelli, 1988a, 1988b, 2008; Haertlein, 1999)	Adults with chronic mental illness who are inpatients or outpatients in a community mental health clinic (CMHC)	Assessment of behavior and skills needed for adequate functioning in the client's living situation	Twenty subtests measuring basic living skills, safety, communication, and transportation	In B.J. Hemphill-Pearson (1999), *Assessments in occupational therapy mental health: An integrative approach* (pp. 245–257).
Performance Assessment of Self-Care Skill: Version 3.1 (PASS; Holm & Rogers, 1999, 2008)	Adults	Assess the types of assistance needed to remain in the community	Mobility, ADL, and IADL from perspectives of independence, safety, and task outcome	In B. J. Hemphill-Pearson (2008), *Assessments in occupational therapy mental health: An integrative approach* (2nd ed.; pp. 101–110)

restrict the scores to the central range of the scale, leaving the impression that the individual being rated has few strengths or weaknesses. Second, results from rating scales obtained from different settings (e.g., individual therapy and large classroom settings) may show very different scores. This is frequently attributable to the client's varied behavior in different settings. Finally, differences obtained on the scales may occur because of the day on which the rating scale was completed (Martin et al., 1986), thereby reflecting the behavioral variability of either the rater or the client. For these reasons, more than one informant should be used to complete the rating scale. If possible, each informant should complete a couple of rating scales over a short period of time.

11.11.2 Physical Dysfunction, Motor Control, Pain, and Independent Living

Tests of functional capacity, vocational aptitude, pain, and independent living assess the degree to which an individual can live and work independently in the community. They assess an individual's ability to perform physical movements as they relate to work, vocational activities, and activities of daily living. These measures are extremely important to rehabilitation research in determining whether an individual can return to work, or live in independent housing.

Functional capacity evaluations are comprehensive and systematic approaches that measure the client's overall physical ability such as muscle strength, endurance, joint range of motion, ambulation, sitting, standing, and lifting.

Outcome Measures and Functional Assessment

There is an ongoing need in health care to demonstrate intervention effectiveness and client satisfaction. Outcome measures have been designed to evaluate the overall functional status of clients who have received services in hospitals, outpatient clinics, rehabilitation centers and home environments. These outcome measures (Keith, 1984) are usually designed for specific populations such as individuals with stroke, brain injury, spinal cord injury, low back pain, psychological diagnoses, or developmental disabilities. The outcome measures evaluate the client's ability to perform functional activities of daily living, the degree of pain intensity, ability to work, to engage in leisure activities, to have restful sleep, to drive, to be mobile in the community, to communicate, to ambulate, to academically achieve, and to perform other activities related to functional abilities. See Table 11–5.

11.11.3 Vocational and Prevocational

In assessing an individual's prevocational ability, an evaluator seeks information on basic ability levels required

for specific occupations. Most prevocational tests involve some aspect of motor coordination. Some tests require the subject to perform tasks using small tools in an assembly operation. Work samples are used to assess an individual's vocational aptitudes, worker characteristics, and vocational interests (Nadolsky, 1974) in areas of vocational potential in various fields, gross and fine manual dexterity, visual and tactile discrimination, and work habits. The tests purport to measure skill proficiencies related to industrial work. Tests have been devised, such as the *McCarron-Dial Systems* (1986) to evaluate work behavior at a sheltered workshop as indicative of vocational aptitude. Other work sampling tests include the *Micro Tower System of Vocational Evaluation* (IDC Rehabilitation and Research Center, 1977) and the *VITAS: Vocational Interest, Temperament and Aptitude System* (Vocational Research Institute, n.d.). More elaborate methods for assessing vocational aptitude in various industrial occupations are available through the Valpar International Corporation (www.valparint.com) and Stout University

11.11.4 Geriatrics

A number of tests have been developed specifically for the geriatric population. Many of these tests can be administered in a hospital, nursing home, or home setting. Table 11–6 describes some of the most commonly used tests administered by occupational therapists.

11.11.5 Pediatrics

The basic assumption underlying all child development scales is that development is vertical, sequential, and hierarchical. Arnold Gesell and associates in the Children's Development Laboratories at Yale University during the 1920s and 1930s used observational analysis of children's behavior to develop norms. Gesell provided the earliest data correlating age with task attainment in such areas as perceptual-motor, language, and personal-social. Since Gesell, other developmental researchers have provided data demonstrating that the growth of human abilities is linked to a biological clock that determines when behavior unfolds at certain critical periods along an age continuum. Differences among child development tests are based on the factors identified and the methods used for assessment. These tests also vary in the time involved in administering a test and in the requirements needed to validly interpret results. For example, the *Denver Developmental Screening Test* (Frankenburg et al., 1990) takes about 15 minutes to administer by non-professional health aides, whereas the *Gesell Developmental Scale* requires at least two hours to administer by a professionally trained psychometrician. Examples of the most widely used child development scales are described in Table 11–7.

TABLE 11–5

FUNCTIONAL ASSESSMENT OF PHYSICAL DYSFUNCTION

	STRENGTH/RANGE OF MOTION	MOTOR CONTROL/ MOTOR SKILLS	PAIN	INDEPENDENT LIVING SKILLS
Purpose	To measure specific joint mobility, grip strength, individual muscle strength	To evaluate a person's functional motor activities	To evaluate a client's pain to determine effectiveness of treatment (Ross & LaStayo, 1997)	To assess activities of daily living (ADL) skills and Instrumental ADL skills needed to live safely in the community (Power, 2000)
Sample of Variables Assessed	• range of motion • muscle strength • grip strength • pinch strength	• muscle tone • postural control • gross mobility • somatosensory function • functional hand skills • ambulation • balance	• pain intensity • pain tolerance • pain location	• social skills • self-care • safety and health • communication • transportation • money management • home making • leisure activities • fall risk
Examples of Widely Used Instruments	*Goniometric Range of Motion* (Gilliam & Barstow, 1997) Available from: Rehab Outlet or Performance Health Grip Dynamometers (Gilliam & Barstow, 1997; Bohannon, Peolsson, Massy-Westropp, Desrosiers, & Bear-Lehman, 2006) Available from: Rehabilitation Outlet or Performance Health Manual muscle tests (Radomski & Trombly Latham, 2014; Daniels & Worthingham, 2013, 9th ed., by Hislop, Avers, & Brown) Pinch meters and gauges: Available from: Performance Health or Abledata	*Assessment of Motor and Process Skills* (AMPS; Fisher, 1994, 2016) *Bruininks-Oseretsky Test of Motor Proficiency, 2nd ed.* (BOT–2; Bruininks, 1978; Bruininks & Bruininks, 2005) *Fugl-Meyer Assessment* (Fugl-Meyer et al., 1975; Gladstone et al., 2002) Rivermead Mobility Index (Collen et al., 1991; Wade et al., 1992)	*Short-Form McGill Pain Questionnaire–2* (SFMPQ–2; Melzack, 1987; Dworkin, 2009) *Visual Analog Scale* (VAS; Carlsson, 1983; Cork et al., 2008)	*Barthel Index* (Mahoney & Barthel, 1965; Collin et al., 1988; Sainsbury Seebass et al., 2005) *FIM* ™ Formerly known as Functional Independent Measure Granger et al., 1977; Keith et al., 1987; *Performance of Self-care Skills* (PASS; Rogers & Holm, 1989; Chisolm et al., 2014) Fall risk: *Berg Balance Scale* (Berg, et al., 1992) Measures mobility and balance *Falls Efficacy Scale* (Tinetti et al., 1990) Measures fear of falling to the extent of avoiding activities

TABLE 11–6

GERIATRIC TESTS

TEST	PURPOSE	VARIABLES ASSESSED	FORMAT	PUBLISHER
COGNITIVE FUNCTION				
Contextual Memory Test (Toglia, 1996)	Measure awareness and strategy use	• awareness of memory • recall of drawn items • strategy use	Interview/questionnaire	Therapy Skill Builders San Antonio, TX Washington University St. Louis, MO baumc@wustl.edu MOCA – Montreal Cognitive Assessment www.mocatest.org/splash/
Executive Function Performance Test (EFPT; Baum et al., 2008)	Executive function	• initiation • organization • sequencing • safety • task completion	Performance of real-world tasks	
Montreal Cognitive Assessment (MOCA; Nasreddine, 1996)	Screening for cognitive impairment	• memory • visuo-spatial • executive function • attention/concentration • language • orientation to time and place	Oral questionnaire administered by examiner; performance tasks	
Allen Cognitive Level Screen (ACLS; Allen, 1985; Allen et al., 2007) Independent Living	Screening for cognitive impairment	Six cognitive levels: • automatic actions • postural actions • manual actions • goal-directed actions • exploratory actions • planned actions	Performance tasks	S & S Arts www.ssww.com/therapy-and-rehab/allen-diagnostic-module/

(continued)

TABLE 11-6 (CONTINUED)

GERIATRIC TESTS

TEST	PURPOSE	VARIABLES ASSESSED	FORMAT	PUBLISHER
COGNITIVE FUNCTION				
Assessment of Living Skills and Resources–Revised-2 (ALSAR-R2; Williams et al., 1991; Clemson et al., 2008)	Assess the living skills and resources in a community dwelling of elderly residents to determine treatment protocol and assist in problem-solving	Assesses areas of IADL including • use of community resources • leisure time • medication • finances • home management	Rating scale, with scores combined to determine risk	Available from: www.sydney.edu.au/health-sciences_documents/assessment-living-skills.pdf
Instrumental Activities of Daily Living (IADL Scale; Lawton & Brody, 1969; Graf, 2007)	Assess skills needed by elderly individuals to live independently	Eight categories of IADL (e.g., housekeeping, food preparation, finances) rated according to level of independence	Rating scale, with higher scores indicating need for more assistance	*Gerontologist* (1969), 9, 179–186.
Older Adults Resources and Services (OARS; Duke University Center for the Study of Aging and Human Development, 1978; 2005)	Multidimensional instrument to obtain information in basic and instrumental activities of daily living for elderly clients living in the community	• social resources • economic resources • mental health • physical health • activities of daily living	Structured interview, now available online exclusively.	Available from: OARS Center for the Study of Aging and Human Development Box 3003 Duke University Medical Center Durham, NC 27710, USA
Performance Assessment of Self-Care Skills (Rogers, 1984) General Well-Being Screen	Tool to measure occupational performance of daily life tasks	• Functional mobility • BADL • IADL (physical) • IADL (cognitive)		Available at www.shrs.pitt.edu/performance-assessment-self-care-skills-pass
Rapid Geriatric Assessment (Little, 2017) Quality of Life	Package of four screening tools covering frailty, nutrition, cognition, strength	Indicates risk of several geriatric syndromes and need for further assessment	Structured interview	Available at www.aging.slu.edu
World Health Organization Quality of Life-BREF (Harper et al., 1996) Fall Risk Assessment See Table 11-5	Measure of quality of life across world cultures	• physical • psychological • social • environmental	Self-administered questionnaire	The WHOQOL Group, Programme on Mental Health, WHO, CH-1211 Geneva 27, Switzerland www.who.int/mental_health/media/en/76.pdf

TABLE 11-7

PEDIATRIC TESTS

DEVELOPMENTAL	BEHAVIOR	SENSORY PROCESSING AND INTEGRATION	VISUAL, AUDITORY, AND MOTOR PROCESSING	SCHOOL AND HOME
Bayley Scales of Infant and Toddler Development, 4th ed. (Bayley-IV®; Bayley & Aylward, 2019)	*Adaptive Behavior Assessment System-3* (ABAS-3; Harrison & Oakland, 2015)	*Sensory Profile™-2* (Dunn, 2014)	*Bruininks-Oseretsky Test of Motor Proficiency-2* (BOT-2; Bruininks & Bruininks, 2005)	*Roll Evaluation of Activities of Life* (REAL; Roll & Roll, 2018)
Pediatric Evaluation of Disability Inventory (PEDI; Haley et al., 1992)	*Behavior Rating Inventory of Executive Function-2* (BRIEF-2; Gioia et al., 2015)	*Sensory Processing Measure 2* (SPM-2; Kuhaneck et al., 2007; Glennon et al., 2017)	*Beery-Buktenica Developmental Test of Visual-Motor Integration-6* (BEERY™ VMI; Beery et al., 2010)	*Participation and Sensory Environment Questionnaire (Home and Teacher Version)* (PSEQ; Piller & Pfeiffer, 2016)
Pediatric Evaluation of Disability Inventory—Computer Adaptive Test (PEDI-CAT; Haley et al., 2011)		*Sensory Integration and Praxis Tests* (SIPT; Ayres, 1989) Soon to be replaced with EASI and SP3D (2023)	*Motor-Free Visual Perception Test-4* (MVPT-4; Colarusso & Hammill, 2015)	*Classroom Sensory Environment Assessment* (C-SEA; Kuhanek & Kelleher, 2015)
Peabody Developmental Motor Scales-3 (PDMS-3; Folio & Fewell, 2023)			*Test of Visual-Motor Skills-3* (TVMS-3; Martin, 2006)	*Children's Kitchen Task Assessment* (CKTA; Rocke et al., 2008)
Movement Assessment Battery for Children-2 (Movement ABC-2; Henderson et al., 2009)			*Test of Visual-Perceptual Skills (Nonmotor)-4* (TVPS-4; Martin, 2006, 2016)	*Goal-Oriented Assessment of Lifeskills* (GOAL; Miller & Oakland, 2013)
Miller Function & Participation Scales (M-FUN; Miller, 2006)				*Children's Assessment of Participation and Enjoyment & Preferences for Activities of Children* (CAPE/PAC; King et al., 2017)
				Canadian Occupational Performance Measure (COPM; Law et al., 1990)

11.11.6 Special Populations

In addition to general tests in psychosocial function and physical disabilities, assessments have been developed for specific populations such as individuals with arthritis or stroke. These tests have been standardized with these specific populations and should not be used with typical individuals.

11.11.7 Neuropsychological Batteries

Clinical neuropsychology is a relatively new field that attempts to relate behavior to brain functioning. Neuropsychological testing is requested by clinicians, therapists, and educators in special cases. For example, neuropsychological testing is usually requested when a client has sustained a traumatic or acquired brain injury. Neuropsychological testing may also be requested when a more specific understanding of an individual's strengths and weaknesses is desired. Although individual neuropsychological tests can be given, frequently neuropsychologists use a specific battery of tests generated by their particular philosophical stance.

11.12 REVIEWING AND EVALUATING TESTS

For the researcher, the selection of a valid and reliable instrument is critical. Knowledge in assessing the adequacy of a measuring instrument is extremely important in view of the literally thousands of tests that are published by test corporations. Before the researcher chooses a test to use in research, the purpose for the test must be determined. Does the researcher need to screen participants for normal intelligence or average achievement? Is adaptive behavior a concern? If the purpose of the investigation is to evaluate the effect of a treatment on reducing low back pain, the researcher will want to make sure that all subjects have clinically significant low back pain (see Figure 11–4).

The next step in determining which test to use is to review the appropriate tests that are available, taking into account the psychometric properties, including the reliability, validity, and measurement scales of each test. If there are special qualifications in administering the test, the researcher must know who is able to administer the test and how long it will take to administer. The following outline and examples of reviews of tests will illustrate the manner in which tests are analyzed (Stein, 1988).

11.12.1 Outline for Reviewing Tests

1. **Title**
2. **Date published, date(s) revised**
3. **Authors**
4. **Publisher**: Distributor of test or where test is available
5. **Target population**: What was the original sample from which data were collected in terms of age,

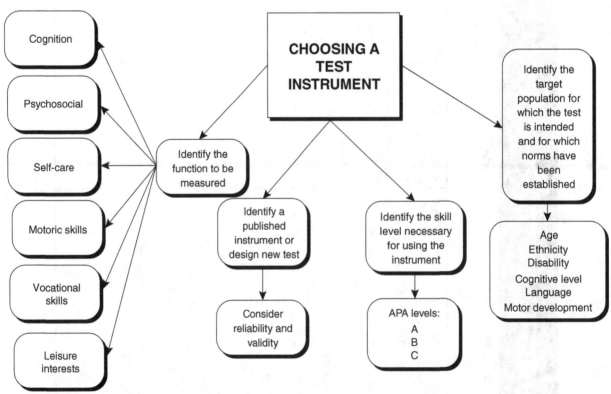

Figure 11–4 Factors in choosing a test instrument.

diagnostic group, and geographical location? Is there a specific target population for which the test is appropriate?

6. **Variables assessed**: What are the specific areas of function, behavior, or skills that are being assessed? What are the major stated purposes of the test?

7. **Measurement scales**: What is the level of measurement in the test?

    a. Discrete

       i. Nominal scale of measurement refers to evaluating variables using independent categories such as *can* or *cannot perform a specific task.*

       ii. Ordinal scale of measurement refers to evaluating variables using magnitude and ranking such as *completely dependent in task, needs assistance,* or *independent functioning.* Variables can also be rated on a numerical scale from 1 to 5, for example, where 1 indicates *no self-care* and 5 *indicates cares for self independently.*

    b. Continuous

       i. Interval scale of measurement refers to scoring variables on a continuous scale with equal distances between score values. Pulse rate, blood pressure, joint ROM are usually measured on interval scales.

       ii. Ratio scale of measurement incorporates an absolute zero.

8. **Administration of instrument**: Who administers the test and when is it administered? How long does it take to administer? Is there special training to administer the test? Are special materials or environments required?

9. **Scoring and interpretation of results**: Are there overall scores or subtest scores derived from the test results? Are there norms available to interpret raw scores? How are the results used in treatment planning, documentation of progress, and discharge recommenddations?

10. **Test reliability and validity**

11. **Other comments**: Included in this section are miscellaneous comments such as the theoretical orientation or conceptual framework of the test and its appropriateness for the clinical researcher.

12. **References**: Includes books, journals, test manuals, and other sources where the test has been published or critically evaluated.

11.12.2 Example of Test Review

1. *Kohlman Evaluation of Living Skills* (KELS; Thompson, 2016)

2. Originally published in 1978, revised in 2016 (4th edition)

3. Linda Kohlman Thomson, MOT, OTR, OT(C), FAOTA

4. American Occupational Therapy Association, 6116 Executive Boulevard, Suite 200 North Bethesda, MD 20852-4929

5. Clients with acute psychiatric disorders, elderly patients in acute care hospitals; adolescent through elderly. Must be used cautiously with individuals hospitalized for more than 1 month.

6. Thirteen living skills categorized into five main domains: self-care, safety and health, money management, transportation and telephone, and work and leisure are measured.

7. Measurement scales: Nominal and ordinal scales.

8. The test can be given by an occupational therapist or occupational therapist assistant when supervised by the occupational therapist.

9. Each of the 13 living skills are scored for either "independent" or "needs assistance" with a score of 1 (*Vi* for the work and leisure category) given if the client needs assistance. Items scored as independent are given a score of 0. Individuals obtaining an overall score of *5Vi* or less are considered able to live independently; scores above $5^1/i$ suggest the client needs assistance to live in the community.

10. Inter-rater reliability ranges from $r = .84$ to 1.00. Concurrent validity has been measured at $r = .78$ to .89 with Global Assessment Scale; –.84 with BaFPE. The test has successfully predicted which geriatric patients could live independently.

11. The test provides a quick assessment to provide information about a person's ability in everyday functioning in daily living skills, independent living, and work/leisure.

12. Kohlman, L. (2020) Kohlman Evaluation of Living Skills (KELS). In B. J. Hemphill, *and C. K. Urish Assessments in Occupational Therapy Mental Health: An integrative approach* (pp. 397–405). SLACK.

Thompson, L. K. with Robnett, R. (2016). *The Kohlman Evaluation of Living Skills* (4th ed.). American Occupational Therapy Association.

Thompson, L. K. (1999). The Kohlman Evaluation of Living Skills. In B. J. Hemphill-Pearson (Ed.), *Assessment in occupational therapy mental health: An integrative approach* (pp. 231–244). SLACK.

(continued)

Pickens, S., Naik, A. D., Burnett, J., Kelly, P. A., Gleason, M., & Dyer, C. B. (2007). The utility of the KELS test in substantiated cases of elder self-neglect. *Journal of the American Academy of Nurse Practitioners, 19*, 137–142. doi: 10.1111/j.1745–7599.2007.00205.x

Burnett, J., Dyer, C. M., & Naik, A. D. (2009). Convergent validation of the Kohlman Evaluation of Living Skills as a screening tool of older adults' ability to live safely and independently in the community. *Archives of Physical Medicine and Rehabilitation, 90*, 1948–1952.

11.13 CRITERION-REFERENCED TESTS AND NORMATIVE-REFERENCED TESTS

Until recently, most tests were norm-referenced tests, or NRTs. These tests, described previously, were developed to classify individuals into levels of instructional groups. The scores obtained by the normative sample on a norm-referenced test are distributed along a normal curve. Raw scores obtained by individuals taking a norm-referenced test are compared with the normative sample and can be converted into standard scores and percentiles.

There are several advantages to NRTs. Individuals taking the test are compared with the general population, thus the performance of a student or patient can be judged to be typical or atypical. Because NRTs are usually commercially published, psychometric characteristics such as reliability and item analysis are carefully considered in the development. Additionally, standardization of an NRT includes administering the test to large samples of individuals stratified across many socioeconomic groups, ages, ethnic backgrounds, and educational levels. In this way, raw scores obtained from a given individual can be compared to the raw score obtained from a population containing individuals with similar demographic characteristics.

At the same time, there are disadvantages to an NRT. Because the tests are broad measures of a subject and contain a limited number of items from many areas within that subject, they are often referred to as survey tests. It is not uncommon for an NRT designed to be used in grades 1 through 12 to include only 100 sight words. Because there is no national or state curriculum, the content found on the test may not match the curriculum of a particular school or community. Finally, because the number of items in each area is limited, the test results cannot be used to measure small gains in progress. Likewise, there is limited value for using the results of an NRT in determining an instructional or therapeutic program.

The purpose of NRTs is (a) to compare an individual's achievement or performance with other individuals of the same age, educational level, and socioeconomic status, and (b) to obtain information regarding the normal population. When these tests are used with atypical populations,

there may be a bias, which results in systematic error. In spite of these disadvantages, NRTs are useful in research.

In testing circles during the last 30 years, there has been a growing interest in devising criterion-referenced tests (CRTs) in lieu of norm-referenced tests (Deno, 1985). CRTs, first proposed by Glaser (1963), use content or curricular domains to set the standard of performance. They compare the performance of an individual with a specified level of mastery or achievement rather than with a normative population. Because the performance is compared with a criterion, performance on these tests allows the therapist or teacher to suggest specific classroom goals and objectives to use in program planning. Progress can be monitored more effectively and more discretely.

CRTs are based on a comprehensive theory that generates ideas for a specific content domain. In CRTs, items are selected systematically to represent the content domain. For example, if an investigator is interested in determining the visual perceptual skills of individuals, the first task would be to determine the dimensions of visual perception from the theoretical and experiential perspectives. The investigator would use the theoretical framework to guide the writing of test items, making sure that each aspect of the framework is covered by test items in the CRT. Operational performance standards, obtained by surveying a representational sample of the general population, are used in writing test items. For example, a survey of ten-year-olds would reveal that most of them have no difficulty with activities involving visual closure or visual figure ground. The operational performance standard, therefore, might be set at a criterion level of 90% accuracy for recognition of figures in tasks involving visual figure ground or visual closure.

One example of criterion-referenced testing occurs when measuring an individual's independent living skills. For instance, in the criteria of dressing completely, we might include the act of putting on all clothes right-side out and frontwards, tying shoes, and fastening all fasteners. The individual's ability to perform this activity is measured by a given standard. Until the individual has mastered the expected standard, the individual is not considered to have reached competency. Social skills and self-help skills are often evaluated by CRTs.

CRTs are sometimes referred to as curriculum-based measures (CBMs) or curriculum-based assessments (CBAs). CBAs and CBMs establish a student's instructional needs in relationship to the requirements of the actual curriculum being used. Just as with CRTs, the CBAs and CBMs assess mastery of learning by providing an operational performance criterion as a necessary standard for passing. Although commercial CRTs are available, teachers and occupational therapists frequently develop the measurement instrument based on their own criteria.

In summary, a CRT is constructed to obtain measurements that can be interpreted in terms of specific criteria or performance standards. Scores obtained on NRTs, however, are interpreted in terms of comparison to a population. The choice of which test to use depends on the outcome desired. If a researcher is interested in the progress of a particular student over time, a CRT is more appropriate; however, if the researcher is interested in the differences between two groups of participants, then an NRT may be more appropriate.

A summary of the differences between criterion- and norm-referenced tests is given in Table 11–8. This summary may help in deciding which type of test to use.

11.13.1 Applying Criterion-Referenced Concepts to Research

The major content areas for researchers in evaluation include basic living skills, interests, work behavior, and skill attainment. If one uses a criterion-referenced approach to these areas, one should look for the following factors:

- The theory underlying these concepts is identified.
- Research evidence supporting any assumptions of the test is stated.
- The content domain of the test that considers a comprehensive view of skills, interests, and behavior is discussed.

- The specific target population is operationally defined in terms of age, intelligence, education, and degree of disability.
- The test items are generated by selecting representative samples of behavior.
- Performance standards in the test are based on systematically collected data from representative samples of the target population.
- Test items are pilot-tested for clarity and ease of administration.
- Scoring methods are devised that are operationally defined.
- Reliability and validity data are established.
- A test manual for administering, scoring, and interpreting data is provided.
- The degree of competency needed for administering the test is included in test descriptions.

11.14 Test Publishers

The development of new tests and measuring instruments is a relatively recent event in the occupational therapy professions. The nature of these fields and the service-oriented process of intervention have led to an emphasis in the past on developing new treatment techniques rather than measuring outcome variables. However, as the need for accountability and validation for treatment continue on federal and state governmental levels (e.g., through laws such as Individuals with Disabilities Improvement Education Act [IDEIA-2004] and Americans with Disabilities Act [ADA]), the use of tests and measuring instruments to justify therapeutic and educational intervention has become more important. Many tests have been developed for use by occupational

TABLE 11–8	
COMPARISON OF CRITERION-REFERENCED TESTS AND NORM-REFERENCED TESTS.	
CRITERION-REFERENCED TESTS	**NORM-REFERENCED TESTS**
Absolute standards of competence or mastery are established based on theory	Relative standards are based on normal standards
Scores are derived from standards or behaviors or competency	Scores are compared to established norms
Scores are interpreted based on what the student can or cannot do and then used diagnostically	Scores are interpreted by percentile ranks, standard scores, and organized along a normal curve
Content or items are comprehensive of domain	Content of items are a sample of domain
Cut-off score for passing is based on minimal standards of competency	Cut-off score for passing is based on pre-established percentile rank
Theoretically all can pass or all can fail	The number of failures is predicted before test is administered

therapists in the past ten years. In addition to publishing their own tests, most test corporations distribute the most widely used tests. Thus, in general, a researcher is not limited to one corporation to obtain a specific test.

The following list includes test publishers that are frequently used by occupational therapists and other clinicians.

American Occupational Therapy Association (AOTA): https://myaota.aota.org/shop_aota/search.aspx#q=assessments&sort=relevancy

Consulting Psychologists Press, Inc.: https://shop.themyersbriggs.com/products/index.aspx

Curriculum Associates, Inc.: www.curriculumassociates.com

Educational and Industrial Testing Service (EdITS): www.edits.net/

Flaghouse Rehabilitation: www.schoolspecialty.com/shop-flaghouse

Lafayette Instrument: www.licmcf.com

Par, Inc.: www.parinc.com/

Pearson Assessments (also PsychCorp): www.pearson-assessments.com/professional-assessments.html

Pro-Ed, Inc.: www.proedinc.com/

Riverside Publishing: www.riversidepublishing.com/

Stoelting Publishing: https://stoeltingco.com/

Stout Vocational Rehabilitation Institute: www3.uwstout.edu/scri/index.cfm

Trace Research and Development Center: http://trace.wisc.edu/

Valpar International Corporation: www.valparint.com/

Western Psychological Services (WPS): www.wpspublish.com/

11.15 Ethical Considerations in Testing

Competence in test use is a combination of knowledge of psychometric principles, knowledge of the problem situation in which the testing is to be done, technical skill and some wisdom.

American Psychological Association (1974, p. 6)

This quote is from the Standards for Educational and Psychological Tests published by the American Psychological Association. To protect psychological tests from abuse, standards fall into three areas: guidelines for devising a new psychological test, qualifications for administering tests, and the guidelines for interpreting results. The following guidelines should be adhered to in using tests:

1. The researcher publishing a new test should provide reliability, validity, normative data, scoring procedure, and qualifications for using the test in an accompanying manual.

2. A standardized test procedure should be carefully followed by the tester.

3. Results should be reported that can be compared to specified populations.

4. The researcher using psychological tests should obtain informed consent from the participant and assure the participant's confidentiality.

11.16 Summary

In the last 50 years, literally hundreds of tests have been developed for use with individuals with and without disabilities. In this chapter, the authors have presented descriptions of tests that are the most commonly used in occupational therapy practice. These tests are available to use by occupational therapists knowledgeable in the administration, scoring, and interpretation of test results. These tests can be used as outcome or descriptive measures in research. The use of a specific test is a key component in the research process and could affect the results if the test selected is not sensitive to changes in individuals or is not reliable or valid; therefore, the researcher should have knowledge of reliability and validity of the test before using it. When using a test in research, the researcher must be aware of the level of qualification needed to administer and interpret it.

Because new tests are developed frequently, the researcher should keep informed. Annual catalogs obtained from the test publishers listed in section 11.14 are helpful in locating new tests. Before developing a new test, occupational therapists should search the literature, references in testing, textbooks, publishers' catalogs, and websites for locating new tests.

12

Scientific Writing for Thesis and Capstone Projects

Vigorous writing is concise. A sentence should contain no unnecessary words, a paragraph no unnecessary sentences, for the same reason that a drawing should have no unnecessary lines and a machine no unnecessary parts. This requires not that the writer make all his sentences short, or that he avoid all detail and treat his subjects only in outline, but that every word tell.

Strunk Jr. and White (1979, p. 23)

OPERATIONAL LEARNING OBJECTIVES

By the end of this chapter, the learner will be able to:
1. State ways to prepare for writing a scientific research paper
2. Proofread for errors in language mechanics and style in scientific writing
3. Identify and discuss the important divisions of a research paper
4. Outline a literature review
5. Compose a reference list or bibliography using the *Publication Manual of the American Psychological Association* (APA) (7th edition)
6. Prepare an oral or poster presentation for a conference
7. Compose a manuscript to submit for publication
8. Critically evaluate a manuscript
9. Design a research (thesis) proposal

DOI: 10.4324/9781003523154-12

12.1 Preparation for Writing a Scientific Manuscript

Scientific writing is a type of technical writing that uses neutral language that is backed by empirical evidence. The main purpose of scientific writing is to communicate with peers in a specific field, new findings that build upon published evidence, or to convey research that replicates or extends a previous study. Effective scientific writing is a skill that becomes more refined as it is practiced. Clear, simple, and direct language is the hallmark of good scientific writing. For some individuals, a major block to writing is the first step of initiating the writing and organizing ideas on paper. The desire to write as if whatever one first puts on paper is chipped forever in granite sometimes can prevent the flow of ideas. Effective scientific writing requires self-criticism and continual revision.

The time and setting in which one writes are important initial considerations. Some individuals do their best writing during the morning in a quiet, sunny room with a large table where they can spread out their computer, reference books, scrap paper, and notes. Others work better in the late evening. Some individuals can work 12–14 hours for several days, followed by several days of complete rest. Some writers report that they work at a set time every day. Setting aside enough time is important, so that the writer does not feel rushed, allowing the writer to feel that something can be accomplished. Scientific writing takes discipline and mental energy and therefore requires concentrated effort. Some students do their best work in a college library, cafeteria, or even in a coffee shop, despite many distractions. Some can write using paper and pencil on a yellow pad, while others prefer working directly on a computer, or dictating by using speech recognition software. It is helpful for writers to discover for themselves, individually, the environment and the means which best facilitate writing a scientific paper.

Writing a capstone project, thesis, or research article for a publication requires self-discipline. In a way, the individual should prepare for writing much as an athlete would train for a sporting event. A period of "conditioning" for mental rigor prior to writing can be important. Some individuals take long walks in nature, ride bicycles for miles, listen to music or take part in physical sports in preparation for writing. Others prepare mentally by playing chess, doing crossword puzzles, solving arithmetic problems, reading prolifically, or doing intricate manual work. Sleeping on an idea or letting it brew beneath the surface for a while also may be helpful. For the author of a research project, completing the document is a creative process. Writing is a continuous open-ended process with much editing and revision. After the first draft, there will be ample time for revision.

The thesis or the capstone project includes an explanation of why the undertaking was initiated and how the methodology serves as an outline for data collection. In completing the study, the writer summarizes the relevant literature, describes the methodology used, presents the results using tables and graphs, discusses the findings, and makes specific recommendations based on these findings in relation to previous research. In this way, the final scientific paper becomes a part of the body of literature, placing the research findings within the context of previous published studies. A well-conceived paper requires critical thinking and analysis by the writer. The conceptual relationships between previous research and present findings must be considered. The hypothesis or guiding question(s) proposed by the writer must be concisely and clearly stated and should cover all the points included in the paper. The arguments used in the paper to advance one's conclusions should be compared with previous results from other researchers. On the other hand, a writer may present new findings that may be contradictory to prior findings or to accepted beliefs in the scientific community.

Another essential component for writing a scholarly paper is to understand as fully as possible the literature encompassing the topic. This is accomplished by completing an exhaustive literature review. The writer will review much more literature than will be discussed in the paper. This fact does not minimize the need for an extensive literature review; rather, it emphasizes the need for the writer to understand the relationship of a specific question to the entire body of knowledge. For an understanding of the occupational therapy methods used to treat individuals with a stroke, the writer would identify the most up-to-date research on the topic through, for example, a Cochrane Review (www.cochranelibrary.com) that evaluates the effectiveness of the interventions through systematic reviews.

The writer would search the medical literature by using PubMed (https://pubmed.ncbi.nlm.nih.gov/). PubMed comprises more than 35 million citations for biomedical literature from MEDLINE, life science journals, and online books. Citations may include links to full text content from PubMed Central and publisher websites.

Other databases related to occupational therapy include:

- OTseeker (www.otseeker.com/Search/BasicSearch. aspx). Since mid-2002, work has been underway to locate, collect, and rate randomized controlled trials and systematic reviews relevant to occupational therapy.
- CINAHL (www.ebsco.com/products/research-databases/cinahl-database). CINAHL indexes the top nursing and allied health literature available including nursing journals and publications from the National League for Nursing and the American Nurses Association.
- REHABDATA (www.naric.com/?q=en/content/cf-rehab-adv-search). The REHABDATA database spans almost 50 years of disability and rehabilitation research. More than 200,000 abstracts are available

through this database, including approximately 115,000 records originally indexed in the Center for International Rehabilitation Research Information and Exchange (CIRRIE) database.

- ERIC – Education Resources Information Center (https://eric.ed.gov/). ERIC is an online library of education research and information, sponsored by the Institute of Education Sciences (IES) of the US Department of Education. This database provides access to information from journals included in the Current Index of Journals in Education and Resources.

It is not uncommon to revise the initial hypothesis or guiding question several times as one's knowledge base increases through reading and reviewing the literature. Writing and reviewing literature is an organic process that helps scholars modify their thinking while extending their knowledge. It is a creative process that calls upon one to be neutral and self-critical. This process is sometimes referred to as "cognitive dissonance" (the state in which there is conflict between one's attitudes and one's behavior, generally resulting in changing one's thinking so that there is equilibrium between the two), or reflective decision making (the process of making decisions by critically examining all sides of the issue). For example, one may change one's attitude toward trans gendering as one becomes more knowledgeable about the subject and perhaps becomes acquainted with someone who is transgendered. The "Socratic method" of learning is another method which is based on the scholar raising critical questions from many perspectives regarding a subject. All these methods rely on the individual's ability to be reflective and open-minded in reviewing the literature and accepting results that may be contrary to the scholar's initial assumptions.

12.2 Outlining the Project

The overall organization of the project, outlined in Table 12–1, is dictated by tradition. Each of the major sections in the research paper contains specific content.

12.2.1 Introduction to the Topic and Establishing the Need for Research or Capstone Project

The first part of the research study or capstone project contains a brief introduction, including the need for the study, and the research or guiding question(s). A pivotal part of this portion of the research paper, capstone article, or manuscript is a clear statement of the hypotheses or guiding questions such that they are (a) well understood, (b) lead the reader to anticipate the major sections of the paper, and (c) indicate the direction in which the paper will be written. For example, a researcher interested in studying aging in place would first state the guiding question such as: What are the factors that enable a person over 80 years old to live a healthy life in the community? In this example, what evidence—such as economic, quality of life, and psychological factors—would justify the study?

Evidence for the need for a study could include epidemiological statistics such as the number of people in the US who are living with a specific disability or the number of homeless persons in a population. For example, in a capstone project, "Developing and implementing a wellness recovery program for people with depression," the student-researcher would state the magnitude of the problem by citing how many people annually in the US are treated for clinical depression, and what costs the condition and the intervention cause society to incur.

Finally, this part of the paper should include definitions for any specific terminology that is used. For example, terms such as sensory integration disorder, cognitive deficit, social skills, and self-care skills should be operationally defined so that a reader can better appraise the paper and so that a subsequent researcher can more closely replicate the study.

Below is an excerpt from the introduction on a study of occupational therapy and stroke, exemplifying the definition of important terms and the citation of the social magnitude of the problem.

> By stroke or cerebrovascular accident (CVA) we refer to those sudden circulatory system episodes that compromise the stability of an affected brain area, either permanently or temporarily. As a result, we will use the defined terms to refer to cerebral infarction, as well as intracerebral and subarachnoid hemorrhages. Stroke is a cerebrovascular disease with great health and social impacts due to its high incidence and prevalence, and for being the leading cause of acquired disability in adults in developed countries. Its incidence in Spain is 187.4/100,000 inhabitants/year. It is a great burden, not only from a health point of view, but also from a personal and family point of view, due to its impact on the lives of the people who suffered it and their caregivers. It is also one of the main causes of hospital stay and death in Spain.
>
> (García-Pérez et al., 2021)

12.2.2 Review of the Literature

The second part of the paper, which contains the literature review, is to some extent a measure of what the student has learned from primary (empirical research studies) and secondary sources (theory papers, systematic reviews, and textbooks). In some papers, this section and the previous section are written as a single part. In a thesis or dissertation, this section is traditionally identified as Chapter 2 or, if written with the introduction, as Chapter 1.

TABLE 12–1

ORGANIZATION

Title Page

Abstract
150   250 words

Introduction Paragraph
Introduces the study
Introduces the purpose

Background
General studies (Independent Variable, pop, Dependent Variables, Results, your interpretation)
Specific studies (shows need) (IV, pop, DV, Results, your interpretation)
Purpose statement
Rationale statement for Hypothesis(es), independent variable
Hypothesis(es)

Method
Participants
Sample size, Gender, mean, and standard deviation of age, inclusion/exclusion criteria,
recruitment method power analysis to justify sample size
Apparatus/Instruments
Procedure
Informed consent, randomization, dates of data collection, research set-up and protocol
Statistical Analysis
Research design, description of dependent variables

Results
Statistical
Descriptive
(figures & tables)
Housekeeping stats

Discussion
Review of purpose
Statement of the results with regard to the hypotheses
Why you got the results (your interpretation)
Comparison with other studies (originally found in literature review background)
Application to OT
Limitations
Future directions

Conclusions
Summary statement of the precise finding of the study as well as your conclusions (what do you
conclude from the study?)

References

Tables

Figures

A good literature review selects relevant papers in a balanced way and cites them to justify the current project. The first task of the scholar is to find the related studies through a search of databases. The second step is to sort through these studies by evaluating their actual relevance, in addition to the reliability and validity of their results. The quality of some published research has been called into question because of the number of predatory journals that publish research without quality peer review. Researchers should consult the Bealls List of Predatory Journals, which is updated frequently (http://beallslist.weebly.com).

Knowledge in a scientific field is part of a cumulative process in which information expands, based on the previous work of researchers. "If I have seen further," Isaac Newton wrote in a 1675 letter to fellow scientist Robert Hooke, "it is by standing on the shoulders of giants" (Newton letter to Hooke, 1675). Breakthroughs in knowledge do not occur spontaneously. The scientist exploring solutions to problems first investigates the previous literature to determine (a) what has been accomplished, (b) what questions still remain, and (c) what research is recommended based on the findings in the literature.

A search of the literature involving the selection of relevant studies is a critical part of the research process. It is impossible to conceive of a researcher devising a research plan without first examining previous findings. The literature search is not only a method of uncovering, it is also a way for the researcher to attain a historical perspective and overview of a problem.

Scientific research is a methodical procedure that advances knowledge. For many scientists, discovery of new information is a process of juxtaposing research from diverse fields in relation to an identifiable problem. In his pioneering work on cybernetics (1948), which had profound influence on modern computers, Norbert Wiener, a mathematician, attained success by brainstorming with engineers, psychiatrists, educators, and physicists. These specialists shared their ideas, and their collaboration enabled the examination of a problem from many perspectives. Wiener, from this experience, developed a theory of thinking based on the integration of physical science theory with behavioral observations. The lesson from Wiener's research is that investigators exploring the literature should not only examine studies directly related to a problem, but also try to find studies from other fields that have an indirect or implied relationship to their question.

If, for example, a researcher is interested in examining the relationship between therapist morale and intervention effectiveness, it could be warranted to search the literature in management psychology, if a preliminary search reveals few studies on the topic in the occupational therapy literature. A diversity of findings would add strength to a study, especially if corroboration derives from different disciplines. The Hawthorne effect (Landsberger, 1958), which was first noted in factory workers, is now widely accepted as a factor in client response to intervention as well.

For example, McCartney (2007) found that there was a moderate Hawthorne effect in a study of patients diagnosed with Alzheimer disease. Spinoffs from research in the space programs (https/spinoff.nasa.gov), such as the advances in nutrition, specialized clothing, computer programming, temperature control, and monitoring of vital body functions, serve as examples of applying data generated from a seemingly unrelated field.

The main goals of the investigator in searching the literature are to:

- make an exhaustive search for the most up-to-date related studies
- identify the landmark studies that had an important impact on the topic of investigation
- evaluate the rigor and internal validity of the research findings
- synthesize the results into subject content areas
- summarize the findings from previous studies
- highlight areas where results are either inconclusive or controversial, and identify limitations of the published findings and recommendations for further research
- justify the current study based on the literature review.

These goals are part of the overall preliminary process of research that precedes the initiation of data collection.

Conceptual View of a Literature Search

The steps involved in a conceptual view of the literature search are listed below:

1. The first step in initiating a literature search is to identify the key words in the study. The key words may be identified through (a) reading a secondary source, (b) professional experience with a particular population, (c) reviewing a journal article, or (d) examining a thesaurus of terms such as the Medical Subject Heading (MeSH; www.ncbi.nlm.nih.gov/mesh) to find key words to build a literature search strategy. ERIC (Education and Resources Information Center; www.eric.ed.gov/), is another database that publishes a thesaurus. These key words can be linked to the independent variable (e.g., intervention technique), dependent variable (e.g., how the desired outcome is measured), outcome measuring device or test instrument (e.g., Allen's Cognitive Level), target population (e.g., individuals with cognitive difficulties from a traumatic brain injury), contextual setting (e.g., assisted living center), age range (e.g., 65 years old and older), or frame of reference (e.g., occupational behavior).

2. Key words are important for scholars when initiating a literature search because they selectively differentiate between similar topics. For example, if a scholar wants to examine the literature on sensory integration, use of the key word phrase "sensory

integration" may exclude studies concerning sensory processing approaches. This exclusion may or may not be desired by the researcher.

3. The next step in a literature search is to locate a recent textbook or review article in which the researcher can obtain an overall summary of the major research on the specific topic. For example, a scholar may be interested in the effectiveness of occupational therapy on improving academic achievement of students with learning disabilities. The scholar would examine a recent textbook on pediatric occupational therapy such as *Case Smith's Occupational Therapy for Children and Adolescents* (8th ed., 2020) by O'Brien and Kuhaneck to gain an overall view of intervention and to identify contemporary references. The textbook may help in the identification of key words and in narrowing the focus of the study.

4. Next, the researcher proceeds with an internet search of recent articles in the field. PubMed®, Google Scholar, MEDLINE, EMBASE, Cochrane Library, OT Seeker, CINAHL, and ERIC are useful for the initial search. Another way to discover recent articles is to scan current issues or yearly indexes of occupational therapy journals. Examining the reference lists of relevant articles may also help to locate other articles. After identifying relevant articles, it is important to save the bibliographic citations and abstract for later use.

5. The next step is the categorization of the articles into types of publications, such as theoretical paper, review, or empirical research (see Table 12–2). Articles can also be categorized into subject areas for easier access later.

6. The researcher must critically evaluate each article for internal validity (i.e., rigor of the methodology)

TABLE 12–2

TYPES OF PUBLICATIONS

TYPES OF PUBLICATIONS	EXAMPLES OF PUBLICATIONS
Primary data research	Journal articles Dissertations Theses Conference proceedings Government documents Statistical surveys
Review articles	Journal articles Monographs
Evaluation findings	Joint Commission on Accreditation Results Special commissions
Conceptual or theoretical papers	Journal articles Monographs Conference proceedings
Position papers	Journal articles Associational and organizational statements Monographs Editorials
Secondary and tertiary information	Popular magazines *Scientific American* Encyclopedias College texts
Other publications	Test manuals Reference books for test instruments Book reviews Software programs and reviews Manuals for self-help devices
Bibliographic references	*Books in Print* Information retrieval system Directories of reference

and external validity (i.e., applicability or generalizability of results). The researcher examines how the variables were defined and controlled, participant selection, randomization, reliability and validity of the outcome measures, and the operational definition of the independent variable, if the study used a quantitative methodology. For an article using a qualitative methodology, corresponding examination would take place. The study's dependability, authenticity, confirmability, and data-gathering and analytic rigor would be appraised.

7. A descriptive tabulation of research studies identified by the literature review is the next step. The researcher designs a table that includes the title of the study, date of publication, authors, number of participants, methodology, intervention used, outcome measures, results (statistical or thematic), and conclusions. Reference management software such as RefWorks, EndNote, or Zotero can be particularly helpful in this stage of the review. For writers who are required to create an annotated bibliography, such reference applications allow for the insertion of the article abstract and provide fields for a brief critique of each study.

8. ChatGPT has become a significant source for information in 2024—"GPT" stands for generative pretrained transformer. It has become a widely used internet site. Over 100 million people worldwide signed up ChatGPT in one month! It is based on artificial intelligence that uses an immense amount of data to answer questions and converse with the user. It differs from a Google search, for example in asking ChatGPT "Is occupational therapy effective?" ChatGPT came up with the following response:

Default (GPT-3.5)

Is occupational therapy effective?

ChatGPT

Yes, occupational therapy (OT) is generally considered effective in helping individuals with a wide range of physical, mental, and developmental conditions to improve their functional abilities and overall quality of life. Occupational therapists work with people of all ages and tailor their interventions to address specific challenges individuals may face in performing activities of daily living (ADLs) and instrumental activities of daily living (IADLs).

Here are some ways in which occupational therapy can be effective:

1. **Rehabilitation:** Occupational therapists help individuals recover and regain independence after injuries or surgeries, such as those resulting from accidents, strokes, or joint replacements. They work on improving physical function and mobility.

2. **Mental Health:** OT can be effective in treating various mental health conditions, including anxiety, depression, and post-traumatic stress disorder (PTSD). Therapists use techniques to help individuals manage stress, develop coping strategies, and engage in meaningful activities.

3. **Pediatrics:** Occupational therapists work with children who have developmental delays or disabilities to improve their fine and gross motor skills, sensory processing, and social interaction. Early intervention can have a significant impact on a child's development.

4. **Geriatrics:** For older adults, OT can help maintain independence and improve their ability to perform daily tasks. This includes strategies to prevent falls, adapt to age-related changes, and manage chronic conditions.

5. **Neurological Conditions:** Occupational therapists assist individuals with neurological conditions like multiple sclerosis, Parkinson's disease, and traumatic brain injuries in managing their symptoms and optimizing their functional abilities.

6. **Autism Spectrum Disorder:** OT is often used as part of a comprehensive approach to help individuals with autism develop social skills, sensory processing abilities, and self-care skills.

7. **Workplace Ergonomics:** Occupational therapists can provide guidance on creating ergonomic workspaces to prevent work-related injuries and improve overall productivity.

8. **Home Modifications:** They can recommend home modifications and adaptive equipment to make living spaces more accessible for individuals with disabilities.

The effectiveness of occupational therapy depends on various factors, including the individual's specific needs, the therapist's expertise, the goals set for therapy, and the individual's willingness to actively participate in the process. In many cases, occupational therapy is integrated into a broader healthcare or rehabilitation plan to achieve the best outcomes.

It's important to note that the effectiveness of occupational therapy is supported by research and clinical evidence. If you or someone you know could benefit from occupational therapy, it is advisable to consult with a qualified occupational therapist who can assess specific needs and develop a personalized treatment plan.

The same question to Google will result in the citing of related articles.

The main advantage or disadvantage of ChatGPT is that it is a secondary source of information. For a scholar or researcher, it is only helpful in initiating a literature search. ChatGPT cannot be used as a primary source of evidence. There is also the threat of plagiarism:

> The use of artificial intelligence tools does not automatically constitute academic dishonesty. It depends how the tools are used. For example, apps such as ChatGPT can be used to help reluctant writers generate a rough draft that they can then revise and update.

> (Eaton, 2023)

The researcher now has the resources to write the literature review section of the paper. The "Funnel Model" described below may assist in guiding the writer.

Funnel Model for the Literature Review

There are many ways to write up a literature review. It can be daunting to the writer to begin. The funnel model, described below, may be useful in many instances.

The top of the funnel—the widest part—is where the section begins. This entails a description of the definition and magnitude of the problem for society. It can include data on the incidence and prevalence of a disease, injury, or condition (henceforth, "condition"), or on the severity of the impact on individuals who are affected. It may also include an estimate of the financial cost to society of this condition. For example, if the study concerns CVA, there would be information on the number of new cases in the US in the most recent year (incidence), the number of people living who have had a stroke (prevalence), how widely and deeply the occupational performance is affected in people who have had a stroke (ADL, IADL, social participation), and the costs accrued by society for the cumulative expenses for medical treatments and rehabilitation, as well as lost earnings by the person with the stroke and the family or caregivers for that person. Public health statistics could be cited here.

The next step in the funnel—a somewhat narrower region—is a description of the effects of the condition on a specific population. In the CVA example above, this narrowing might come from the study's focus on people who had a right CVA. Specific symptoms, such as spatial disorientation and visual field cut leading to left neglect, and their impact on occupational performance would be concisely discussed. Spatial disorientation and visual field cut should be defined. General medical references or an occupational therapy textbook might be cited as the source for this information.

The next narrowing occurs as a discussion is pursued about those effects that are within the scope of occupational therapy practice. Frequently the OT Practice Framework, latest edition, is cited here. Recent studies by occupational therapists on interventions that were investigated can also substantiate that these issues are within the scope of the profession's practice. In the right CVA example, the symptoms fall into the categories of perception and motor planning, and thus they have been established as within the scope of occupational therapy practice.

Next the funnel narrows to the specific effects of interest for the current study, from among all the effects for this specific population that would be within the scope of occupational therapy practice. For example, the scholar might be specifically interested in spatial disorientation.

The next part of the funnel—somewhat narrower again—contains a discussion of the impacts of these specific challenges on occupation. Narrowing again, the writer may focus next on the effects of spatial disorientation on the person's ability to safely perform transfers. Past research studies investigating this relationship, if any have been published, would be cited here.

The next stage in the funnel is the transition to those interventions which have been studied in the past, and how effective they were shown to be. It could be that a new intervention is now available (the one of interest in the current study) or it could be that prior interventions have never been tried on the specific population of interest. In the example, the new intervention may be a set of color-tagged visual cues. Here, the writer might cite any report on the existence of the new intervention (for people with CVA or for any other application of the cuing system), or the writer may be left asserting that "no pertinent example of such an intervention was found in the review conducted."

The funnel has now narrowed all the way down to the spout. Out of the spout flows the purpose of the current study. "Therefore, the purpose of the current study will be [was] to determine the effectiveness of using a color-tagged, visual cuing system for improving the safe and independent performance of wheelchair to toilet transfers in persons 65 years of age or older with a right CVA." (Note: this study theme was fictionally constructed as an example.)

Pertinent literature has been organized, sequenced, and critically reviewed as it is cited in turn during the logical funneling, from social impact down to the statement of the current study's purpose.

It is not necessary for the writer to cite every article or book that was found on the topic of the study. First, the writer can assume that the reader has some knowledge of the subject. Second, redundant citations are simply not necessary. Major, oft-cited relevant studies should be covered, though, and if there is disagreement as to outcomes from an intervention, both sides must be fairly presented in the literature review.

Scholars may be tempted to review and incorporate articles after only reading their abstract. After all, one may think, the abstract does contain all the major elements of the study. Good research protocol, though, is for each article cited to be read by the writer in its entirety. Frequently there is crucial information in the article text that was not reflected in the abstract. This information may have to do with the demographics of the clients who actually ended up in the study (e.g., that the sample was 75% male), or an attrition rate of 40% which is higher than desirable for strong internal validity, or the fact that the intervention was only provided 70% of the planned time, due to participant illness. Any such detail can reveal critical factors in the appraisal of the validity of the study.

Using the funnel model, or whichever parts of it are appropriate, may help the writer present the source material critically and in a logical flow, leading to why this particular study is being or was proposed.

Research studies need to be selected and discussed fairly, citing both positive and negative research findings that relate to the present study question. In this way, one can avoid writer bias, as shown in the following example from literature on treating depression. A researcher may be interested in the effect of using cognitive-behavioral therapy (CBT) with individuals with depression. A review of literature identified the following categories of studies involving the use of CBT to treat individuals with depression: (a) those where there was no improvement (Jacobson et al., 1996; Twisk, & Maes, 2009), (b) those where there was improvement (Clarke et al., 1999; Pinninti et al., 2010), and (c) those where there was mixed success (McIntosh et al., 2010). These differences in conclusion need to be carefully analyzed. Did the samples in the various studies have markedly varying demographics? Was the CBT that was applied operationally the same in all studies? Was the length of time or the intensity of the intervention equivalent in all studies? Did providers delivering the intervention have essentially equivalent expertise and experience with CBT?

Sometimes the content of the intervention or the delivery method may make a difference. In a meta-analysis of the effects of CBT on people with depression, López-López et al. (2019) found:

Cognitive-behavioural therapy (CBT) is an effective treatment for depressed adults. CBT interventions are complex, as they include multiple content components and can be delivered in different ways. We compared the effectiveness of different types of therapy, different components and combinations of components and aspects of delivery used in CBT interventions for adult depression. We conducted a systematic review of randomised controlled trials in adults with a primary diagnosis of depression, which included a CBT intervention. Outcomes were pooled using a component-level network meta-analysis. Our primary analysis classified interventions according to the type of therapy and delivery mode. We also fitted more advanced models to examine the effectiveness of each content component or combination of components. We included 91 studies and found strong evidence that CBT interventions yielded a larger short-term decrease in depression scores compared

to treatment-as-usual, with a standardised difference in mean change of –1.11 (95% credible interval –1.62 to –0.60) for face-to-face CBT, –1.06 (–2.05 to –0.08) for hybrid CBT, and –0.59 (–1.20 to 0.02) for multimedia CBT, whereas wait list control showed a detrimental effect of 0.72 (0.09 to 1.35). We found no evidence of specific effects of any content components or combinations of components. Technology is increasingly used in the context of CBT interventions for depression. Multimedia and hybrid CBT might be as effective as face-to-face CBT, although results need to be interpreted cautiously. The effectiveness of specific combinations of content components and delivery formats remains unclear…

(López-López et al., 2019)

In some cases, it may be that the variations among study results cannot be explained, at least for now. Reporting this state of affairs clearly and honestly is in the interests of the entire research and practitioner communities.

12.2.3 Method

The third section of a research paper or capstone project includes a description of the methodology used in the study. This portion of the study should be written in a detailed yet concise manner, with enough information available so that others can replicate the study.

Traditionally, there are three subdivisions in the method section: (a) a profile of the participants sought for the study, (b) the measurement apparatus or tests used to collect data, and (c) the procedures used for data collection and analysis. Detailing demographic factors sought by the design, such as number of participants, age range, gender, and ethnicity, and exclusion criteria, is critical. For quantitative studies, a statistical power analysis (such as with the free application G*Power) should be used, when possible, to calculate the number of participants required, given the expected effect size of the intervention, in order for the study to have a selected percentage probability of being successful (rejecting the null hypothesis). Additional demographic information that may be important for the study might include education level, socioeconomic level, handedness, disabilities, prior testing, and previous need for therapies, especially occupational therapy. If a control group is used, the demographics of the control group must at a later point be compared with those of the experimental group. The manner in which participants were chosen (e.g., stratified random sample, voluntary response to a social media posting) is also described in this section. Eventually potential participants will be screened by the researcher for eligibility to enroll in the study. If eligible, the participant volunteer undergoes the informed consent process. An attestation by the researcher that informed consent was conducted for all participants must be reported in the final paper, usually in the Method section.

A description of the tests or measurement apparatus includes the names of the tests or surveys used, any laboratory or clinical equipment needed, and any specific directions or adaptations to the test or procedure that might not be found in a test manual. For example, if only part of a perceptual motor test is used, one must name the subtests chosen and justify the modification. When a standardized test is used, the reliability and validity of the test (or test portions) used must be indicated. If a survey or questionnaire has been developed for the study, a copy is put into the appendix following the major sections of the paper.

Finally, the researcher describes the methods of data collection and the statistical or other procedures that will be used to analyze the data. For example, will the researcher collect data alone, in person, or by telephone? Will others be trained to collect the data? Will the data collectors be blinded as to the purpose of the study and the group assignment of the participants (if applicable)? If a questionnaire will be used to collect data, will it be mailed or left in a public place for people to fill out as desired? Will a second letter be sent as a follow-up? How long will data collection occur? Will it be collected in one or more sessions? Will it be gathered by outcome measures (pre- and post-testing)? What types of statistical procedures will be used to analyze the data? In the excerpt below from the method section of a study on occupational therapy and dementia the author described the participants and study design.

> For this study, 35 dementia patients with a mild stage of AD who were attending an adult daycare center were recruited and then randomly divided into the experimental and control groups. The majority of the users for both institutions were AD patients, as were the selected subjects. Before the intervention, the two groups' general characteristics and cognitive functions were first examined to confirm homogeneity. All assessments and interventions were performed by a therapist who had over five years of occupational therapy experience. The experimental group joined a recollection-based occupational therapy program constructed by the author where they were asked to engage in one activity every day from Monday to Friday. By contrast, the control group participated in the regular activities provided by their existing daycare centers. Regular activities included physical and recreational activities, arts and crafts, music activities, and rest... The program for the experimental group was offered for a total of 24 sessions, five times per week for an hour per session, and the initial evaluation and reevaluation were conducted prior to and after the intervention, respectively. The program was offered in both institutions, but at different times in order to avoid overlap.

(Kim, 2020, p. 2)

The Method section will close with a paragraph or two on the planned data analysis. If the study is quantitative, this section should contain a justification for the specific statistical test(s) chosen to be performed. If the study follows qualitative methodology, a plan of analysis should be described, even though some analytic procedures may not be determined until after the data collection is underway.

12.2.4 Results

The fourth section of the research paper presents the results from the study without attempting to interpret them. Usually, the first information reported are the pertinent demographics of the sample of participants who were enrolled in and completed the study. These descriptive statistics should be separately presented for each distinct group in the study (e.g., control group and intervention group). If any demographic variable appears to show a difference between the groups, a statistical test is conducted to determine the likelihood of that much difference occurring by chance. If the probability reported by the statistic is greater than 5% ($p > .05$), then the two groups are deemed "essentially equivalent."

Each hypothesis or guiding question is then addressed separately. First, descriptive statistics on the outcome variables are presented. These would include a measure of central tendency (mean, median, mode) and an indication of variability (standard deviation, variance, range, or interquartile range). In this way the researcher is establishing for the reader whether the variable distributions are normal or not. If they are not normal (either skewed, or leptotic or kurtotic, or very different from one group to the other) then using non-parametric statistics in the next step may be warranted.

Finally, inferential statistics are reported. Typically, the attention is on overall differences in the mean values between the various groups in the study (the main effects). The statistical output will indicate whether these differences are distinct enough to be unlikely to have happened by chance more than 5% of the time ($p < .05$). If there is a statistically significant difference between the two groups, the effect size of this difference should be reported. Then if there are two or more dependent variables, it is possible and may be relevant to calculate interaction effects among the dependent variables. The interactions, if any are statistically significant, should be clearly reported. Tables and figures depicting important relationships between variables often make the presentation more understandable. They should, however, be self-explanatory and add to the information in the text of the paper rather than repeat it.

The following excerpts from Izadi-Najafabadi et al. (2022) show how the authors implemented this reporting scheme.

> Results

> ...from a total of 80 children recruited for this study, 37 children with developmental coordination

disorder [25 male, 12 female; mean (SD) age: 9.7 (1.5) years] and 41 children with developmental coordination disorder with co-occurring attention deficit hyperactivity disorder [38 male, 3 female; mean (SD) age: 10.2 (1.4) years] participated in this study…

most frequently read (Best & Kahn, 1997), it is crucial that the researchers summarize the results and critically review these findings in the context of prior studies. The usefulness of the research paper, whatever the findings, is influenced by the way in which the discussion section is written.

VARIABLE	DCD ($N=37$)				DCD + ADHD ($N=41$)			
	PRE-TEST MEDIAN (IQR)	POST-TEST MEDIAN (IQR)	EFFECT SIZE	MEDIAN 95% CI	PRE-TEST MEDIAN (IQR)	POST-TEST MEDIAN (IQR)	EFFECT SIZE	MEDIAN 95% CI
COPM Performance	2.7 (2.2)	7.0 (1.0)	0.62*	3.00–4.33	2.3 (1.7)	7.0 (1.5)	0.61*	3.83–4.67

…the pre-post analysis demonstrated a statistically significant ($p < 0.001$) improvement in self-rated performance and satisfaction of motor goals on the Canadian Occupational Performance Measure and Performance Quality Rating Scale, but not the Bruininks-Oseretsky Test of Motor Proficiency – 2nd ed.

(Izadi-Najafabadi et al., 2022)

12.2.5 Discussion, Including Implications of the Findings and Limitations

In the final section, the writer summarizes the findings and attempts to interpret them in the context of previous results. Acceptance or rejection of hypotheses are stated in this section. Although statements of generalization can be made here, one must be careful not to over-generalize or overstate the applicability of the findings. The writer should be aware of the limitations of the study and state them in a separate section such as small sample, unknown test reliability, or inexplicable results. There is no need here to state the inherent limitations in this type of study design (such as, "the pre-existing groups were not randomly assigned"). Implications for further research, professional practice, or policy changes are advanced. The internal and external validity of the study should be discussed. Internal validity concerns whether the study design, methodology, reliability and validity of test instruments, participant selection and attrition, and neutrality of the data collectors were favorable.

According to Best and Kahn (1997), the discussion section of the research paper is the most difficult part to write. Inexperienced authors tend to over- or under-generalize, thinking their results less or more important than the data would support (Winkler & McCuen, 1998). The discussion section should be a critical and analytical summary of the findings, rather than a superficial overview of the results. Because this part of the full research paper is the

Below is an excerpt from the discussion section on a research study examining the variable social functioning in clients with severe mental illness (SMI).

Discussion

We examined the social functioning effect of people with SMI by home-visit OT using the MTDLP [Management Tool for Daily Life Performance]. We verified the presence of significant differences in the effectiveness of the MTDLP compared to the control group, over four months on the social functioning improvement of individuals with SMI. A previous meta-analysis on social functioning [2] reported, that minimum follow-up times of 12 months for schizophrenia and 6 months for depression are recommended. Therefore, as a study duration of four months is a relatively short time frame to observe clinically meaningful change, improvements in social functioning for those with SMI within four months support the strength of the intervention effect.

(Mashimo et al., 2020)

12.2.6 Reference List and Appendices

In the last section of the research paper, the writer lists all of the cited references. The writer must be careful not to leave out any reference, to include all information in the citation, and to check for accuracy and correct spelling and formatting of the information. An incomplete or inaccurate citation risks instilling frustration in a reader who wishes to obtain the original article. (Refer to section 12.5 for further information.)

Sometimes a writer wishes to place a bibliography along with the reference list into the research paper. (Most journals do not permit this, though.) A bibliography contains any article, book, or chapter that might be helpful in understanding the topic. A reference list, on the other hand, includes only those journal articles, books, or other sources used in the research and preparation of the paper and cited within the article (American Psychological Association, 2020). Any additional information (e.g., copy of the survey or test protocol, drawing of specific apparatus) can be placed in an appendix following the list of references and any tables or figures included.

12.2.7 Abstract

The abstract of a research study, which is written last and then placed at the beginning of the study, contains summary statements of each section of the paper (i.e., introduction, method, results, discussion, and includes a conclusion). The abstract should contain enough information so that the reader will know the purpose of the study, the specific variables and groups studied, the number of participants, the measuring instruments used, the main results, and the conclusions presented. An abstract of a research study is usually limited to between 150 and 300 words. When preparing an abstract, it is useful to extract key sentences from each part of the study and then integrate the sentences through transitional phrases. Abstracts are extremely important to investigators reviewing literature; therefore, it is vital to present as complete a summary of the total study as possible within the number of words permitted. Abstracts are not merely a summary or discussion of the results as perceived by some investigators. An abstract should be a complete statement representative of the total study. Key words or key phrases are usually placed below the abstract. These key words are very important for researchers in identifying relevant studies found in databases.

Below are two examples of abstracts, the first is from a systematic review and the second is a good example from a randomized controlled trial.

Abstract

Importance: Parkinson disease is the most common form of parkinsonism, a group of neurological disorders with Parkinson disease-like movement problems such as rigidity, slowness, and tremor. More than 6 million individuals worldwide have Parkinson disease.

Observations: Diagnosis of Parkinson disease is based on history and examination. History can include prodromal features (eg, rapid eye movement sleep behavior disorder, hyposmia, constipation), characteristic movement difficulty (eg, tremor, stiffness, slowness), and psychological or cognitive problems (eg, cognitive decline, depression, anxiety). Examination typically demonstrates bradykinesia with tremor, rigidity, or both. Dopamine transporter single-photon emission computed tomography can improve the accuracy of diagnosis when the presence of parkinsonism is uncertain. Parkinson disease has multiple disease variants with different prognoses. Individuals with a diffuse malignant subtype (9%–16% of individuals with Parkinson disease) have prominent early motor and nonmotor symptoms, poor response to medication, and faster disease progression. Individuals with mild motor-predominant Parkinson disease (49%–53% of individuals with Parkinson disease) have mild symptoms, a good response to dopaminergic medications (eg, carbidopa-levodopa, dopamine agonists), and slower disease progression. Other individuals have an intermediate subtype. For all patients with Parkinson disease, treatment is symptomatic, focused on improvement in motor (eg, tremor, rigidity, bradykinesia) and nonmotor (eg, constipation, cognition, mood, sleep) signs and symptoms. No disease-modifying pharmacologic treatments are available. Dopamine-based therapies typically help initial motor symptoms. Nonmotor symptoms require nondopaminergic approaches (eg, selective serotonin reuptake inhibitors for psychiatric symptoms, cholinesterase inhibitors for cognition). Rehabilitative therapy and exercise complement pharmacologic treatments. Individuals experiencing complications, such as worsening symptoms and functional impairment when a medication dose wears off ("off periods"), medication-resistant tremor, and dyskinesias, benefit from advanced treatments such as therapy with levodopa-carbidopa enteral suspension or deep brain stimulation. Palliative care is part of Parkinson disease management.

Conclusions and relevance: Parkinson disease is a heterogeneous disease with rapidly and slowly progressive forms. Treatment involves pharmacologic approaches (typically with levodopa preparations prescribed with or without other medications) and nonpharmacologic approaches (such as exercise and physical, occupational, and speech therapies). Approaches such as deep brain stimulation and treatment with levodopa-carbidopa enteral suspension can help individuals with medication-resistant tremor, worsening symptoms when the medication wears off, and dyskinesias.

(Armstrong & Okun, 2020)

Abstract

Background: Mild stroke can cause subtle cognitive-behavioral symptoms, which although might be hidden, can restrict community reintegration and participation. Cognitive rehabilitation programs exist for stroke but not specifically for mild stroke and the research evidence varies. The Functional and Cognitive Occupational Therapy (FaC$_O$T) intervention was developed specifically for this population.

Objective: To examine the effectiveness of FaC_oT intervention for improving daily functioning and participation compared with standard care.

Method: A single blind randomized controlled trial with assessments pre (T1), post (T2) and 3-month follow-up (T3). Individuals in the FaC_oT group received 10 weekly sessions practicing cognitive and behavioral strategies. The Canadian Occupational Performance Measure (COPM) was the primary outcome measure, IADL-questionnaire, Reintegration to Normal Living questionnaire (RNL) were secondary measures.

Results: In total, 66 community-dwelling individuals with mild stroke were randomly allocated to FaC_oT (n = 33, mean (SD) age 64.6 (8.2), 33% women), or control group (n = 33, mean (SD) age 64.4 (10.8), 45% women). Time X Group interaction effects were found for the COPM performance ($F(1.4,90.3) = 11.75$, $p < 0.000$) and satisfaction ($F(1.5,96.8) = 15.70$, $p < 0.000$), with large effect size values. Significant between-group effects were found for RNL ($F = 10.02$, $p < 0.002$, $\eta_p^2 = 0.13$). Most participants in FaC_oT achieved a clinically important difference in COPM between T1–T2, T1–T3, and in RNL between T1 to T3 compared with the control group.

Conclusions: FaC_oT intervention is effective to improve daily functioning, participation and satisfaction of individuals with mild stroke compared with standard care, therefore FaC_oT should be implemented in community rehabilitation settings.

Keywords: PROMs; cognitive–functional interventions; participation; stroke rehabilitation.

(Adamit et al., 2021)

12.3 Writing the First Draft

Writers begin the first draft of the project proposal after completing the outline. As stated above, the outline aids in organizing the literature review, but the outline is not set in stone. After the first draft has been written, the organization may need to be revised. Nonetheless, having an outline allows the writer to have a sense of the direction in which the paper is going.

A difficult skill for inexperienced writers is using notes effectively. There is a tendency to quote extensively rather than paraphrase the cited author's words. Frequently, this is caused by a lack of understanding about what the author meant. If this is the case, scholars must do additional reading until they completely understand the material. Although quotes from the original source can be an effective means of relating information, too many quotations make the research paper difficult to read and leave "the impression that students have done [no more than] 'cut and paste' from books and articles they have read" (Winkler & McCuen, 1979, p. 114). It is better to use quotations sparingly, intermixing the quotations with summaries and paraphrases of the original sources. When quoting or paraphrasing, one must document the source (APA, 2020).

The literary and scientific styles used for citations are determined by each particular journal. The four most commonly used systems are The Chicago Manual of Style, University of Chicago Press, 17th edition, 2017, the Modern Language Association (MLA, 9th edition, 2021), the American Medical Association Manual of Style (AMA, 11th edition, 2020), and the Publication Manual of the American Psychological Association, 7th edition (APA, 2020). The APA style (which is used in this book) is the most frequently used style in occupational therapy, psychology, education, and social and health sciences journals and books.

12.4 Making Revisions

Once the final paper has been written, revisions will be necessary. Revising the paper five or six times is not uncommon. Each time that writers review their paper for accuracy and cohesiveness, they may discover additional ways to improve clarity.

The function of revision is to make sure that specific editing requirements have been followed. These editing requirements are summarized in Table 12–3.

12.4.1 Avoiding Bias

First, the writer will want to make sure that no type of bias (gender, sexual orientation, racial or ethnic, disability, age, or historical and interpretive inaccuracies) has been introduced into the paper. Several guidelines have been established by the APA for avoiding bias in one's writing. "Part of writing without bias is recognizing that differences should be mentioned only when relevant. Marital status, sexual orientation, racial and ethnic identity, or the fact that a person has a disability should not be mentioned gratuitously" (APA, 2020, p. 136).

"Gender" refers to role (APA, 2020, pp. 120–121) while sex is biological (APA, 2020, p. 138). Both gender and sexual bias can be avoided by specifically describing participants, rather than using a general term to describe the population. For example, bias occurs when the writer uses the term "man" to mean the human race rather than using a more inclusive term such as person, people, or individuals. Additionally, use of specific gender words (e.g., his, her) or using terms that end in man or men (e.g., postman, chairman, policemen) must be avoided. Stereotyping (e.g.,

TABLE 12-3

CHECKLIST FOR PROOFING ONE'S ARTICLE

1. GENDER AND ETHNIC BIAS
- Is the article free of language that might be ambiguous or stereotypical?

2. PEOPLE FIRST
- Is the manuscript written with the individual emphasized rather than the disability?
- Have all references to a disability been written in the form "individual with..."?

3. GRAMMAR
- Are there run-on sentences or sentence fragments?
- Are there split infinitives, dangling modifiers, errors in verb-subject agreement?
- Is the writing in parallel structure?
- Are relative pronouns used appropriately?
- Has a grammar program been used to check the language?
- Has past tense been used rather than presence tense (e.g., the author *said*)

4. SPELLING/PUNCTUATION
- Has a spell check been used to check spelling?
- Has the article been reviewed for commas, quotation marks, hyphens, and apostrophes?

5. ABBREVIATIONS
- Is the abbreviation placed in parentheses following the full term the first time it is used?
- Are the Latin abbreviations used correctly and according to APA style?
- Are abbreviations invented by the author kept to a minimum?

6. TRANSITIONAL WORDS, PHRASES, AND SENTENCES
- Are there transitional statements or words between ideas?
- Is there a sense of unity and integration in the paper?
- Do words such as "however," "although," or "nevertheless" need to be added?

7. CLARITY
- Is the language clear and simple?
- Do any unusual terms need to be explained or defined?
- Would a figure or table help explain the information?
- Has the material been reviewed by a 2nd reader?

8. ORGANIZATION
- Do the hypotheses or guiding question(s) drive the content of the research paper?
- Is there consistency between sections?
- Are unnecessary repetitions removed?
- Is the sequence of the research paper logical and coherent?

the psychologist… he; the nurse… she) can be avoided by using specific language (e.g., these boys enjoyed playing with Legos while the participant girls enjoyed reading), by using parallel language (e.g., men and women rather than men and girls), or by changing the term to a plural (e.g., their instead of his or her, while respecting individual's preferred pronouns). Compounds, such as "his/her," or "(s)he" should be avoided (APA, 2020). The term sexual orientation is recommended and not the phrase sexual preference.

There are certain groups who wish to be referred to in a manner that affirms their identity (e.g., "autistic individuals" versus "individuals with autism"). The American Psychological Association has a well-written section on "bias-free" language with regard to people groups in particular (APA, 2020). Bias involving disabilities occurs when the writer attributes to a specific group something that has no supporting data (APA, 2020). An example of this stereotyping occurs when someone writes "Individuals with traumatic brain injury have psychosocial difficulties."

Ethnic or racial bias can be avoided by using commonly accepted designations, such as the census categories, while being sensitive to the preferred designations. For example, many persons of Hispanic background in New Mexico prefer to be called Hispanic or Spanish, while many persons of Hispanic background in southern California or southern Texas consider themselves Mexicans or Mexican-Americans (see www.pewresearch.org/short-reads/2022/09/15/who-is-hispanic/). Latinx (gender neutral) is another recent term that some people use to describe Latino people.

Avoid terms that are either dated or derogatory. Finally, terms used to refer to racial or ethnic groups are proper nouns, and therefore should be capitalized. By asking the study participants their preference in naming, ethnic or racial bias can be avoided. APA suggests that an informal test can be completed by substituting another group (e.g., your own) for the group being discussed. If the writer perceives offense in the revised statement, then bias is probably present. Other important considerations may also apply (Kendi, 2023).

When referring to individuals by age, specific ranges should be used. APA suggests that individuals under 12 should be referred to as girls or boys, while young men or young women is used for individuals between 13 and 18. Individuals older than 18 are referred to as women or men. Terms such as elderly or senior are generally not acceptable, as some participants will find these terms pejorative. Other guidelines can be found in the APA manual on page 135.

12.4.2 People First Language

Another reason for revision is to make sure that the writing is in people first language. Because of the Individuals with Disabilities Education Act (1990), all references to disabilities must be written with the individual placed first. Thus, woman with a spinal cord injury is accepted, while spinal cord injured woman is less desirable. This convention emphasizes the value of the human being and delegates the disability to secondary importance. Note that as an effect of the disability rights movement and other self-advocacy efforts, some groups of people wish to be identified by their diagnosis, when that diagnosis plays a profound role in their identity vis-à-vis society. For example, some people may wish to be addressed as "an autistic teenager," or "a deaf adult." The writer must grant participants the right to designate their preferred descriptor.

The writer should also distinguish between the terms handicap and disability. A handicap can be thought of as a disadvantage imposed on an individual by the environment or by another person or society, whereas a disability is something that an individual is unable to do, a lack of a body part, or physical or psychosocial impairment. For example, an individual with a spinal cord injury may not be able to walk; the inability to walk is a disability. However, this disability becomes a handicap if there is no wheelchair access in public spaces. The presence of a disability does not necessarily make an individual handicapped.

12.4.3 Mechanics of Writing

Clear writing requires use of a formal writing style and using grammatically correct language. A third reason to revise the manuscript is to ensure that there are no grammatical errors. Errors such as lack of subject-verb agreement (e.g., using "the woman with many talents are…" rather than "the woman with many talents is…"), punctuation and capitalization, run-on sentences, sentence fragments, and dangling modifiers are common among less experienced writers. Run-on sentences and sentence fragments can be an indication that the research paper has not been proofread. Other common errors include (a) failing to use parallel structure for grammatical units (e.g., using different parts of speech in a series or in connecting phrases), (b) having dangling modifiers (e.g., sentences in which a modifying phrase has no subject anchor, such as, "Growing up as a child, my grandmother used to bake me cookies on Saturdays," (c) improper number agreement (singular/plural) when using relative pronouns (e.g., "a young man must keep their head" rather than, "a young man must keep his head"), (d) using the passive tense rather than the active tense (e.g., "seven measurements were made" instead of "the researchers made seven measurements"), and (e) placing prepositions at the end of sentences ("ethical and legal obligations that occupational therapists are faced with" rather than "ethical and legal obligations that occupational therapists face"). For checking proper grammatical structure, a basic grammar resource is indispensable.

Many excellent sources are available to help writers avoid grammatical errors and improve their writing. The following list provides major references and online programs:

- Strunk, W., & White, E. B. (1999). *The elements of style* (4th ed.). Allyn & Bacon. A classic containing a gold mine of writing ideas, including rules of usage, principles of composition form, and writing style. The epitome of concise, effective writing.
- American Psychological Association. (2020). *Publication manual of the American Psychological Association* (7th ed.). APA. An exhaustive guide to organizing a journal article for publication. Includes content areas such as headings, quotations, references, tables, figures and graphs, and other matters of style that can keep a writer up all night.
- Booth, W. C., Columb, G. G., Williams, J. M., Bizup, J., Fitzgerald, W., & University of Chicago Press Editorial Staff. (2018). *A manual for writers of research papers, theses, and dissertations*, 9th ed. University of Chicago Press. This is a helpful resource for citing in Chicago style format.

- Kipfer, B. A. (2010). *Roget's international thesaurus* (7th ed.). Collins Reference. An invaluable guide to the writer for selecting the most appropriate word. It is helpful both in locating a specific word and in varying one's language.
- Anonymous. (2021). *Taber's cyclopedic medical dictionary* (24th ed.). F. A. Davis.
- An essential guide for those researchers needing medical terms defined and clarified. Taber's also has an online version at www.tabers.com/tabersonline/
- Anonymous. (2019). *Merriam-Webster's collegiate dictionary* (12th ed.). Merriam-Webster. Having a dictionary is a must, both for finding meanings of words or using correct spelling. This is also available online at www.merriam-webstercollegiate.com.
- Purdue Online Writing Lab (OWLS), available at https://owl.english.purdue.edu. This online resource provides over 200 resources for writing, including format and style guides for MLA and APA, help with writing and grammar, English as a second language, and ways to avoid plagiarism.

Another reason for revision is to check for spelling and punctuation errors. It is critical to check one's spelling with a spell checker to ensure that there are no errors. One must be careful, however, to read the article and proof for errors, rather than relying on the computer speller to find all errors. It cannot find errors when the words are spelled correctly but misused. For example, if the words to and too are used incorrectly, many spell checkers will not identify the error. A checklist for proofing one's manuscript is outlined in Table 12–3.

In scientific articles, it is common practice to abbreviate terms used repeatedly (e.g., cerebrovascular accident as [CVA], cognitive behavioral therapy as [CBT], learning disability as [LD], multiple sclerosis as [MS], and quality of life as [QOL]). Abbreviations invented by the writer should be kept to a minimum and used only for terms that are long and frequently repeated in the paper. Tables of statistical data containing abbreviations should contain a footnote defining any abbreviations.

Latin abbreviations are useful for shortening sentences. The following are the most commonly used abbreviations in scientific articles. Notice that they are not italicized.

- a posteriori: after the fact; procedure used in generating a new theory from new data
- a priori: procedure used in testing an existing theory
- ca. (circa): about a certain time, e.g., ca. 130 BCE
- e.g. (exempli grata): for example
- et al. (et alia): and others
- et seq. (et sequens): and the following
- ibid. (ibidem): in the same place
- i.e. (id est): that is to say
- viz. (videlicet): namely, used to introduce lists

Be sure to refer to the APA manual for the proper way to use abbreviations. For example, many abbreviations (including i.e. and e.g.) must be used only within parentheses.

12.4.4 Transitional Words, Phrases, and Sentences

Another reason for revision is to make sure that transitional statements are present so that the flow of ideas is smooth. Writing a well-organized, integrated manuscript requires the use of words and phrases that connect ideas and summarize a section of a paper. In reviewing scientific literature, it is important to group the citation of studies into topical areas and to develop a logical sequence (e.g., using the funnel model described above). Writing should be coherent. Transitional words, such as however, although, or nevertheless, can be used to make the connection smoother and the paper unified. (Note that many style guides frown on beginning a sentence with however.) In addition, sentences can be used to facilitate the smooth transition from one idea to another. The reader should have no difficulty following the train of thought or the arguments used to build a case. Additionally, reading the research paper as a whole will uncover any inconsistencies in terminology or repetitions between sections. Often, having someone unacquainted with the topic read the manuscript can help in improving clarity and grammar.

12.4.5 Clarity of Thought

A researcher should try to communicate ideas simply and rigorously. Some of the most profound ideas can be expressed in clear, direct language. It is not a sign of intellectual prowess to present ideas so that they are difficult to understand. Therefore, a sixth reason for revision is to ensure that the paper is written clearly. Scientific writing is particularly prone to abstruseness and ambiguity, especially when language is used loosely without precise operational definitions. One method of ensuring clarity is to include an operational definition for unusual terms or for jargon specific to a certain discipline. Even if the writer chooses not to create a glossary, uncommon terms must be explicitly defined. Use of well-thought-out tables or figures can facilitate the clarity of the research paper. It is not unusual for readers to look at the tables and figures before reading the text, especially when these visual aids provide an overall summary of the principal findings.

12.4.6 Organization

Finally, the author should examine whether the background information is represented accurately, whether ideas unrelated to the topic have been deleted, and whether the hypotheses or guiding question(s) have directed the writing. Each statement of results should be supported by data. Differences or contradictions in the findings compared to those of previous studies need to be discussed and, when possible, explained. The whole paper should be reviewed for sequence of ideas. Even though there may be future editorial changes to the paper, the author must stand behind the manuscript as presented.

> [T]he secret of good writing is to strip every sentence to its cleanest components. Every word that serves no function, every long word that could be a short word, every adverb which carries the same meaning that is already in the verb, every passive construction that leaves the reader unsure of who is doing what—these are the thousand and one adulterants that weaken the strength of a sentence.
>
> (Zinsser, 1990, pp. 7–8)

12.5 QUOTATIONS, REFERENCED MATERIAL, AND BIBLIOGRAPHIC CITATIONS

Whenever one uses material written by another person, whether the material is directly quoted or only paraphrased, one must make reference to the original author(s). Failure to do so is plagiarism. Some authors (Winkler & McCuen, 1998) have suggested that plagiarism is common in everyday language. One might use in speech an example stated in a lecture by a professor and in that moment fail to give that professor the credit. In another case one may use a proverb such as "A stitch in time saves nine" and fail to give Benjamin Franklin the credit. Although these examples are not routinely considered plagiarism and are generally acceptable in everyday speech, plagiarism is not acceptable in a scholarly paper.

Plagiarism occurs when scholars intentionally or unintentionally take another person's ideas and incorporate them into their own writing without giving proper credit to the original author. Examples of plagiarism include the following: (a) taking another's research ideas and submitting them as one's own, (b) paraphrasing an idea in an article without giving credit to the author, or (c) directly copying part of an article without citing the authors or without putting the quotation in quotation marks. Using any copyright material without giving credit to the original author is considered plagiarism (Winkler & McCuen, 1998).

If the material used is a direct quote from another author or authors, the writer must cite the author(s), year of publication, and page number of the quotation in the text. There must be no change in spelling, phrasing, capitalization, or punctuation from the original. The exception to this rule is when the first word of a quotation needs to be capitalized

or placed in lower case to make the statement grammatically correct. When it is necessary to make changes (e.g., when a pronoun must be clarified or a word added to make the content more understandable), the change must be put in square brackets ([ ]). When a word is misspelled or the grammar is incorrect in the original, [sic] follows the misspelling or grammatical error to show that the quotation is reproduced exactly. For example, "The article was written by an england [sic] author."

A quote can be introduced as part of a grammatical sentence, or it may stand alone as a sentence or passage of several sentences. When material is omitted from the quotation, then an ellipsis (…) replaces the material that is left out. When the quote is more than 40 words, it should stand out as a separate paragraph without quotation marks. In this case, the quoted material is extra indented from the paper's margins, punctuated, and the reference for the quoted material is placed after the paragraph, in parenthesis and with no ending punctuation. Examine the following:

> Slang, hackneyed or flippant phrases, and folksy style should be avoided. Since objectivity is the primary goal, there should be no element of exhortation or persuasion. The research report should describe and explain, rather than try to convince or move to action. In this respect, the research report differs from the essay or the feature article. (Best, 1977, p. 317)

When the quoted material has fewer than 40 words, it is placed within a paragraph. The reference is placed in parentheses at the end of the quote. For example, … according to experienced writers of scientific papers, "The research report should be presented in a style that is creative, clear, and concise" (Best, 1977, p. 317).

When the writer wishes to paraphrase another author's material, then the writer must cite the author(s) and date of publication. Examine the following two examples:

> 1. Best and Kahn (1997) suggested that when writing a research article, one must be careful to write concisely and clearly.
> 2. When writing a research article, one must be careful to write concisely and clearly (Best & Kahn, 1997; Winkler & McCuen, 1998).

Notice that no page numbers are used in either reference and that the author's name is put within parentheses at the end of the sentence if it has not been used as part of the sentence structure.

Whether the writer has quoted the source directly or paraphrased the material, a complete reference must be placed in the reference list at the end of the research paper for every citation made in the paper. (The only exception is when a personal communication has been cited.) Further information regarding the appropriate style for capstone projects, theses, dissertations, secondary sources, movies, or films can be found in the APA manual. Regardless of the type of publication, all references in the list must include enough information so that the reader can locate the original source.

12.6 FORMAT OF A PAPER

The format of the paper is dictated by the style of writing used. For journal publications using the APA style, the size of the margins, line spacing, and font size are specified. Individual professors and journals using other style guides may have different requirements. In a thesis or dissertation, additional sections may be required by the student's department or university. A typical organization of the sequence for a thesis or dissertation is listed below.

1. Title page
2. Approval page indicating names and titles of thesis or capstone readers
3. Acknowledgments, including individuals who aided in the study and any grant support accepted
4. Table of contents, including chapter and section headings, appendix, and bibliography
5. List of tables
6. List of figures
7. Abstract
8. The content of the text
   a. Introduction including purpose and need for the study
   b. Review of the literature
   c. Method
   d. Results
   e. Discussion, including implications of the findings and limitations of the study
   f. Conclusions and recommendations for further research
9. References (optional bibliography)
10. Tables
11. Figures
12. Appendices
13. Vita, listing professional education, work history, and previous publications

A running title, consisting of no more than 50 characters including punctuation and spaces, is placed in capital letters in the upper left-hand corner of each page. One-inch margins are used for the top, bottom, and both sides. APA style dictates the position of page numbers (usually below the running title), the use of Roman and Arabic numbers, the type of paper, the levels of headings, spacing, and use of quotations.

12.6.1 Outline of a Research Proposal

1. Title of study
2. Investigator
3. Date
4. The research problem
   a. statement of problem in question form
   b. justification of the need for the study
   c. implications of anticipated results in relation to clinical intervention, or professional, educational, or administrative problems
5. Literature review
   a. outline of major areas to be reviewed
   b. plan for search of related literature
   c. annotated bibliographical notation organized under major areas reviewed
6. Research design
   a. research model (e.g., experimental, descriptive, qualitative)
   b. operational definitions of variables
   c. statement of hypotheses or guiding questions
   d. identification of presumed independent or dependent variables (quantitative studies)
   e. theoretical explanation underlying study
7. Method
   a. procedure for selecting sample and screening criteria for participant inclusion
   b. setting for study and procedure for collecting data
   c. tests, questionnaires, or instruments used in the study, including the evaluation of their reliability and validity
   d. tentative time schedule for study
      i. time period for literature review
      ii. collection of data: number of hours required
      iii. date for completion of research
   e. projected costs for study
      i. clerical
      ii. instrumentation
      iii. travel
      iv. other
   f. Plan for statistical or qualitative data analysis

12.7 WHY ARE RESEARCH PROPOSALS NOT APPROVED

The following list of major reasons for the disapproval of research proposals is based on the authors' experiences as raters on governmental and university committees.

- **The research problem is insignificant, and the results will have little impact on clinical practice currently or in the future.** An example of an insignificant problem is an investigation of the relationship of low birth weight with the incidence of cerebral palsy. A literature search in this area already confirms that low birth weight is one among many risk factors for cerebral palsy. Nonetheless, not all infants with cerebral palsy are born prematurely nor are all infants with low birth weight destined to have cerebral palsy. This study will have little impact on our understanding of the causes of cerebral palsy and will not provide insight into prevention and treatment. The projected results from this type of study would have a splintering effect where one variable is linked to a disability that has already been found to have multiple causes. A better study in a related area would be to examine the effects of low birth weight on one area of development, such as motor function. In this way, the investigator can narrow the research and control for extraneous variables that could have a potential effect on the results.

- **The hypothesis presented is not supported by scientific evidence and seems speculative.** As a hypothetical example, a researcher proposes that a computer application for cognitive rehabilitation is effective in treating individuals with brain injuries. The investigator equates improvement with the client's ability to learn a computer game. The investigator does not demonstrate through a literature review that there is a carryover of this computer skill to the learning of functional skills in independent living. A better study is to investigate the types of skills that are facilitated while learning with a computer.

- **The research problem is more complex than the investigator presents, and it needs to be narrowed down.** For example, a researcher proposes to examine the effects of sensory integration therapy on children with Attention Deficit Hyperactivity Disorder (ADHD). Both variables are complex and must be operationally defined. Sensory integration therapy includes a number of components in treatment, whereas ADHD is a complex disorder with multiple causes. A better study is to identify one aspect of sensory integration therapy, such as vestibular stimulation, and evaluate its effectiveness with a measurable variable, such as motor proficiency, as assessed by the *Miller Assessment for Preschoolers* (MAP; Miller, 1988).

- **The anticipated results from the study will be of only local significance and lack external validity or generalizability.** An example of a flawed proposal is when a researcher designs a survey of job satisfaction for occupational therapists in a local school district without considering the generalizability to a larger sample or population. The data collected from this study would have only local interest and could not be generalized to teachers in other schools. In a better study of job satisfaction among occupational therapists, the researcher would determine first the demographics of an average occupational therapist, considering age, gender, and educational level. These variables could be used to determine if the occupational therapists are representative of a larger population. The survey would be designed with the intention of applying it to a more general sample. Questions would be generated that examine the broad issues of job satisfaction among occupational therapists in general, rather than looking at local issues that affect job satisfaction in that particular school district.

- **The research proposed has too many uncontrolled elements.** For example, a researcher wants to study the effects of in utero exposure to alcohol on children born with fetal alcohol syndrome. The amount of alcohol exposure is unknown and is dependent on the mother's self-report, which is often unreliable. In addition, the home environment and genetic makeup are variables that may play a part in the child's behavior. These variables are difficult to measure and are often neglected by the researcher. A better approach is a retrospective case study analysis of an infant with fetal alcohol syndrome and the child's mother, exploring the dynamics of the case.

- **The research methodology seems overly complex and difficult to replicate.** For example, a researcher wants to examine the relationship between the onset of a depressive episode and an individual who is vulnerable. The interactions between family relationships, work situations, and personal attitudes are complex and make it difficult to identify the interactive factors that result in depression. Because of the individuality of each episode, replication of the study using a group method or survey would be difficult and might distort results. A better study would include a qualitative research method using an in-depth case study approach to identify within each individual the interactive effects that trigger depression.

- **The proposed outcome measures are either inappropriate, unstandardized, unreliable, or invalid.** A researcher investigating the effects of exercise on depression creates a scale for depression without testing for its reliability or validity. A better approach to measurement is to use more than one instrument to measure outcome (triangulation). For example, the investigator can use a physiological measure, a standardized test, and a client self-report. These three measures will increase the internal validity of the study in assessing outcome.

- **Extraneous variables are left uncontrolled and may have an influence on the results.** For example, a researcher wants to examine the effect of a specific treatment method on improving motor skills.

Although the researcher is careful to administer pre- and post-tests, extraneous variables, such as practice at home, additional interventions, or sessions per week, are not included in the analysis. These variables will most certainly affect the results. A better study would be to take frequent measures of performance, perhaps at the beginning and end of each therapy session, to determine changes in skill level. Another possibility is to have the client and researcher keep a log describing motor performance.

- **Overall design of the study seems incomplete and not well conceived.** In this example, elements of the research proposal are missing, such as controlling for extraneous variables that could possibly influence the results, or a large section of the literature review is omitted. It is important for the researcher to work with an outline that lists the essential components of a research proposal.

- **The statistical tests suggested for analyzing the data are not appropriate.** An investigator has collected ordinal data, such as ranking of students on an achievement test. Rather than using a nonparametric test, such as the Spearman Rank Order Correlation used for ordinal type data, the researcher inappropriately applies a parametric test, such as the Pearson Correlational Coefficient statistical test used for interval scale data. The statistical test applied should be based on the measurement scale of data. The assumptions of parametric statistics, such as normality of data distribution, should be followed. The appropriate statistics are based on the assumptions underlying the statistical tests.

- **Selection of subjects for the study is not representative of a target population.** If it is known that the incidence of traumatic brain injuries (TBI) is higher for males than females by more than 2 to 1 and that more than 50% of clients with TBI are between the ages of 15 and 24, then the investigator should try to select participants who reflect these statistics. This is especially true for studies where the investigator intends to generalize results to a representative sample. Nonetheless, there are studies in which the investigator is interested in examining a non-representative sample that is a portion of the target population, such as females or children with TBI. Then the investigator must delineate clearly the target population in the title of the study.

- **The treatment procedure under investigation has not been adequately defined in enough detail to replicate.** An investigator identifies the independent variable as counseling; however, not enough detail is given regarding the type, frequency, and duration of counseling. Therefore, this study cannot be replicated.

- **The literature review seems outdated and lacks landmark studies in the area of investigation.** In reviewing the literature, it is wise to first examine current secondary texts or to survey articles in the area to identify the major landmark studies that are cited frequently. An up-to-date literature review also can be found by scanning the current journals in a subject area and by looking at the journal's yearly index.

- **The equipment identified in the study is outmoded or unsuitable.** For example, a test that has been standardized on adults is used for children. This is inappropriate and unsuitable for the study.

- **The investigator has not proposed adequate time for completion of the study.** In outlining the proposal for a study, the researcher should set up a time line graph that breaks down the components of the study into time periods. (See Box 12–1.)

- **Resources are inadequate to complete the study.** For example, a research plan includes a request for funds to pay assistants to collect data. The funds requested for support are insufficient to complete the study.

- **The setting and environment for the study are unsuitable.** In this instance, the investigator attempts to complete a complex study without securing an appropriate environment for the study, such as a fully equipped laboratory or testing area that is free from distracting noise.

- **The investigator has not considered the ethical nature of the study, such as stating the potential physical and psychological risks to subjects in an informed consent form or has not received approval from an institutional review board (IRB) regarding human subjects.** For example, a researcher begins to collect data for a study on apraxia and its relationship to students with learning disabilities before the IRB has approved the research design. This is unethical, and data collected cannot be used in the final analysis.

12.8 PREPARATION FOR A CONFERENCE PRESENTATION

12.8.1 Poster Session

A poster display is an opportunity for researchers to present their research in a less formal environment. At many conferences, a portion of the conference area is set aside for poster displays. Usually, the researcher stays with the poster and discusses the data analysis and procedures with the conference participants. This is an opportunity for the participants to ask questions related to the research.

BOX 12-1. WORKSHEET GUIDE FOR SELECTING A RESEARCH PROBLEM

1. What is the target population? (e.g., group with disabilities, or student or clinician from the allied health profession)

2. What are the perceived needs of the population? (e.g., investigating causes of disability; evaluation and diagnostic methods; student performance; evaluation of therapists' effectiveness; investigation of treatment techniques; evaluation of personnel factors).

3. What are the primary and secondary sources relevant to responses 1 and 2?

• Journal articles	1
	2
	3
	4
	5
• Annual reviews	1
	2
	3
• Textbooks	1
	2
	3
	4
	5
• Statistical compendiums	1
	2
	3

4. Are independent and dependent variables identifiable?

• Independent variables: (presumed causes)	1
	2
	3
• Dependent variables: (presumed effects)	1
	2
	3
	4

(continued)

Box 12-1. Worksheet Guide for Selecting a Research Problem (continued)

5. How can the research impact on···	
• Treatment	
• Education	
• Administration	
6. Can research variables be operationally defined?	
7. What explanation or theory accounts for the presumed relationship between variables?	
8. What research model(s) are relevant to the study? Identify model and state research question relative to research model.	
Quantitative	
• Experimental (pretest/posttest)	
• Methodological (construction of instrument	
• Evaluation (evaluation of health care system)	
• Correlation (relationship between variables)	
Qualitative	
• Survey (description of population)	
• Historical (reconstruction of events)	
• Clinical or naturalistic observation (dynamic analysis of subject)	
• Heuristic (discovery of relationships)	
9. Research problem/question	
• State the research problem	

(continued)

Box 12-1. Worksheet Guide for Selecting a Research Problem (continued)

• State the hypothesis in null or directional form	
• State the guiding question	
10. To which groups are the research findings directed? (e.g., Clinicians, individuals with disabilities, students, academicians, program administrators)	
Feasibility check	
• Where can participants be obtained?	
• How many participants are necessary?	
• What tests, instruments, or apparatuses will be necessary to measure outcome?	
What are financial costs?	
• Travel	
• Mailings	
• Tests	
• Protocols	
• Clinical time	
• Apparatus	
• Computer analysis	
• Books and duplicating	
• Clerical and typing	

(continued)

BOX 12-1. WORKSHEET GUIDE FOR SELECTING A RESEARCH PROBLEM (CONTINUED)

• Laboratory analysis of findings	

11. Analysis of time (list the projected time sequence or dates for completion of research phases)

Initiation of study	Review of literature	Preparation for data collection	Approval from IRB	Collection of results	Writing discussion chapter	Completion of study

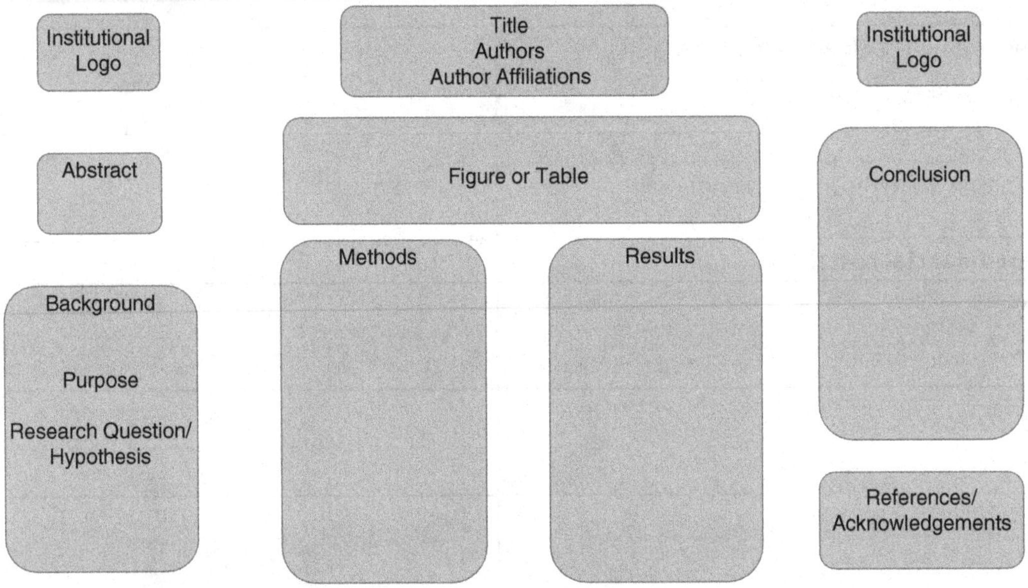

Figure 12–1 Sample of the layout of a poster session.

The poster should be presented in a clear and comprehensive manner. Components of the poster itself include (a) an abstract written in 25 to 50 words, (b) the purpose or aim of the study, (c) the methodology including sample selection, measurements, procedures or intervention approaches, (d) results presented in graphic form, and (e) a summary of the conclusions. In addition to the poster, a handout is usually available that may include all the components, plus a summary of the literature review and a means of contacting the researchers.

Key points in preparing a poster:

- Size of print: The print size should be large enough for participants to read it at a distance of 4 feet, generally a font size of 18- to 24-points.
- Layout: The layout is determined by the space provided at the conference and directions from the conference committee. Try different designs within the space specifications. The material should be arranged to facilitate understanding, generally top to bottom in a left-to-right sequence (see Figure 12–1).

- Amount of information: Information should be written in bullets (three-to-four-word phrases) rather than in sentences. Include essential information about the design, procedure, and results. Figures, charts, or photographs are essential for making the findings visually attractive and accessible. Additional information can be included in the handout.
- Color: Use color in highlighting the results and conclusions. A light color (e.g., yellow) printed on a dark paper is frequently easier to read.
- Background: Use of a contrasting color or border behind the individual components will make the poster visually attractive.

12.8.2 Conference Paper (Oral Presentation)

Researchers are encouraged to present the results of their findings at local, state, national, and international conferences. A call for papers is issued in many occupational therapy publications, journals, and websites. Paper proposals are considered through a peer-reviewed process and not all are selected. When presenting a paper, it is important to recognize that those in attendance are adult learners with a professional knowledge base.

YouTube is another way for researchers to present their findings. Some universities require that occupational therapy doctoral (OTD) students present their research on YouTube. (For example, see Ohio State University 2020 OTD students and advisors presenting their findings here: https://u.osu.edu/osuot/doctoral-capstone-poster-presentations-2020/doctoral-capstone-mental-health-topics-all-ages/). Capstone projects are also presented on Voice Thread (see https://voicethread.com/workshop-categories/workshop-archive/).

> What is VoiceThread? VoiceThread is an interactive collaboration and sharing tool that enables students to build online presentations by adding images, documents, and videos, and other media to which other users can add comments for discussion.
>
> Anonymous. (2023b)

Key points of presenting a paper:

- Rehearse the presentation, considering time available for the presentation. If a presenter has only 10 to 15 minutes, focus the discussion on one or two major points.
- Consider the possible range in the number of people and the size of the room. Be prepared to present the paper in a less formal way if attendees turn out to be few in number. If a large room is full of many attendees, plan to move more briskly through the talk. Leave ample time for questions.
- Consider who will be in the audience (e.g., parents, professionals, new graduates, experienced practitioners) and plan your presentation's depth accordingly.
- If the paper is to be read verbatim, use conversational expression and make frequent eye contact with members of the audience.
- When presentations are more than 15 minutes long, prepare a visual presentation (PowerPoint, Keynote), that can be used to discuss the paper rather than reading it verbatim.
- Allow 5 to 10 minutes for questions from the audience.
- Speak loudly and clearly enough for everyone in the audience to hear.
- Prepare the visual presentation so that people in the last row can see the slides. If possible, provide handouts of the images.
- When preparing slide presentations, be sure that the font is large (36 points or above) and that attendees have handouts (in smaller fonts) of the presentations. For slides a light print with a dark background (dark blue background with yellow print) may be easier to read. A sans serif font (e.g., Arial, Calibri, or Helvetica) is also preferable. Although adding animations can be entertaining, they may distract from the actual content of the presentation.
- Be sure that equipment works prior to the presentation. Go to the room at least ten minutes before the presentation and try out the equipment.
- Include a beginning, middle, and end in your presentation. The beginning should establish rapport and set the purpose of the presentation with the audience. The ending should summarize the presentation. Make your conclusion memorable.
- Generally, the audience will be adult learners. Adult learners are pragmatic, eager to apply what they learn, have a variety of experiences, and often challenge the presenter. Embrace this intellectual richness.
- Include a one-page handout with references.

Audiovisual aids:

- PowerPoint/KeyNote: These are useful tools for the organization of material. Individual points can be displayed as they are discussed, rather than all at once, as they would be on a transparency or slide. Sequencing and timing are also facilitated. Handouts should be used to help the audience follow the program. In addition, speaker notes can be scripted to remind the speaker of specific points. Because presentation applications are updated frequently, the speaker should verify that there are no compatibility issues with the presentation hardware. This is particularly true if the presentation has imbedded video or audio.
- Document monitors: Document monitors will project items (e.g., printed material or other physical objects) onto a projection screen. In general, prepare items with a word-processing program rather than free-hand print. Use contrasting colors if possible. Pictures can be scanned into a document and printed. The print should be large enough for those in the back to see. Graphics should be sharp and uncluttered with no distracting material.
- Flip charts: Use dark-colored markers, write in large lettering, and place the easel on a platform above the audience so those in the back can see the chart.

12.8.3 Publication

Numerous opportunities exist for students and practitioners to publish their research in occupational therapy journals. The following outline lists the steps in selecting a journal and preparing the research study or capstone project for publication. In addition, based on the third author's experience as the editor of a scholarly journal, questions used to evaluate a submitted manuscript to a refereed journal have been included.

Selecting the appropriate journal: The researcher should obtain the journal-specific instructions for submission of a paper before submission. The style (e.g., APA, AMA), margins, page length, manuscript length, and the arrangement of the manuscript are specific to each journal. Most journals require work to be submitted electronically, either by email or through the website of the publisher or an intermediary. Go to https://research.aota.org/ajot/pages/authorguidelines for current instructions when submitting a manuscript for publication to the *American Journal of Occupational Therapy* (*AJOT*).

Classifying the manuscript:

- Research paper, presenting original empirical data (quantitative or qualitative)
- Position paper (e.g., advocating for a change in the health care system or in health care policy)
- Review article (systematic synthesis of research studies)
- Description of service delivery program
- Description of a clinical device
- Book review
- Letter to the editor

Components of manuscript:

- Title: include variables, participants, settings
- Author(s): include degrees, affiliation, email address, and corresponding address
- Abstract: 100–250 word summary of article
- Key words: 4–5 descriptive words
- Introduction and literature review
- Method
- Results
- Discussion, including limitations and recommendations for further research
- Conclusions
- References
- Tables
- Figures
- Appendices (if any)
- Acknowledgements

Process of getting into print:

- Submit the manuscript to only one journal at a time. If the submission is rejected, then consider submitting it to another journal. Revising is usually necessary.
- Keep in mind that approximately 60% of manuscripts are rejected.
- The lag between submitting an article and seeing it in print is often up to 18 months.
- Refereed journals: The types of decisions made are (a) accept as is (rare), (b) accept with minor revisions, (c) reconsider after major revisions, and (d) reject.

BOX 12-2. THE JOURNAL REVIEW PROCESS (QUESTIONS POSED FOR THE REVIEWER)

Is the title representative of the manuscript? For example, is the independent variable identified, such as the intervention? Is the dependent variable identified, such as the desired outcome? Is the population identified? Is the setting for the study identified? For example, a clinical research study could be titled: The effects of constraint therapy (intervention) on functional abilities (outcome) in patients with stroke (population) in inpatient rehabilitation (setting).

- Does the abstract summarize the major points in the study? The abstract should include the objective of the study such as to evaluate the effectiveness of an intervention with a specific population. Are the methods for collecting data included, such as screening criteria for participant selection, assessments used to measure outcome and the design of the study including a control group? The next section of an abstract includes the results stated concisely and the discussion which includes recommendations for further research and possible limitations of the study. The discussion section closes with the main conclusions from the findings of the study.
- Is there justification for the need for the study? The author should introduce the study by citing statistics that demonstrate the importance of the study such as the incidence and prevalence of stroke.
- Is the literature review current and comprehensive? The literature cited should demonstrate that the author has done an extensive review of studies that are current and come from a wide source of journals.
- Does the (quantitative) study have internal validity (control of extraneous variables), or for a qualitative study, confirmability? In the methodology section the author describes in enough detail the procedure used in collecting data. The methods should be operationally defined so that the study can be replicated. The inclusion criteria are found in this section. The assessments for measuring outcome should include reliability and validity data.
- Is the results section objectively presented by the author? Are there tables of data to show statistical analyses of the data?
- In the discussion section, does the researcher interpret the current results and compare them with the results reported in the literature?
- Does the author state the limitations of the study and recommendations for further research? Are the conclusions consistent with the results?

12.9 RESEARCH AND EVIDENCE-BASED PRACTICE

In applying published research evidence to the practice of occupational therapy, careful appraisal and reasoning are important skills in the process. The occupational therapist has to weigh the internal validity (rigor) of each study and its relevance, applicability, and feasibility (generalizability) to practice. Applying evidence to practice may include:

1. Evaluating the effect size and specific applicability of a specific intervention such as tai chi or yoga in stroke rehabilitation

2. Creating a resource for teaching by determining the best published interventions for children with autism

3. Analyzing recent research evidence in light of current practices in occupational therapy through meta-analysis and by so doing making it possible to improve practice

4. Facilitating the transfer of knowledge from research to practice by attending conference presentations and reading journal publications, and discussing them with colleagues with an eye toward implementation

Skills needed to utilize research evidence in practice:

- A critical attitude towards one's own practice
- Intellectual curiosity in staying current with the published literature
- Knowledge of research methodology, statistics and qualitative analytic techniques
- Familiarity with resource databases and Cochrane Reviews for retrieving research studies
- Ability to systematically analyze without bias the published literature
- Ability to transfer research findings to clinical practice

Likewise, professional practice can be more readily kept up-to-date and improved if researchers collaborate closely with practitioners in the selection, design, and implementation of their research. Surveying practitioners for their practice questions is a good place to start. Their continued involvement in the design of a study, lending their perspective on the feasibility of interventions under study, will enhance the transferability of the study's findings. Practitioners should also be involved in the interpretation of the findings, to be presented in the paper's discussion section.

Potential areas for research in occupational therapy in 2024:

- Identifying effective interventions for individuals with long COVID symptoms
- Describing how artificial intelligence may have an impact on occupation and occupational therapy
- Applying ergonomics in adapting home and work environments for those with disabilities
- Evaluating purposeful and meaningful activities in treating individuals who are homeless with mental illness
- Developing standardized teaching activities of daily living to individuals with disabilities who are aging in place
- Evaluating sensory integration as an intervention with children diagnosed with autism
- Using artificial intelligence as an environmental intermediary for individuals with Alzheimer's disease
- Adapting a computerized wheelchair for individuals with amyotrophic lateral sclerosis
- Evaluating and assisting individuals with disabilities to drive a car
- Improving perceptual skills in children with learning disabilities
- Evaluating constraint-induced movement therapy with individuals with hemiparesis
- Maintaining cognitive functions in individuals with dementia
- Preparing individuals who are homeless and with mental illness to work in paid employment
- Applying stress management programs for individuals with post-traumatic stress disorders
- Using biofeedback in interventions for decreasing incontinence
- Developing client-centered exercise programs for individuals post a cardiac event
- Evaluating sensory stimulation programs for infants in neonatal units
- Teaching individuals with amputations to use electronic prosthetic devices

In conclusion, research in occupational therapy in tandem with evidence-informed practice can have a powerful effect on improving the quality of service provision and provide evidence for using interventions that are effective.

12.10 EXAMPLE PAPER

Altruism and Performance of Elderly Women Living in Long Term Care and Assisted Living Facilities

Amanda F. Hatfield
Research Advisor: Martin S. Rice, PhD, OTR/L
Department of Occupational Therapy
Occupational Therapy Doctorate Program
The University of Toledo Health Science Campus
May 2008

Abstract

The purpose of this study was to investigate the performance of female long-term care and assisted living residents who participated in an altruistic occupation. Residents from four long-term care and assisted living facilities were randomly assigned into either an altruistic or non-altruistic group. Residents in the altruistic group colored and filled therapy pillows for donation to a local domestic violence shelter. Residents in the non-altruistic group colored and filled therapy pillows to keep for their own use. Time spent making the pillows (seconds), the number of pillows made, rating the meaning of making the pillows, and rating the meaning of learning to make pillows were all measured after completion of the occupation. Residents who participated in the altruistic group spent more seconds making therapy pillows ($p =.01$), made more pillows ($p =.03$), and rated the occupation as more meaningful ($p =.02$) than did residents in the non-altruistic group. Findings provide support for engaging long-term care and assisted living residents in altruistic occupations to improve performance. Further research is necessary to confirm the beneficial effect of altruism on performance.

Introduction

Overview

In this introduction, a brief history of relevant principles of occupational therapy will be reviewed (Hall, 1910; Dunton, 1931; Levine, 1987), the definition of the words meaning and purpose will be explored (Nelson & Thomas, 2003), and then a literature review will be presented regarding variables pertinent to meaningful and purposeful performance. Examples of such variables include contextual relevance (Ferguson & Rice, 2001) and choice (Oxer & Kopp Miller, 2001; Rice & Nelson, 1988). The possibility of a relationship between these variables and altruism in occupational therapy (Kanny, 1993) will then be introduced. Finally, studies of the effect of social contribution, role acquisition, and altruism (Brown et al., 2005; Duellman et al., 1986; Getz, 1987; Hatter & Nelson, 1987; Hughes, 2002; Mattox, 1995; Schwartz et al., 2003; Yuen, 2002), on the performance of elders will be reviewed.

History

According to Dr. William Rush Dunton (1931) there is therapeutic value in eliciting a patient's interest when engaging in occupations. The patient must understand the value of the occupation for it to be a benefit to their well-being. The foundation for this statement comes from the principles formulated by the National Society for the Promotion of Occupational Therapy (1917), which include: facilitation of courage and confidence, arousal of interest, and establishment of industrial and social usefulness. Another early occupational therapy theorist, Herbert J. Hall (1910), validated the success of a work cure to take the place of commonly prescribed bed rest for patients

with symptoms such as anxiety, fatigue, irrational fears and compulsive behavior. Physicians like Hall (1910) and Dunton (1931) combined ideas from the medical model and the arts-and-crafts movement and helped to create a new profession called occupational therapy (Levine, 1987). Occupational therapy utilizes the curative effects of meaningful doing to benefit patients, including the redirection of wandering minds in elders (Levine, 1987).

Meaning, Purpose, and Performance Definition

According to Nelson and Thomas (2003), an individual encountering a set of physical and socio-cultural circumstances interfaces with an occupational form. Meaning involves interpretation of, and affect towards, the occupational form. Once a person interprets a situation, he or she often wants to do something about it, resulting in purpose. The amount of purpose possessed by an individual provides the desire and the motivation necessary for performance (Nelson & Thomas, 2003). It is thought that by increasing the meaning, and subsequently the purpose of an occupation, the individual will increase their performance. Thus, the patient's valuation of the product and valuation of the process in creating it is an important concept to consider in providing health enhancing occupations. Motivation is facilitated by a positive interpretation of the occupation being performed and positive affect about that occupation.

Meaning, Purpose, and Performance Literature

There have been several lines of research that have investigated the relationship between meaning, purpose, and performance. For instance, the research of Ferguson and Rice (2001) investigated whether practice of a self-care occupation in a contextually relevant environment improved learning and skill transfer. Fifty-six college-aged women were randomly assigned to one of three learning phase groups: tying a necktie onto a mannequin, a wooden pole, or a no practice group. All three groups were measured on movement time, movement units, and knot quality while they tied neckties onto themselves (transfer phase). Those 21 participants learning the occupation in a contextually relevant environment performed the task with significantly lower rates of performance change during the transfer phase than the 18 participants who learned the task in a non-contextually relevant environment. This result is indicative of a learning plateau that occurred faster within the group that learned within a relevant occupational form as opposed to those who learned the occupation without associated contextual cues as well as those who did not learn the occupation prior to testing. Contextual relevance is thought to have enhanced the meaning and purpose experienced by the group learning to tie the neckties onto the mannequins, and therefore benefited that group's performance, as evidenced by a faster approach towards the learning plateau compared to the group tying neckties onto the wooden poles. The effect of contextual relevance on performance is similar to the effect of choice on performance.

In a study of the effect of choice on performance, Rice and Nelson (1988) investigated the performance of 24 adolescent males with developmental delays engaging in a t-shirt ironing task. In one condition they were given a choice of which shirt to iron and in another condition they were not given a choice. Performance was assessed by the amount of water evaporated from the finished shirt. More water evaporated when the participant was given a choice of which shirt to iron and keep compared to when no choice was given. The authors concluded that increased participation can be observed when participants are given a choice. The variable of choice is thought to increase the amount of meaning and purpose experienced by the participants, with the end result being an improved performance by those participants who were given a choice compared to those participants who were not given a choice.

Oxer and Kopp Miller (2001) investigated the effects of choice on 32 adolescents who lived in residential treatment facilities. The task involved painting ceramic figurines. The amount of paint applied to figurines was significantly greater when the adolescents were given a choice of which figurine they wanted to paint than when no choice was provided. The implication of this study is that participants may be expected to perform better when given a choice within the occupation, as opposed to random assignment of an occupation not chosen by the participant. The variable of choice is thought to have enhanced the amount of meaning and purpose experienced by those participants who identified a figurine they would like to paint, resulting in significantly greater performance, as evidenced by significantly more paint applied by those participants who were given a choice, as compared to participants who were not given a choice.

Altruism Definition

Beyond contextual relevancy and choice, an emerging area for enhancing performance involves the concept of altruism. Encyclopedia Britannica defines altruism as a construct in ethics that regards the good of others as the end of moral action (2006). In a paper published by the American Occupational Therapy Association, Kanny (1993) lists altruism as the first of seven basic concepts organizing the core values and attitudes that comprise the base of professional occupational therapy. Kanny defines the value of altruism as the unselfish caring for the welfare of others, and its reflection in attitudes of commitment, caring, dedication, responsiveness, and understanding. Altruism's stated central role in occupational therapy is underrepresented in the evidence-based literature, however, the concept of altruism, as it is hypothesized to affect occupational therapy, has been discussed. Fidler (1996) asserts that achieving social efficacy and feeling personal satisfaction require the ability to contribute to the welfare of others, adding that occupations that are most valued in society have greater meaning in defining social efficacy than less socially significant occupations, and that the end-product or outcome of an occupation verifies competence. A caveat of such statements made by Fidler is that their formal investigation has been lacking in the literature. Although altruism, as an independent variable, has limited exposure in research, the following paragraphs will describe the studies available that either used altruism as an independent variable or as an integral part of the study.

Altruism Literature

Brown et al. (2005) investigated the relationship between social contribution and health in the elderly. Measurements of social support (given and received) were conducted in four ethnic groups living in the Northeastern United States. Data were collected during face-to-face interviews using the Network Analysis Profile (NAP; Cohen & Sokolovsky, 1979; Sokolovsky & Cohen, 1981) to assess social network variables. The NAP is a measurement of the participants' social networks (parents, children, siblings, aunts, uncles, cousins, friends, acquaintances, and neighbors), and has been shown to be valid with elderly and multicultural populations. Participants named each member of their networks with whom they had engaged in material (tangible) or emotional (intangible) support exchanges within the previous three months. Participants then rated each member as either giving support to the participant, receiving support from the participant, or equally exchanging support with the participant. Physical health and functional mobility were measured by using the Comprehensive Assessment and Referral Evaluation (CARE) instrument (Teresi et al., 1984), an assessment that has been shown to possess good construct, concurrent, and predictive validity which has shown that conditions such as sleeping disorders, ambulation impairment, somatic conditions, and heart disease are predictive of mortality one year later. As expected, Brown et al. found that greater giving was negatively associated with conditions previously found by the CARE to be predictive of imminent mortality, but levels of receiving were not associated with those conditions. Any effects of social support given were interpreted as perceived levels of giving rather than actual altruism, as the social network members were not interviewed. The implication of these results is that the perception of giving support to others, an essential part of altruism, may have a beneficial effect on health.

Schwartz et al. (2003) investigated whether altruistic social interest behaviors, such as engaging in helping others, were associated with better physical and mental health in a stratified random sample of 2016 members of the Presbyterian Church throughout the United States. Mailed questionnaires evaluated giving and receiving help and self-reported physical and mental health. Both helping others and receiving help were significant predictors of mental health after adjusting for age, gender, stressful life events, income, general health, positive and negative religious coping, and asking God for healing. Psychospiritual, stress, and demographic factors were controlled. Giving help was a stronger predictor of high mental health scores compared to receiving help, implying that altruism may be a factor in improved mental health performance.

In a pilot study with 20 residents of four long-term care facilities, Yuen et al. (2008) found that the Life Satisfaction Index-A (LSI-A; Neugarten et al., 1961) scores of elderly residents of long-term care facilities improved significantly after participation in a mentoring program for improving language skills of international students. College students whose second language was English met with mentors for conversation once a week for three weeks. The LSI-A served as a measure of subjective well-being and was administered before and after the intervention. Results of an analysis of covariance revealed a higher adjusted mean score in the mentoring group than the non-mentoring group. The participants who were in the mentoring group reported a significantly higher level of "well-being" than those who were not in the mentoring group. Mentoring is giving of the self for others' growth. These results suggest that giving, a factor in altruism, may positively affect an individual's life satisfaction.

In another study, Hughes (2002) investigated the relationship between altruism and the performance of 172 elderly individuals living in a retirement community. These participants were randomly assigned to a group engaging in a can crushing occupation to earn money for donation to homeless children in an impoverished foreign country (altruistic condition) or a group crushing cans for money that would be given to the participants (non-altruistic condition). The participants' perception of the level of purpose and meaning in the occupation was not assessed. The results, determined by counting the number of crushed cans in each condition, showed no significant differences between the number of cans crushed in the altruistic condition and the number of cans crushed in the non-altruistic condition. The meaning of the crushed cans, and their implied monetary value to children in Guatemala, may not have been perceived as being substantially significant to these community-dwelling elders. Investigation of whether participants understand the meaning of their efforts is indicated.

Hatter and Nelson (1987) investigated altruism and performance. Persons living in a home for the aged were invited to participate in a cookie-decorating activity. The invitations for two of the groups (one group from each of two of the wings of the home) stated that the cookies would be a gift for a local preschool. The invitations for the other two groups (one group from each of the other two wings of the home) did not mention giving away the cookies. The results showed greater attendance ($n = 25$) of those invited to engage in occupationally embedded tasks that involved giving (altruism) compared to attendance ($n = 14$) of those who were invited to perform rote exercise (non-altruistic). These results suggest that elders in long term care facilities might be more likely to participate when an occupation benefits others.

Mattox (1995) investigated the relationship between altruism and performance in retired community dwellers ($n = 172$). As in the previously described study, participants were randomly assigned to a group (altruistic or non-altruistic), and then were measured on attendance. The task involved either making Halloween decorations for children at a community agency or making Halloween decorations for participants to keep for themselves, depending on group assignment. Emphasis was placed on the children at a community agency's valuation of the Halloween decorations. The difference between altruistic and non-altruistic groups making Halloween decorations was not significant. The insignificance of these results suggests that the task of making Halloween decorations for children may not have been more meaningful to the participants than making Halloween decorations for themselves, as evidenced by homogenous attendance levels of both groups. Based on these results, further investigation of the meaning of a given occupation to the participants is warranted.

Getz (1987) examined altruism in a population of elderly women in skilled nursing facilities ($n = 33$). Participants were referred to the study after achieving a score of 25 or more on the Paracheck Geriatric Rating Scale (Paracheck & King, 1976), which allowed only those individuals above a particular cognitive level to be included. The participants were randomly assigned to eight groups, four of which made stationery for children who had been abused, stenciling the children's initials on the top of the paper. The other four groups made stationery personalized with their own initials. Participants were given as many breaks as they desired. There was a strong emphasis placed on the children who received the stationery. For instance, pictures of the children were provided and children's initials were stenciled onto the paper. Reminders of the meaning of the occupation were given frequently according to the script provided by researchers, including comments about how much the children needed the gift to write to friends and family. Analyses of both the quantity of stationery pieces and duration of stationery creation revealed that participants engaged for a significantly longer time period and made more pieces of stationery when the product was given to abused children than when the product was kept by the participant. This study supported the use of altruism as a motivating factor for participation in a craft-type occupation.

Purpose

The research is inconclusive regarding the efficacy of using altruism as a motivating factor for participation in occupations. A central tenet of occupational therapy is that the amount of meaning (personal relevancy) a performer attributes to an occupation affects the amount of purpose (motivation) that performer has for the occupation, and consequently the amount of effort exerted for performance is increased when an occupation is experienced as meaningful when compare to when the occupation is experienced as meaningless (Nelson, 2003). Many of the prior studies of altruism use occupational forms that are assumed to have greater meaning, but the impact of altruism on performance is inconclusive. Some of the studies described above support the positive effect of giving or altruism on performance (Brown et al., 2005; Getz, 1987; Hatter & Nelson 1987; Schwartz et al., 2003; Yuen, 2002), while some of the studies did not support the effect of giving or altruism on performance (Mattox, 1995; Hughes, 2002). In other words, despite our current state of knowledge, we still do not have a firm understanding of how altruism can affect performance. Additionally, this study incorporates the level of meaning associated with the occupation expressed by the participants, which has yet to be investigated. The purpose of the current study is to investigate the effect of meaning on performance as a function of both the meaning attributed to an occupation and whether the occupation is considered by the participants to be altruistic. This study is different from other altruism studies, because it includes a measurement of meaning to the participants which may show an effect beyond a significant difference in the number of and time spent on resulting products.

The study at hand sought to investigate the effect of the knowledge of an altruistic contribution upon the performance of elderly women who live in long-term care and assisted living facilities. This study used a handmade craft-making occupation and informed half of the participants that the craft would be given to victims of domestic violence after its creation. The other half of participants were allowed to keep the craft for themselves. It was expected by the investigator that observance of the number of therapy pillows made by each participant and the amount of time spent making therapy pillows would reveal a significant difference between those who donated their therapy pillows compared to those who kept them. In this study, the altruistic occupation involved making therapy pillows for victims of domestic violence and the non-altruistic occupation involved making therapy pillows for oneself. The victims of domestic violence were chosen as recipients of the altruistic occupation because it was thought that they would be viewed as legitimately needful of help.

Elderly women living in a long-term care or assisted living facility were recruited to participate in a task to help or benefit others (altruistic) or in a task to benefit oneself (non-altruistic). The number of pillows produced, the amount of time engaged in the occupation (total time and time per pillow), and the participants' meanings attributed to the occupation were measured. It was hypothesized that:

1. Participants in the altruistic group would perform longer, measured using a computerized stopwatch, and make a greater number of products.
2. Participants in the altruistic group would associate a higher level of meaning, defined using a three point Likert scale, to the product than participants in the non-altruistic group.
3. Participants in the altruistic group would associate a higher level of meaning, defined using a three point Likert scale, to the occupation than participants in the non-altruistic group.

Method

Participants

The sample consisted of 30 female senior citizens (65 years old or older) who lived in a long-term care or assisted living facilities. Studies that had similar sample sizes found statistical significance. Therefore, it was believed that this n provided enough statistical power to avoid risking a Type II error. Exclusion criteria via self report included any type of physical or neurological conditions that would adversely affect the ability to participate in a coloring and pillow stuffing task. Participants were recruited from long-term care and assisted living facilities. Once permission was granted to conduct the study in the facility, a staff person from the facility asked residents (whom the staff person had perceived as appropriate for the study) if they would like to learn more about participating in the study. If the participant agreed to learn more about the study, then the staff person gave the name of the interested persons to the investigator who then met with the interested residents to explain the study and provide materials for completion of the therapy pillows. Competence and cognitive abilities were assessed via verbal self-report by the participant that she had no physical or neurological impairments that might interfere with the study.

Apparatus

The following materials were used: (a) fabric pens, (b) white fabric sown into 4 × 5 inch pockets, (c) templates, (d) rice, (e) a funnel, (f) a bucket, (g) a sewing machine, (h) a stopwatch, and (i) a questionnaire. The questionnaire, administered as a measurement of the participants' meaning attributed to the occupation, included questions about how much the therapy pillow meant to the participant and how much learning to make the therapy pillow meant to the participant. The rationale for this measurement was to identify the level of meaning participants attributed to the occupation and product, and to investigate differences between levels of meaning reported by participants in the altruistic condition and levels of meaning reported by participants in the non-altruistic condition. A custom software program kept track of the time spent on the task and was used to record the number of pillows completed.

This occupation was age-appropriate regardless of whether the creator was the recipient of the product or not. Therapy pillows were products that were potentially useful for younger women, children, and elderly women. The product, a decorated pillow filled with rice, was approximately 1 pound and 4 × 5 inches in size. Drawing on the fabric and stuffing the pillows with rice were chosen as the performances examined in this study. The use of fabric pens allowed for easy application to the fabric, facilitating the occupation for persons living in long-term care facilities. It is a brief occupation that is practical in terms of time and expense. The pillow is small enough that, conceivably, a person would want to have more than one for effective use.

Procedure

This study was approved by the Biomedical Institutional Review Board of the University of Toledo. Before any data were collected, informed consent was obtained. Participants were randomly assigned to the altruistic or non-altruistic group. Randomization occurred using a custom software program that randomly assigned group assignment in a permutated blocked fashion using two blocks of four sessions and four blocks of three sessions. Specifically, the group section (altruistic or non-altruistic) was randomly assigned. It was anticipated that up to four participants would participate in each session. Therefore, to accommodate an *n* of 30, ten sessions were included in the randomization process. The investigator entered the number of the session in a computer program (e.g. 1, 2, etc.) and the computer program assigned the session to one of the two group conditions. Both groups received an explanation of how the therapy pillows would be used, including heat therapy, positioning, or as a game. In the non-altruistic group, the completed pillow was given to the participant to keep for herself. In the altruistic group, the participant was told that the investigator would give the completed pillow to domestic violence victims living in a local shelter, specifically women and children.

The altruistic group was instructed to decorate and fill therapy pillows for victims of domestic violence. A description of the mission of the shelter where the victims of domestic violence lived was given or read to the participants. The completed products were given to the victims of domestic violence by the investigator. The non-altruistic group was instructed to decorate and fill therapy pillows to keep for themselves.

All of the participants were seated at tables in groups of up to four people per table, according to the order in which they arrived. Group size was limited to four in order to optimize instruction. Each group was given the same set of instructions. The occupation consisted of two steps: (a) the decoration of the empty pocket using fabric pens, and (b) the filling of the pocket with rice. Once the pocket was filled, it was sewn shut by the investigator, and an additional pocket was offered to the participant.

If participants asked how long they should continue making the pillows, they were told to continue as long as they would like. When participants stopped performing the occupation, each was given the verbal (closure) prompt: "Would you like to continue making pillows for yourself/child/woman?" If the subject answered "No," a second and final verbal (closure) prompt was given: "Are you sure that you do not want to make another pillow for yourself/child/woman?" If the participant answered "Yes" the duration

was recorded. If the participant answered "No" to the verbal (closure) prompt, the pillow-making activity was resumed.

Rests were allowed. Time was recorded at the beginning and the end of a rest. A rest was suggested if the participant appeared fatigued: "Are you tired? You may take a rest if you would like one. Go ahead and rest for a moment." After one minute, the participant was asked "Are you ready to work again?" in order to reengage the participant in the activity. If the participant did not want to reengage in the activity, the previously mentioned verbal (closure) prompts were used.

The occupation took place at the place of residence of the participants, at approximately the same time of day for each group. Non-participating residents were not present in the room.

Statistical Analysis

A simple experimental design was used. The dependent variables included: time spent working on the pillows (finished time was measured using a digital stopwatch with split timing), number of pillows made (recorded on the same form as the time record), and questionnaire scores. Questionnaire scores were assessed using a three point Likert scale of the meaning of the occupation and the meaning of learning to make the product. Cohen's effect size *d* was calculated for each of the comparisons (1988). Non-parametric measures (Mann Whitney *U*) were used for the ordinal data (number of pillows made and meaning measures), while parametric measures (*t*-test) were used for the continuous data (time).

12.11 Summary

In this chapter the authors discussed the components of effective scientific writing as a key component in a research study. The primary purpose of scientific writing is to communicate the results of a study or theoretical concepts in clear, objective, and logical wording. In this process, the first step is to establish an environment for writing that promotes the writer's best efforts. The components of a research paper include an introduction to the topic including the need for the study and the possible impact of the results of the study, for example on clinical practice. The next component of a research study is the literature review which should be extensive and up-to-date. The third component of a research study is the methodology which includes an operational description of how the study is implemented. The next sections of the study include the results section which is presented in an objective way with figures and tables, the discussion section which compares current results with prior studies, and the limitations of the study. The transmission of the results of the study such as publication in a journal, presentation at scientific conference, and the newer methods through social media were discussed.

13

The Scholarly Capstone

Judith Parker Kent, Martin S Rice, George Tomlin, and Franklin Stein

As modern technological innovations are the direct outcome of scientific research, scientists can no longer afford to stand aloof from social problems.

Rene Dubos (1959, p. 221)

As the culminating piece of the entry-level occupational therapy doctorate, the doctoral capstone provides students the opportunity for in-depth exposure in one or more of the eight areas of focus delineated by ACOTE, ultimately resulting in dissemination of project outcomes, and demonstrating synthesis of the skills and knowledge gained.

Ad Hoc Document Development Committee (2022, p. 1)

OPERATIONAL LEARNING OBJECTIVES

By the end of this chapter, the learner will be able to:
1. Identify the capstone requirements for the occupational therapy doctorate
2. Formulate a feasible capstone project
3. Apply research-based concepts to ACOTE capstone project categories
4. Create relevant questions pertaining to a capstone project
5. Generate ideas on how the capstone project can be utilized to further not only the field of occupational therapy but also the evidence of its value to the client, health care, and society
6. Examine topics, methods, and models appropriate for research-based capstone projects

DOI: 10.4324/9781003523154-13

13.1 INTRODUCTION

The proportion of occupational therapy doctoral (OTD) programs continues to grow amongst entry-level occupational therapy programs in the United States. A unique part of the OTD is the capstone component. The Accreditation Council for Occupational Therapy Education (ACOTE) first published accreditation standards for the OTD in 2006 (*AJOT*, 2007). While there are other aspects differentiating the OTD level entry point from the occupational therapy Master's degree, the capstone component is arguably the most distinguishable. While the title of this text communicates the focus of this book, the authors feel it is essential to include a chapter on the capstone project. The reason being is that many of the strategies, methods, and concepts espoused throughout this text are useful to the planning, development, implementation, and dissemination of the capstone project. Applying these strategies, methods, and concepts to the capstone project will facilitate the capstone project to become more robust and impactful to the many groups of associated people including the student, the mentors, the subject population and the community at large. It has been said that rising seas lift all boats.

In the 2023 ACOTE standards, there are 59 occurrences of the word "Capstone" (ACOTE, 2023). Familiarity with the ACOTE standards yields four major sections, notably identified as being *A*, *B*, *C*, and *D*, and the term capstone is dispersed in all four. However, the *D* section is wholly focused upon and is entitled the "Doctoral Capstone." In that section, the standards identify seven potential areas of focus. These include clinical practice skills, research skills, administration, leadership, program and policy development, advocacy, education, and theory development. At the time of this writing the next iteration of ACOTE standards propose to drop theory development from the list (ACOTE, 2023).

Among the seven surviving areas of capstone areas of focus, research is identified and is most closely aligned with the other chapters of this text. However, it is our contention that the other six areas identified by ACOTE can be enhanced and supported by the fundamental concepts woven throughout this text. For instance, each category of capstone project (as defined by ACOTE) will involve some level of construct identification; all will involve some level of comparison or analysis, hence some form of research design; all will then involve some form of measurement in order to analyze the efficacy of the project; with measurement, all will involve statistics. All will involve a statement of generalizability; Feasibility of the project will need to be considered, and lastly all should include a plan for sustainability. Figure 13–1 illustrates the relationship of these concepts across the seven capstone categories. What follows in this chapter is a discussion of how construct identification, research designs, measurement approaches, statistical/qualitative analyses, generalizability, feasibility, and sustainability are applicable to clinical practice skills, research, program/policy development, leadership, advocacy, administration, and education.

13.2 CONSTRUCT IDENTIFICATION

For any given capstone project, there needs to be an idea behind it. It needs to have a focus. In a research capstone project, the idea or focus is usually centered upon the

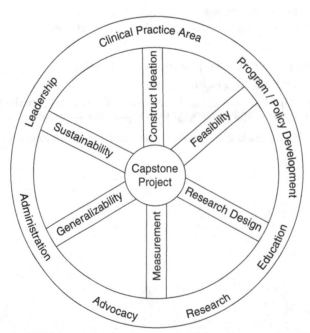

Figure 13–1 Relationship between the ACOTE capstone categories and research-based concepts. Note that each capstone category is linked to each of the research-based concepts.

independent variable. From the independent variable is borne the research question or hypothesis. The independent variable is the lynch pin of the whole research study. Likewise, capstone projects need to have a focus or a central theme. It is what the capstone is about. This is what construct identification is. An example may be how the environmental context (independent variable) affects the ability of clients with TBI to engage in community activity. It is the formal process of naming, defining, and explaining what the central focus of the capstone project is. This is an essential step in designing and developing the capstone. It will drive the types of studies that are included in the bibliography. It is the fulcrum upon which a needs assessment balances. Regardless of the type of capstone project to be completed, construct identification is one of the initial steps to be taken. And once identified, the whole capstone project will revolve around that central idea.

13.3 FEASIBILITY

Feasibility is all about the likelihood that the project can actually occur. A feasibility study must occur during the planning phase of the capstone project. There are many aspects that play into whether a project is feasible or not. There are financial implications. Questions to ask related to finances are: What are the associated costs to carry out the study? Will participants receive a gift of some sort as a thank you for participating? Will there be items consumed in the course of the project? Will there be fees associated with any of the measurement tools? Will travel costs be incurred? And the list goes on. Time is another constraint that must be considered. Unlike many research projects (often, dissertation phases of PhD programs last years), the capstone experience is determined, minimally, by ACOTE standards; typically, OTD programs schedule the capstone experience within a university semester (currently 14 weeks). As such, careful planning is essential for all of the capstone objectives to be completed within that defined timeframe. Other constraints include availability of human resources, an adequate number of participants, the availability and access to space, the knowledge base/skill set of the faculty mentor, and institutional imposed limitations such as the institutional review board. During every research project and capstone experience, unexpected challenges will occur. Depending on the magnitude of the challenge, a variety of potential solutions can be employed to overcome, adapt, or otherwise deal with the challenge. Some challenges are minor and limited in scope, such as a conflicting schedule that comes up. Perhaps simply rescheduling is all that is needed. Other challenges can be catastrophic. An example of this may be the unexpected death of a key member of the capstone team or participant, or an international pandemic that forces the closure of facilities and communities. The point is that while some challenges can be planned for, there are other challenges that come as a complete and total surprise, some of which may be significant and formidable to overcome. The best preventative measure, however, is good planning. Additionally, it is important to build in some redundancies so that it is more likely that alternative plans can be employed to overcome the unexpected. The old saying of having a plan "B" is apropos here.

13.4 RESEARCH DESIGN

A student on capstone who has chosen to design a project in any of ACOTE's capstone areas except research may think that a research design is not necessary. However, in all capstone projects, there will be a need to determine whether the intervention, the program development, or the leadership growth was effective in meeting the goals that the student established prior to the implementation. As such, a research design needs to be employed in order to enhance the integrity of the capstone project outcome. For instance, this might involve a pre- and post-test questionnaire to determine if growth has occurred, or in the case of a case study, whether the client(s) met their goals. At the very least, projects will likely involve some level of a descriptive research design upon which the needs assessment data are communicated in order to establish a genuine need to implement a program. Qualitative research designs may also be employed if a focus group is recruited to discuss their lived experience based upon the project's identified construct.

13.5 MEASUREMENT

What follows on the heels of research design is measurement. As mentioned above, all projects will involve some form of outcome evaluation. This necessitates the need for some form of measurement. It is not enough for the student or mentor to just "think it turned out okay!" There needs to be some data behind it and that data needs to be measured. This is actually directly tied to the ACOTE standards D.1.2, D.1.3, and D.1.7. Specifically, D.1.2 requires that individualized objectives and plans be established and D.1.3 requires that the "...capstone project includes a literature review, needs assessment, goals/objectives, and an evaluation plan" (*AJOT*, 2018, p. 45). Moreover, D.1.7 requires that the student's performance across the capstone experience is formally evaluated. Inherent in these three standards is some form of measurement. Variables need to be measured throughout the capstone experience; the capstone project itself as well as the student's performance through the capstone. The type of measurement is not specified in the ACOTE standards, but rather the measurement and/

or the measurement tools are to be determined during the planning phase of the capstone. These may include self-determined objectives that the student specifies, they may involve some norm-reference standardized assessments, they may involve some measurement tool that the site or site mentor uses that may be unique to that site, or it might be a widely used measure across multiple settings and geographical locations. A good example of the latter is quality of life measures. There are a number of examples, however the World Health Organization developed the WHOQOL-BREF, which is a 26-item questionnaire that measures quality of life (World Health Organization, 1996). A well-known quality of life measure for pediatrics is the Pediatric Quality of Life Inventory (PedsQL) which is a 23-item survey (Varni & Limbers, 2009).

13.6 STATISTICS

The majority of chapters in this text are focused on one form of statistical analysis or another. Suffice it to say, that since it has been established that objectives need to be measured and that this will occur within the defined research design, some form of statistics will be necessary. These may be descriptive in nature, they may involve a correlation, or they may involve two or more comparisons. In this latter example, depending on the type of data involved, a *t*-test or analysis of variance may be employed. Or in the case of counting the number of times something happened across time and/or across different conditions, perhaps a chi-square should be calculated. Regardless of whether the design is quantitative or qualitative, statistics are necessary to support the interpretation of the results. Using statistics can be a very effective way of documenting how those capstone objectives turned out. Statistics can produce solid evidence that substantiates the efficacy of the capstone's identified construct. In other words, the authors of this chapter may be biased, but they think statistics are "pretty cool" and they can go a long way in validating a student's capstone experience to the world.

13.7 GENERALIZABILITY

Speaking of the world, the importance of generalizability cannot be understated. Generalization speaks to the ability to apply the findings to a larger population beyond those involved in the study or project. How can this happen in practical terms? In fulfillment of ACOTE standard D.1.8, the capstone project must be disseminated. This can occur in any number of forms; however, many students may not realize that beyond their presentation day, whether it be a poster presentation or a platform presentation, their capstone project may be archived in their institution's library. Many of these libraries are searchable through the

internet. In fact, in preparing this chapter, many university libraries were searched and there are currently thousands of capstone examples available in the United States. There have also been many capstone projects that were published in occupational therapy peer-reviewed journals. The value of having these capstone projects available for the public to read is that any given capstone project might have an influence over other occupational therapists around the world. Yes, any student who has their capstone project in a searchable library or published in a journal or trade magazine has in essence preserved their capstone project for future generations. How well the project was designed and how strong the external validity of the project is will determine how applicable or generalizable the project is for other populations.

13.8 SUSTAINABILITY

The difference between a typical project that is tied to an OTD assignment and the capstone project is that it should be a plan for the continuation or "next steps" to be taken once the capstone project is completed. In research, there is often a statement about what future research should entail with a recommended direction. This might be to extend the study to a larger population, or to a different population of participants, or it might be a call to replicate the study while imposing greater experimental controls. A capstone project can be heuristic in that it can generate future studies. In the capstone, the sustainability plan will be unique to the type of capstone project—that is, a clinical practice skills (case-study), research, administration, leadership, program/policy development, advocacy, or education project.

13.9 SPECIAL CONSIDERATIONS FOR THE RESEARCH PROJECT

13.9.1 Single Case Study Design

In a single case study design one subject or group is either followed through their care or a variable is introduced to induce change, such as a method of intervention. The single case study for a capstone needs to be a unique, exceptional, or otherwise beyond the day-to-day typical case or treatment. An example is looking at an adult who has experienced trauma watching a family member being shot to death in front of them, and then using trauma-informed care to work with the client from an occupational therapy perspective focusing on engagement in activities that have meaning to the client now that the family member is accepted as gone. Another example is a family member with a profound disability and the impact it has upon other siblings' emotional development.

13.9.2 Multiple Single Case Study Design

In this type of study, each subject is their own control, usually in a "baseline" and "measurement" phases. There are variations of this involving multiple baseline and measurement phases. See Chapter 7 for more detail on this type of design. An example is working with visually impaired children, monitoring their time on task in a classroom without the intervention to get a baseline measurement, then exposing them to toys with various sensory inputs in a systematic way measuring the same outcome as in the baseline measurement. In this way a comparison can be inferred between the baseline and measurement phases. The outcome measure in this example may be their time on task; during the baseline phase the child would be measured on their time-on-task for ten minutes, however, in the measurement phase the child is given a choice on which toy to play with and the time-on-task is measured in the same fashion during the baseline phase.

13.9.3 Modified Replication

A modified replication involves replicating a project done by a student in previous years with updated modifications. An example might be where the experimental controls are improved from the original project. One student evaluated the forces involved in performing pivot transfers (one chair to another) but there was no method for measuring the forces at the lower back. In a subsequent study, newer technology was implemented that afforded this important calculation (Bartnik & Rice, 2013; Larson et al., 2018).

13.9.4 Data mining

Data can exist in many repositories, such as charts of clients, data collected by universities, schools and governmental bodies, health organizations, as well as research groups. The Centers for Disease Control and Prevention offers several large and extensive databases (CDC, 2023) and the World Health Organization offers several comprehensive health-related databases as well (WHO, 2023). Data mining involves searching the variables within the database to answer a question. An example is investigating the relationship between socioeconomic status and the physical and emotional health of adults within a defined region in the United States.

13.9.5 Faculty Research

Faculty research has the student joining a current project that a faculty member may be conducting to add to their data pool. This supports not only the faculty research and collection of data but also supports the student's knowledge of an ongoing project. For instance, let's say a faculty member has been studying the effects of sleep deprivation on college students' academic performance. A student can join this project at multiple points taking on such roles as the literature review, the initial questionnaires on sleep and finally collecting data on an academic performance measure. Each step is linked to the original research but the individual student is participating in a portion of the research project that supports the research as a whole (Benham et al., 2022). In the sleep deprivation study, the outcome of this study may evolve into ways to help students increase sleep time and improve academic performance.

13.9.6 Research with Control and Experimental Groups

As discussed in earlier parts of the text, experimental research designs involve a control group and an experimental group. This type of design was created to avoid confounding experimental error when comparing the performance of the two groups. As mentioned in Chapter 8, this type of design is often challenging given a number of factors including limited availability of special populations, the setting in which potential participants are located, and ethical considerations surrounding offering or withholding best practice. Regardless, it is possible that a capstone student can carry out a whole study. One of the most challenging factors is the limited time the capstone student has to carry out the study. Because of this, careful planning is essential that needs to occur prior to the actual capstone semester. It is the recommendation of these authors that the project have IRB approval prior to the capstone semester. That way, the student can focus on data collection, analysis, and final write up during the capstone experience semester.

13.9.7 Combining Projects

Combining projects is a unique way to not only have the students undertake individual projects as defined by ACOTE, but this strategy allows all of their data to then be combined by the faculty advisor(s) for faculty independent research. For example, if each student does the exact same project in the exact same way, and inter-rater reliability is validated, with a different population, then comparisons can be made between the various populations' performance. This can be a powerful way to gain an adequate sample size in a manageable amount of time. For example, the research question is whether a specific handwriting program makes a difference in students' performance in the classroom. The capstone student researchers are trained in the specific handwriting method and they are placed in a wide range of settings including preschools, public schools, charter schools, and other settings where individuals with cognitive disabilities as well as autism are located. The students each carry out the project in the exact same way with journaling added to ensure they pick up the nuances of their site and any challenges with the site or the subjects. This type of research design involving multiple capstone students ensures that each student has their own unique project and at the same time a large data set is developed. At the time of this writing, this type of project is currently being conducted with approximately 200 subjects participating as single case studies. This will result in 17 individual capstone projects and data for the faculty investigators to analyze and validate this particular method in a three-month project that has been IRB approved.

The lack of large data sets to verify the effectiveness of occupational therapy methods has been a long-term weakness for the research done in occupational therapy, although there is plenty of rich qualitative data collected from one-on-one interactions. Our profession and universities could look beyond just their own site and sites of multiple universities could be combined to gather data to validate the approaches of our profession in this evidence-based world of science and education. This can be done on a single case study design model or specific methodologies that each student would be trained in. Potentially this type of project could collect data from all over the country, possibly the world. Areas of investigation could include: a specific evaluation tool to be validated, information on populations served, the impact of occupational therapy interventions on long-term mental health, and the list goes on. The students, the faculty, and the site mentors would all become researchers, adding to the evidence base of our profession!

What to do with the data?

Frequently projects conducted by clinical doctoral students have languished within the departments where these studies were conducted or at best shared on a state and national level as posters providing brief glimpses into the unique contributions of the clinical doctorate. Some universities have created archives of their projects as Google documents available to the next year's group of students. Other universities disseminated the projects on YouTube. We as a profession have the opportunity to create a centralized repository for these individual projects, such as in the Wilma West Library. The body of knowledge can be expanded by building upon previously archived capstone projects.

13.10 SUMMARY

The capstone experience and project are daunting for both the students and the faculty yet they provide a rich environment for student learning and application of their skills and knowledge in unique settings. Each step in the learning process guides the student to their place of growth and ultimately a completed project. The key steps are identifying the faculty mentor and site supervisor, doing a needs assessment to identify the topic of choice, a strong literature review and development of the question, followed by methodology that is a good match, completion of the project and ultimately dissemination of the project itself. Each step is a place of growth and potential and at the end of the project students have developed skills that have prepared them to be beginning researchers as well as having stronger professional skills in understanding research and its application to practice.

There are remarkable similarities between the planning, implementation, and sustainability between traditional quantitative and qualitative research with capstone projects. Conceiving of the construct, research designs implantation, using measurement approaches, basing analyses on statistical methods, generalizations to sustainability—all of these are essential components of both research and capstone projects. Incorporating these principles can only strengthen and facilitate the impact that the capstone can have upon future society. Examples of the research-type of capstone have been explored. Also mentioned is the genuine contribution that a disseminated capstone can have upon society. Indeed, the capstone experience is not only a profound expression of the doctoral work that the OTD student creates and participates in; it has the potential to profoundly impact and improve the lives of others, locally, nationally, and internationally.

A Short History of Medicine, Rehabilitation, and Occupational Therapy

The history of medicine has been continuously devaluated in medical education but its importance should not be ignored as for other medical humanities. The educational value of the history of medicine could be summarized as follows; it allows the students 1) to understand the humane aspect of medicine by telling them how medicine has dealt with human health-disease phenomena in each era of the human history. 2) to improve the professionalism by recognizing that medicine is a profession with a long tradition that dates back to the Hippocratic era 3) to improve current medical practice by understanding the limitations and uncertainties of medicine. 4) to understanding the historical changes of the disease phenomena 5) to develop the basic competence of learned intellectual. 6) to integrate the tradition of their own institutions with themselves.

Kwon (2022, p. 469)

OPERATIONAL LEARNING OBJECTIVES

By the end of this chapter, the learner will be able to:
1. Describe seven stages in the history of medicine
2. Explain the cyclical nature of medical progress into the 21st century
3. Recognize the important contributions of medical researchers toward eliminating disease and improving the health of individuals
4. Understand the importance of methodological discoveries in diagnosis, assessment, prevention, and intervention
5. Describe the history and growth of occupational therapy, the allied health professions, and special education
6. Outline occupational therapy's role in the school system and other community settings
7. Identify trends in rehabilitation research

DOI: 10.4324/9781003523154-14

14.1 HISTORICAL REVIEW OF MEDICINE

The rise and development of occupational therapy as a health care profession over one hundred years ago in 1917 has greatly benefitted from the progress in medical practice that came before. The rehabilitation professions (i.e., occupational therapy, physical therapy, speech pathology, and audiology) emerged from the scientific findings in medicine that began in the 19th and 20th centuries. In this chapter, we review seven stages in the history of medicine that are the forerunners of scientific inquiry in the rehabilitation professions.

Before the beginnings of modern medical science in the latter half of the 19th century, relationships between causes and effects still retained explanations that bordered on the supernatural as we would understand them today. Vitalism, a recurrent movement in medicine, was typified by the 18th-century physician who ascribed life functions to mysterious substances in the blood. This theory was an outcome of the pre-scientific thinking that gave way to the systematic and orderly explanations that we now associate with modern scientific research. The understanding of the disease process began with the laboratory experimentation of Pasteur (1822–1895), who served as a model for the medical scientist. The impact of the scientific method in the treatment and rehabilitation of those with illnesses and disabilities has been a remarkable record in human progress. In only a few other areas of knowledge has mankind made greater strides.

The analysis of the progress in medicine, and rehabilitation, can be divided into seven stages as identified in Table 14–1. These seven stages are progressive, interactive, and dynamic. For example, basic research in biological and chemical processes in Stage I continues to be important as evidenced by the investigations of DNA and RNA as the building blocks in protoplasm. Similarly, methodological research is in the forefront by the integration of biomedical engineering and artificial intelligence with clinical practice, as demonstrated in the areas of ergonomics, assistive technology, driver rehabilitation, telehealth, genetic engineering, robotics, prosthetics, transplant operations, kidney dialysis techniques, and artificial replacement of bodily organs. Medical scientists are constantly refining treatment interventions and preventive methodologies. Immunologists who formerly sought chemicals to destroy harmful bacteria and viruses have led the way for

TABLE 14–1		
SEVEN STAGES IN THE HISTORY OF MEDICINE, HEALTH, AND REHABILITATION		
STAGE I		**STAGE II**
Biological Description		*Methodological Advances*
Accurate description of anatomical structure and physiological processes, producing a basic understanding of the bodily organs and systems.		Development of instruments, procedures, and tests to produce valid and reliable methods in evaluation, diagnosis, and treatment.
STAGE III	**STAGE IV**	**STAGE V**
Etiology	*Prevention*	*Treatment*
Understanding of the disease process and cause-effect relationships to produce a science of medicine and universal agreement in diagnosing diseases.	Development of medical technology to prevent initial onset of disease, resulting in the science of immunology and public health.	Application of treatment techniques based on a theoretical understanding of disease processes, leading to the growth of chemical intervention, antiseptic surgery, and nursing care in hospitals.
STAGE VI		**STAGE VII**
Rehabilitation		*Habilitation and Special Education/ Programming Interventions*
Development of therapeutic techniques and restoration of maximum function for individuals with chronic disabilities, leading to the evolution of allied health professions.		The identification of treatments for the developmental and social disabilities applying specialized educational and psychological techniques to populations at risk.

present-day investigators searching for vaccines to prevent cancerous growths and life-threatening diseases, such as acquired immune deficiency syndrome (AIDS) and coronavirus disease (COVID).

14.2 Biological Description—Stage I

14.2.1 The Growth of Scientific Anatomy and Physiology

The earliest medical research started with the discovery of the physiological processes and anatomical systems of the body. Biological description: Stage I, the evolution of medical research, is outlined in Table 14–1.

Centuries before, the ancient Greeks brought rational thought to an evaluation of health and disease. The Hippocratic writings reflect the depth of Greek thought.

14.2.2 The Hippocratic Writings

The first stage in the history of clinical medicine was based on human observation. The healer applying Hippocratic naturalistic methods used himself as a measuring instrument, carefully noting what he saw, felt, smelled, and heard. He used rational thought regarding the causes and treatments of diseases based on these observations. In the ancient Greek civilization, scholars were allowed the freedom to explore all aspects of human life. Thus, a model for the Western physician was emerging. Hippocrates, who is traditionally called the Father of Medicine, was probably in fact several individuals. It is more accurate to speak of the "Hippocratic writings" than to attribute all ancient Greek medicine to one individual. The Hippocratic writings cover many areas of medicine, including ethics, disease etiology, anatomy, physiology, and treatment. These writings are not a consistent work linking theory to practice, but a compendium of clinical histories and a description of Hellenistic medicine.

We know little about Hippocrates' life, except that he lived during the 5th century BCE in Cos, an island off the Greek mainland, and that he was a famous practitioner and teacher of medicine. The following excerpt from the Hippocratic writings, *On the Articulations* (ca. 400 BCE/1952) translated by Francis Adams, demonstrates the method of clinical observation used to diagnose a dislocation of the shoulder joint and the importance of individual differences in human anatomy:

A dislocation may be recognized by the following symptoms: Since the parts of a man's body are proportionate to one another, as the arms and the legs, the sound should always be compared with the unsound, the unsound with the sound, not paying regard to the joints of other individuals (for one person's joints are more prominent than another's), but looking to those of the patient, to ascertain whether the sound joint be unlike the unsound. This is a proper rule, and yet it may lead to much error; and on this account it is not sufficient to know this art in theory, but also by actual practice; for many persons from pain, or from any other cause, when their joints are not dislocated, cannot put the parts into the same positions as the sound body can be put into; one ought therefore to know and be acquainted beforehand with such an attitude. But in a dislocated joint the head of the humerus appears lying much more in the armpit than it is in the sound joint; and also, above, at the top of the shoulder, the part appears hollow, and the acromion is prominent, owing to the bone of the joint having sunk into the part below; there is a source of error in this case also, as will be described and also, the elbow of the dislocated arm is farther removed from the ribs than that of the other; but by using force it may be approximated, though with considerable pain; and also they cannot with the elbow extended raise the arm to the ear, as they can the sound arm, nor move it about as formerly in this direction and that. These, then, are the symptoms of dislocation at the shoulder.

(Hippocrates, as cited in Hutchins, 1952, pp. 94–95)

The Hippocratic writings with their emphasis on diet, exercise, and natural methods were a holistic guide for the ancient physician.

14.2.3 Galen

Greek medicine provided a foundation for medical practice in the Western world. Galen, a product of the Roman civilization, was the next link in the chain of medical progress. He was born in Pergamum, Greece, in the 2nd century ACE when Roman civilization controlled much of the Western world. Galen was educated in philosophy, mathematics, and natural science. He learned medicine by traveling to places where the great physicians practiced. After acquiring knowledge steeped in the Hippocratic tradition, he became a doctor to the gladiators who performed in the Roman arenas. Galen became an acclaimed practitioner in Rome and later spent his time writing extensively. Galen's genius was in his ability to integrate prior knowledge with his clinical observations of disease. Unfortunately, his writings on medicine became authoritative dogma from the Middle Ages to the time of the rebirth of scientific inquiry in the Renaissance. The following excerpt from Galen (ca. 192 ACE/1971) typifies his skill in teaching anatomy, as well as his careful methods of observation.

I therefore maintain that the bones must be learnt either from man, or ape, or better from both, before dissecting the muscles, for those two (namely bones and muscles) form the ground-work of the other parts, the foundations, as it were, of a building. And next, study arteries, veins, and nerves. Familiarity with dissection of these will bring you to the inward parts and so to a knowledge of the viscera, the fat, and the glands, which also you should examine separately, in detail. Such should be the order of your training.

(Galen, as cited in Wightman, 1971, pp. 32–33)

14.2.4 Medieval Medicine

Arabic and Judaic medicine had an important influence in Europe during the Middle Ages. Avicenna's *Canon of Medicine* which incorporated the work of Galen became the standard for medical care. Medical practice in Europe during the Middle Ages (500–1500) centered around the Monastic Orders and the Catholic Priests. "Christianity originally held its own theory of disease, disease was either punishment for sins, possession by the devil or the result of witchcraft. It also had its own therapeutic methods—namely prayer, penitence and the assistance of saints. Every cure, under these circumstances, was basically regarded as a miracle" (Ackerman, 1982, p. 81).

It is to be noted, however, that in the Middle Ages the first medical school in Europe emerged:

the very first recorded medical school was the Schola Medica Salernitana, in Salerno, Italy—now defunct—which had its heyday from approximately the 11th to 13th centuries. The school is important in that it merged the knowledge of the Greek-Latin medical tradition with the Arabic and Jewish medical traditions of the time. Also, in addition to having female students, the school achieved much of its importance from books published by teachers there. Other medical schools were established in Spain, Denmark, and Sweden in the 14th and 15th century.

(*30 of the oldest medical schools in the world*, 2022).

Additional insights into medieval medicine are offered by Pajević et al. citing Avicenna:

Medical works of Avicenna (Ibn Sina) 980–1063:

Ibn Sina represent a pinnacle of most important medical achievements of his time. These works contain synthesis of all Greek, Indian and Iranian medical schools, but also new breakthroughs achieved by Muslim scholars through their own experimentation and practice. Although he wrote many medical works, his most important one is El-Kanun fit-tib, which can be translated as The

Canon of Medicine. It's made out of five books which systematically show everything known in the area of medicine up until that point in time. In it, Ibn Sina discusses, among other things, the structure of psychological apparatus of human being and the connection of psychological functions with the brain as well as the role of psyche in etiology of somatic diseases. He also describes certain psychiatric diseases along with the explanation of their etiology and recommended therapy. He considered psychology to be very important for medicine, so in his psychological works he discusses, in great detail, the essence of human soul, consciousness, intellect and other psychological functions.

(Pajević et al., 2021, p. S1219)

14.2.5 Renaissance Medicine in the 16th and 17th Centuries

The history of medicine parallels, in many ways, the rise of Western civilization. With the onset of the Renaissance, scientists carried out experiments in human dissection under great risk of public denouncement and physical punishment. Despite this, more liberal attitudes were established in the 16th century that allowed medical scholars and scientists to seek the truth by experimentation.

Renaissance physicians rekindled the torch of medical science that had been stagnant for approximately 1,000 years. The scientists of the Renaissance were scholars familiar with Greek, Arabic and Roman writings who questioned all knowledge and accepted little dogma. Furthermore, they re-examined the anatomical knowledge of Galen, experimented in chemistry, and sought explanations for the life processes in humans. In short, their work marked the beginning of the science of physiology.

14.2.6 Andreas Vesalius and the Refinement of Human Anatomy

The most important medical anatomist of the Renaissance was Andreas Vesalius. Along with Leonardo da Vinci he was one of the first to systematically experiment with and dissect human cadavers. By critically examining the work of Galen, he realized that Galen's observations of anatomy were not based on human dissection but were mainly descriptions of the bodily structures of monkeys, pigs, and goats. From 1537 to 1542, Vesalius worked on an anatomical atlas, *De humani corporis fabrica libri septea*, which was published in 1593. The book contained 663 folio pages. Vesalius' research on human anatomy became the basis of anatomical science and provided the necessary knowledge for surgeons. The interplay between laboratory observations and clinical practice provided scholars with the data they needed for readjusting theory to practice and practice to theory. The model for obtaining anatomical knowledge in the medical sciences in Europe was forged in the 16th century.

14.2.7 Paracelsus the Medical Chemist

The next great development in medicine was in physiology. Chemistry and physics are the bases of physiology. The understanding of human physiology awaited great discoveries in these areas. The first physician to apply chemistry to an understanding of biological processes was Paracelsus. He advocated using pharmaceutical agents singly or in combination to treat specific illnesses. He used sulfur, lead, antimony, mercury, iron, and copper as therapeutics. Paracelsus emphasized the relationship between practical clinical experience and scientific experimentation.

14.2.8 William Harvey

William Harvey in 1628 in the publication *Exercitatio* described accurately for the first time the circulation of the blood. Harvey, an English physician, was trained in Padua, Italy, where Vesalius had taught human anatomy. After mastering the physiological theories of his time, he proposed questions such as: What is the pulse? How does breathing affect the actions of the heart? How does the blood move? These questions directed Harvey's experimental procedures. First, he systematically stated a testable hypothesis on the circulation of the blood, and then he proceeded with rigorous experimental observation. He used precise measurements in recording pulse rate and the volume of blood ejected by the heart over time. He observed the movements of the heart and blood in living animals. He also analyzed the blood circulation of the fetus to support his theory. By using the scientific method, Harvey discovered the most vital process in human life. He did this by (a) presenting a researchable question, (b) mastering the published literature on blood flow, (c) using accurate observations, (d) being guided by predictive hypothesis, (e) using rigorous procedures for collecting data, (f) applying measurement to the process of blood flow, and (g) making a deductive analysis and conclusions.

Harvey's achievement in describing the circulation of the blood ranks with Newton's discovery of gravity as one of the greatest scientific accomplishments in the 17th century. Harvey's work at first was met with the jealousy and suspicion which many times accompany an important discovery or change of thinking. In the first chapter from Exercitatio entitled "The Author's Motives for Writing" (1628/1952), Harvey explained his reasons for publishing his findings and his desire to bring objective criticism to his work.

I have not hesitated to expose my views upon these subjects, not only in private to my friends, but also in public, in my anatomical lectures, after the manner of the Academy of old.

These views as usual, pleased some more, others less; some chide and calumniated me, and laid it to me as a crime that I had dared to depart from the precepts and opinions of all anatomists; others desired further explanations of the novelties, which they said were both worthy of consideration, and might perchance be found of single use. At length, yielding to the requests of my friends, that all might be made participators in my labors, and partly moved by the envy of others, who receiving my views with uncandid minds and understanding them indifferently, have essayed to traduce me publicly. I have moved to commit these things to the press, in order that all may be enabled to form an opinion both of me and my labours.

(Harvey, 1938, pp. 273–274)

By the end of the 17th century, the medical scientist was emerging. At this point in history, medical practice was not at all consistent, yet there was a body of knowledge being created that served as the basis for later discoveries and practices. Many medical schools were founded in Europe during the 17th century, but it was not until the latter half of the 19th century that medical education was rigorously evaluated. With the flourishing of medical schools, discoveries occurred in a comparatively short period of intense activity during the 19th century to the present. Medical schools served as laboratories and models for research and clinical practice. The early research describing the anatomy and physiology of the human organism served as a foundation of scientific knowledge that was later expanded and incorporated into clinical practice.

14.3 METHODOLOGICAL PROCESS—STAGE II

14.3.1 Development of Medical Technology Starting in the 18th and 19th Centuries and Continuing into the 21st Century

The second stage in medical research was the development of precision instruments and test procedures that enabled the medical scientist to examine and measure the internal processes in the body. Typical among early scientific inventors in medicine was Laennec (1781–1826) who, by watching children playing with hollow cylinders, invented the stethoscope. Methodological research over the centuries has brought about technological advances such as the electroencephalogram, electrocardiogram, X-Ray, procedures for urine analysis, positron emission tomography (PET), single photon emission computed tomography (SPECT), computed tomographic X-Ray (CT or CAT scan), magnetic resonance imaging (MRI), and other important instruments and procedures that have become basic diagnostic tools in clinical medicine. Moreover, technology is continually being refined and updated.

Methodological research is unique in its application of industrial technology and biomedical engineering to clinical medicine. Initially, the great advances in methodology coincided with the rise of the industrial revolution in the 18th century. Medical scientists working with engineers were able to create objective medical tests which are the basis of modern medicine. Many of these advances were examples of interdisciplinary research where investigators from diverse professions applied their special knowledge to a specific research problem.

Norbert Wiener (1948), who proposed the theory of cybernetics that led to computer technology, used interdisciplinary seminars at the Massachusetts Institute of Technology (MIT) as a means of generating new ideas and stimulating creative thinking. Presently, bioengineers are working in conjunction with medical scientists in applying artificial intelligence to robotic surgery and to create man-made artificial materials and devices that can replace organs in the body. Biomedical engineering is a direct application of methodological research to medicine. Prosthetics, orthotics, assistive devices, driver rehabilitation adaptations are examples of recent methodological research applied to the fields of medicine and rehabilitation.

Since the COVID pandemic in 2020 medical technology has been changing dramatically. For example, telehealth with the health professional communicating directly with a patient through computer applications such as Zoom, Skype, or Google, mobile devices and remote monitoring systems has in some rural areas replaced the in-person office visit.

Electronic health records (EHRs) have revolutionized medical records. All of the patients' records such as doctor visits, vaccinations, pharmaceuticals, and visits to emergency care are available in one file that is accessible to the health care providers and the patient.

Another innovation in health care is the continuous monitoring of physical variables such as heart rate, blood pressure, sleep quality and physical activity using fitness trackers on your wrist or smart phone technology. These instruments can be monitored by a health professional and indicate any changes in health status. For example, a person can monitor changes in blood pressure that occur during daily activities and while sleeping.

Medication management devices have been developed to help the patient to be compliant with taking the proper medication in a timely fashion. Automatic pill dispensers,

artificial intelligence health care assistants, and mechanical reminders for the caregiver and patient are available.

3D printing is another innovation that dentists and physicians are using in designing tooth crowns, implants, and joints for surgical procedures, prosthetics, and prescriptive drugs.

The development of virtual reality (VR) is being used in medical schools to recreate medical scenarios such as surgery, diagnostic examinations, and practice procedures.

TECHNOLOGY IN MENTAL HEALTH

It is estimated, that by 2030, depression will be the leading cause of disease burden globally, making the need for new therapies more crucial than ever. Over the last year, many new technologies have emerged that can help address patients ongoing mental health needs.

Increasingly some apps are able to complete patient intakes and provide an initial diagnosis before a patient ever meets with a provider and AI powered tools are transforming the way mental health treatments are delivered. AI chatbots, like Woebot, that can help patients practice their cognitive behavioral therapy (CBT) strategies to smartphone apps, and voice recognition software Ellipsis, can analyze a patient's voice and speech patterns for warning signs of emotional distress. In addition to this digital symptom tracking is proving crucial for optimizing efficient mental health care for the future. Online symptom tracking prompts patients to share data daily. An AI algorithm then analyses that data to identify patterns and alert providers in real time of any warning signs.

Another technology newly being utilized for mental health is the use of video games. Approved in 2020, EndeavorRx is the first and only FDA-cleared video game treatment. The game is used to help improve the attention span of children aged 8–12 years old with ADHD and requires a prescription. In clinical studies, 73% of participants reported an increased ability to pay attention.

After this success, video games are set to become a more popular, affordable and accessible treatment for a range of health conditions. It was recently announced, DeepWell Digital Therapeutics would be launching a first-of-its-kind video game publisher and developer dedicated to creating gameplay that can simultaneously entertain and deliver, enhance, and accelerate treatment for an array of illnesses and conditions.

(Burke, 2022)

Table 14–2 summarizes the major methodological inventions that have impacted medical care.

TABLE 14–2

THE EMERGENCE OF THE MEDICAL SCIENTIST—STAGE I

MEDICAL EVENTS	DISCOVERY DATES	SCIENTISTS	IMPLICATIONS
Hippocratic writings	400–500 BCE	Hippocrates (500 BCE)	Provided a model for medical practitioners based on ethical and humane treatment
Systematic study of bodily processes	169–180 CE	Claudius Galen (129–199 CE)	Influenced medical practice for 1300 years, presenting an eclectic synthesis of prior knowledge
The Canon of Medicine	Translated 1187	Avicenna (980–1037)	Significant figure of Arabic medicine whose work was dogma during the Middle Ages
Paragranum: The four pillars of medicine: philosophy, astronomy, chemistry, and virtue	1530	Paracelsus (1493–1541)	Created the foundation for general medical practice based on a knowledge of pharmaceutical chemistry
Atlas of Anatomy *De humani corporis fabrica*	1543	Andreas Vesalius (1514–1564)	Made descriptive anatomy the basis of medicine and replaced aspects of Galen's work
Manual of Surgery	1543	Ambroise Pare (1510–1590)	Generated surgical innovations based upon accurate anatomical knowledge
Discovery of the circulation of the blood: *Exercitatio*	1628	William Harvey (1578–1657)	Integrated anatomy with physiological knowledge of blood circulation
Digestive system: *Experiments and Observations of Gastric Juice and the Physiology of Digestion*	1833	William Beaumont (1785–1853)	Used objective observation in discovering the process of digestion

14.3.2 The Practice of Medicine in the 19th Century

The latter half of the 19th century was a golden period in the history of medicine. During this time, medical schools were given the legal authority to certify physicians. Examinations were required for anyone who practiced medicine in the United States and Europe. In England, for example, a Medical Register was established in 1858. Atwater (1973), in an article documenting the medical profession in Rochester, New York, from 1811–1860, described the current state of medical knowledge available to general practitioners. Table 14–3 contains an abstracted description of the advances in medicine made during the prior three centuries according to (Atwater, 1973)

Although medicine had achieved great gains up until this period, most contagious diseases except for smallpox were either untreatable or preventable. Surgeons also worked at a great disadvantage without antiseptic techniques,

and hospitals did not provide the care we associate with excellent nursing. Medical advances would have to wait for Pasteur, Lister, Semmelweiss, Morton, and Florence Nightingale to provide the revolutionary innovations in anti-septic medicine and sanitary conditions in hospitals…

14.4 ETIOLOGICAL ADVANCES— STAGE III: MEDICAL RESEARCH IN THE LATTER HALF OF THE 19TH CENTURY

The third stage in medical research was the integration of physiology and pathology with the use of a reliable methodology to arrive at an accurate and valid diagnosis. The evolution of the dynamic understanding of the disease process is described in Table 14–4.

TABLE 14-3			
METHODOLOGICAL ADVANCES—STAGE I			
MEDICAL EVENTS	**DATES**	**SCIENTISTS**	**IMPLICATIONS**
Clinical thermometer	1614	Santotio Santorio (1561–1636)	Physical examination in clinical medicine
Microscopical anatomy	1661	Marcello Malpighi (1628–1694)	Diagnostic studies of the blood
Clinical microscope	1695	Antony Van Leeuwenhoek (1632–1694)	Refinement of microscope
Technique of thoracic percussion	1761	Leopold Auenbrugger (1722–1809)	Diagnosis of respiratory disorders
Stethoscope	1819	Rene Laennec (1781–1826)	Diagnosis of circulatory disorders
Hypodermic syringe	1853	Alexander Wood (1817–1884)	Blood transfusions
Method for testing the quantity of sugar in urine	1848	Herman von Fehling (1811–1885)	Diagnosis of diabetes mellitus
X-Ray	1895	Wilhelm Roentgen (1845–1923)	Detection of tuberculosis, fractures, and dislocations
Ophthalmoscope	1851	Hermann von Helmholtz (1821–1894)	Detection of morbid changes in the eye
Cystoscope	1890	Max Nitze (1847–1907)	Disease of urinary system
Electrocardiograph (EKG)	1903	Willem Einthoven (1860–1927)	Coronary functioning
Electroencephalograph (EEG)	1929	Hans Berger (1873–1941)	Cerebral dysfunction
Magnetic resonance phenomena used in magnetic resonance imagery	1952	Edward M. Purcell (1905–1983) Felix Bloch (1912–1997)	Diagnostic assistance
Computed axial tomography (CAT)	1972	Allan Cormack (1924–1998) Sir Godfrey Hounsfield (1919–2004)	Diagnostic assistance
Pulsed neuromagnetic resonance (NMR) and magnetic resonance imagery (MRI)	1975	Richard Ernst (1933–)	Diagnostic assistance
Positron emission tomography (PET)	1970s	William H. Sweet (1930–2001) Gordon Brownell (1922–2008)	Diagnostic assistance
Single photon emission computed tomography (SPECT)	1970s	R. Q. Edwards (1921–1976) D. E. Kuhl (1929–2017)	Diagnostic assistance

TABLE 14-4

PROGRESS IN SURGERY, CLINICAL MEDICINE, AND PUBLIC HEALTH UP TO PASTEUR'S FORMULATION OF THE GERM THEORY IN 1878

SURGERY	DIAGNOSIS AND TREATMENT	PUBLIC HEALTH
Use of ether and chloroform as anesthetics	Use of microscope, auscultation, and stethoscope in diagnosis	Construction of municipal sewers
Setting of broken bones and reduction of dislocated joints	Dynamic understanding of anatomy and physiology	Recording of vital statistics
Removal of superficial diseased tissue and kidney stones	Isolation of patients with contagious diseases	Custodial care of people who were "insane, retarded, poor, or homeless" (terms used in the 19th century, which are considered to be improper in the present).
Widespread practice of obstetrics and gynecology	Relief of local pain pharmacologically	Prevention of smallpox through vaccination

During this stage, an understanding of the etiology of a disease through experimental laboratory research was used to verify cause-effect relationships. This breakthrough in treating disease on a scientific basis started with Pasteur's discovery of the germ theory. From Pasteur's work, laboratory scientists were able to investigate disease processes by identifying and isolating a specific microorganism. The age of chemotherapy was initiated. For every microorganism causing a disease (that was isolated in the laboratory), researchers sought a chemical substance, harmless to the body to counteract the germ. From 1850 to 1910, the process of identifying a germ responsible for a disease and the discovery of a chemical to eliminate the germ was the basis for the rapid conquest of many communicable diseases. The elimination of many communicable diseases would not have occurred without the microscope and the laboratory techniques of microbiology and biochemistry. The technology for protecting the individual from infectious diseases was a direct result of the understanding of human physiology and cellular theory. Septic techniques for surgery were later developed by Lister (1827–1912), who was greatly influenced by the work of Pasteur, and by Semmelweis (1818–1865), an obstetrician who recognized the importance of hospital surgeons using prophylactic techniques during childbirth to prevent infection.

The understanding of cellular activity by Virchow (1821–1902) was another line of evidence verifying the germ theory of disease. According to Virchow, the cause of a specific disease was a result of changes at the cellular level. Virchow's cellular theory of disease encouraged pathologists to use microscopes in searching for lesions and abnormalities within the cells. Metchnikoff (1845–1916) discovered phagocytosis, recognizing that white blood corpuscles in the body counteract disease. The understanding of the dynamics of disease led to the science of clinical medicine.

Physicians were then able to diagnose disease through laboratory microscope techniques, thus replacing vitalism and metaphysics as explanations for the onset of communicable diseases. Probably the most important work on medical research in the 19th century was Claude Bernard's *Introduction to the Study of Experimental Medicine* published in 1895. Pasteur acknowledged Bernard as an important influence in his own work. Bernard's major contributions to understanding disease included physiology of digestion, neurophysiology, pharmacology, and organic chemistry. Bernard's work has had a profound influence in medical science. Concepts such as homeostasis and stress introduced by Cannon (1932) and Selye (1956) respectively are based on Bernard's experimental findings on the internal gastrointestinal environment. Bernard, through his experimental methodology, established the future direction of medical research based on rigorous observation, repeated replication, and the acceptance or rejection of a hypothesis. "Scientific generalization must proceed from particular facts or principles" (Bernard, 1957, p. 2). This simple statement is the foundation of 20th and 21st century medical research.

With a refined scientific methodology and a comprehensive theory of disease, medical researchers from about 1880 to 1910 made dramatic progress in identifying disease agents. This advance is exemplified by Koch's work in tuberculosis in 1890, von Behring's work in diphtheria in 1900, and Ehrlich's persistent search for a chemical to counteract syphilis, culminating in the discovery of the drug Salvarsan in 1910, after 606 experimental clinical trials.

14.5 PREVENTION—STAGE IV

14.5.1 Preventive Medicine Beginning in the 20th Century

The advances in medical research that have had the most dramatic effect in eliminating diseases, can be attributed to primary prevention, including public health techniques and mass vaccinations. Public health measures, such as purification of water, proper processing of human waste products, and protection against food spoilage, were also employed by ancient civilizations such as the Egyptians, Greeks, and Romans without an understanding of microorganisms. When superstition prevailed over using prophylactic methods, as during the Middle Ages in Europe, epidemics and widespread disease occurred. Throughout the world, the potential for epidemics still exists as exemplified by the Ebola epidemic in Africa (2013–2016) and the COVID pandemic of 2020–23 and in times of war and natural disasters. The near elimination of typhus, cholera, bubonic plague, polio, and eradication of smallpox in areas with access to modern medicine has been accomplished through the combination of medical advances in vaccinations and public health technology. Vaccination as a means of preventing disease has provided the means to control widespread epidemics that dramatically reduced populations in the past.

One of the first physicians to conceive the use of vaccinations to prevent disease was Edward Jenner, a country doctor (1749–1823) who noted that dairymaids who contracted cowpox by milking infected cows developed a natural immunity to smallpox. This observation led him to believe that if people were deliberately infected with cowpox, a mild infection, they would escape the deadly smallpox. In 1798, Jenner published his findings, which included 23 successful case histories of individuals inoculated with cowpox.

Initially, Jenner's work was not accepted by the medical community in England. He gradually gained recognition after his work was replicated by other physicians. Jenner's original research on vaccinations remained singularly unique until Pasteur's discovery of the germ theory about 100 years later in 1878. Jenner's method of inoculation to prevent disease was rediscovered by medical researchers who were later able to isolate pathogenic bacteria and viruses. Table 14–5 lists many of the communicable diseases that are now controlled by vaccination.

In the 21st century, CRISPR (Clustered Regularly Interspaced Short Palindromic Repeats), a genetic engineering intervention, is being used experimentally to treat cystic fibrosis, cancer, HIV, and sickle cell anemia and in preventing viral infections (Escalona-Noguero et al., 2021).

The concept of preventive medicine in the 21st century includes the following health and behavioral measures:

- Vaccination to prevent communicable diseases such as in childhood diseases, hepatitis, smallpox, polio, and COVID-19
- Environmental health to reduce atmospheric and water pollution causing chronic obstructive pulmonary disease and cancers
- Prenatal care to prevent birth defects
- Mental health community programs to prevent psychiatric institutionalization and homelessness

TABLE 14–5			
DYNAMIC UNDERSTANDING OF DISEASE PROCESSES—STAGE III			
MEDICAL EVENT	DATE	SCIENTIST	IMPLICATIONS
Clinical physiology	1857	Claude Bernard (1813–1878)	Treatment of physiologic and metabolic disorders through pharmacology
Cell theory	1858	Rudolf Ludwig Virchow (1821–1902)	Cellular pathology as the basis of treatment
Germ theory	1878	Louis Pasteur (1822–1895)	The role of microorganisms in disease established
Bacteriology	1882	Robert Koch (1843–1910)	Treatment of bacterial infections could be controlled by the physician
Role of filterable viruses	1888	Pierre Roux (1853–1933)	Identification of viruses resulted in the search for preventative measures
Immunization process	1892	Elie Metchnikoff (1845–1916)	Understanding of the body's "phagocytosis" defense mechanisms against disease was recognized
Chemotherapy	1899	Paul Ehrlich (1854–1915)	Specific chemical compounds used to treat communicable diseases

- Supervision of food handling and processing of foods to prevent botulism and salmonella
- Prevention of industrial accidents and repetitive motion injuries through ergonomics
- Sanitary engineering to prevent diseases such as typhus and cholera
- Smoking cessation to prevent lung cancer and cardiovascular diseases
- Healthy nutrition such as the Mediterranean Diet to prevent cardiovascular and metabolic diseases
- Prescriptive exercise programs to control diabetes, obesity, cardiovascular diseases
- Health education regarding the abuse of alcohol and opioids

In the 21st century climate change has had a significant effect on the occurrence of communicable diseases.

> Human-driven climatic changes will fundamentally influence patterns of human health, including infectious disease clusters and epidemics following extreme weather events. Extreme weather events are projected to increase further with the advance of human-driven climate change. Both recent and historical experiences indicate that infectious disease outbreaks very often follow extreme weather events, as microbes, vectors and reservoir animal hosts exploit the disrupted social and environmental conditions of extreme weather events.
>
> (McMichael, 2015, p. 543)

Until the 20th century, physicians could do little for a patient who was severely ill. The introduction of chemotherapy, aseptic surgery, and sanitary hospital care changed the course of medical practice.

14.6 DRUG THERAPY, SURGERY, AND HOSPITAL CARE: THE BASES OF TREATMENT—STAGE V

14.6.1 Drug Therapy

As knowledge about anatomy and physiology progressed, technology was developed to improve the diagnoses of illnesses. The foundations, created to produce a body of knowledge underlying therapeutics, resulted in drug therapy, surgery, and hospital care as the bases of modern day treatment. Although ancient civilizations, and indigenous cultures existing today, have used various effective interventions based on natural observation and experience, the causes of diseases and the rationale for understanding the processes were veiled in mystery. For example, rauwolfia serpentine was used in India (100 CE)

as the "medicine of sad men" (Thorwald, 1963, p. 205) without the understanding of the biochemical process of a tranquilizer. Ancient Egyptian doctors used mud and soil in the treatment of eye diseases. This type of "sewerage pharmacology" was not understood until 1948 when Dr. Benjamin M. Dugger, a professor of plant physiology at the University of Wisconsin, discovered the drug aureomycin, a chemical similar to natural substances found near the Nile River. Aureomycin has been highly effective in the treatment of trachoma. For centuries, practical treatment for many disabilities, diseases, and illnesses has been applied by trial and error without an understanding of the physiological and genetic dynamics of the disease processes. Healers, such as shamans and witch doctors, intersperse treatment with superstition, sometimes attaining positive results. The important difference between applying therapeutics in modern science and in prescientific civilizations is in the explanation of why a specific treatment cures a disease. The search for cures to diseases, beginning with the germ theory of Pasteur and continuing through Alexander Fleming's discovery of penicillin in 1928 and Selman A. Waksman's discovery of streptomycin in 1944, spurred the corporate growth of therapeutic pharmaceutics. Modern medicine is heavily dependent on the availability of various drugs to control abnormal physical conditions, such as hypertension, arteriosclerosis, blood clotting, edema, gastrointestinal disorders, and mental illnesses. Hormone therapy (in 1921 Dr. Frederick Banting, a Canadian surgeon, and Charles Best, a medical student, identified the hormone insulin as an effective treatment for diabetes), supplementary vitamins such as vitamin C in the prevention of scurvy, and diet modifications in decreasing salt intake and animal fat in preventing the recurrence of heart disease and prescriptive exercise programs are other common methods akin to chemotherapy as forms of health interventions.

14.6.2 Surgery

Surgery as an advanced medical intervention has a long evolution in the history of mankind. Ancient civilizations such as the Incas of Peru in 200 BCE used trepanation (removing parts of a skull) as a method to relieve epileptic fits and intractable headaches (Ellis & Abdalla, 2019). The ancient Romans (ca. 70 BCE – 200 BCE) used up to 200 different surgical instruments in various operations. In addition, ligature of blood vessels was performed; obstetric surgery, specifically Caesarean section, was known; and even anesthesia was used (Martí-Ibáñez, 1962).

Modern surgery as an effective and safe method was the result of two important events: the development of antiseptics by Lister in 1867, who tested the capacity of carbolic acid in preventing infection in general surgery, and the discovery of ether anesthesia as a practical method by

William Morton, a dentist, in 1846 (Ellis & Abdalla, 2019; Hæger & Edlund, 1988).

Surgical interventions in the 21st century have continued to make dramatic gains in improving health care throughout the world. For example, from 1992 to 2012, the total number of surgeries at community hospitals in the United States increased by 17% to about 26.8 million surgeries. Outpatient surgeries represented a growing share (65%; 17.3 million) of all surgeries at community hospitals in the United States in 2012, up from 54% (12.3 million) in 1992 (Dallas, 2021).

Surgery is increasingly used as an outpatient procedure that has reduced the time in surgery and the time for patient recuperation. There was a 300% increase in the rates of visits to free standing ambulatory surgery centers from 1996 to 2006. However, during the COVID pandemic surgeries in the United States actually went down. There were 678,348 fewer procedures in 2020 than in 2019, representing a 10.2% reduction for 2020.

In 2021 the ten most frequent surgical procedures were (Dallas, 2021):

1. Cataract removal
2. C-section
3. Joint replacement
4. Circumcision
5. Broken bone repair
6. Angioplasty and atherectomy (cardiovascular procedure)
7. Stent insertion
8. Hysterectomy
9. Gall bladder removal
10. Heart bypass surgery

14.6.3 Hospital Care

The third component in the development of modern treatment, parallel to drug therapy and surgery, was the rise of hospital nursing care. Florence Nightingale's role in developing the nursing profession is legendary. She brought global attention to the plight of hospital patients, who were often left to die because of neglect. During the Crimean War of 1854, she organized a group of nurses to tend wounded British soldiers. Her experience gave her the insight into the need for clean, efficient hospitals. Reform in hospital care became a national issue in England after the Crimean War, and social legislation was enacted to provide governmental support. Florence Nightingale also started the first school of nursing at St. Thomas' Hospital, London, in 1860. With hospital reform enacted through legislation and a nursing school started, the foundation for progress in the treatment of the hospitalized patient was established.

Below is a short outline of the historical development of hospitals as documented by Sand (1952):

1. Ancient Greece, 6th century, BCE: A large open building was provided for the Greek physician. It comprised a waiting room, consulting room, and theater for operations and dressings.
2. Ancient Rome, 1st century, CE: Sick bays were attached to the family estates of the wealthy.
3. Early Medieval Europe, 4th century, CE: Early Christians established "hospitia" for travelers, abandoned children, and the sick who were traveling on their way to pilgrimages. Care was under the direction of monastic and sisterly orders.
4. Middle East, 12th century, CE: Moslems in Baghdad founded the first hospitals where physicians cared for the ill. Special wards for mental illness, blindness, and leprosy were established.
5. Later Middle Ages, Europe, 5th to 14th centuries: Hostelries under the jurisdiction of the Roman Catholic Church provided care for the sick. Brothers and sisters of the Roman Catholic Church in attached ecclesiastical hospitals provided treatment remedies, performed simple operations, and attended those with serious illnesses.
6. Renaissance Europe, 15th century: For the first time in the Western world, physicians and midwives treated the sick in hospitals. Terminal patients were segregated from the acutely ill.
7. Europe, 18th century: Gradually hospitals began to treat emergency care patients, outpatient departments grew, and hospitals served as training facilities for medical students.
8. Europe and America, 19th century: Nursing care was established in hospitals. Antiseptic surgery, anesthesia, and improvement in general care of the hospitalized patient were initiated.
9. Worldwide, 20th–21st century: The growth of specialized hospitals, regional planning, and national health services. A world movement exists in extending health care to underdeveloped countries under the auspices of the United Nations' World Health Organization (WHO).

Current medical treatment is based on the principle of healing—stopping the progression of a disease and promoting natural bodily processes. Drug therapy, surgery, and nursing care are the three basic methods that have made medical practice effective in treating many communicable diseases and physiological disorders and anatomical defects. However there are still limitations of medical treatment for individuals with severe chronic disabilities, such as dementia, schizophrenia, depression, arthritis, spinal cord injuries, multiple sclerosis, cerebral palsy, muscular dystrophy, chronic obstructive pulmonary disease, cardiovascular disease, and cerebral vascular accident. Medical treatment is most effective when the disease process can be narrowed down to a specific etiology. Chronic diseases present problems of multiple etiologies and interventions requiring complex solutions and interdisciplinary efforts. The search for solutions to helping individuals with chronic disabilities led to the rehabilitation movement in the early 20th century.

14.7 REHABILITATION MOVEMENT—STAGE VI

The emergence of the rehabilitation professions as distinct entities in the health care system began in 1916 during World War I. The aftermath of World War I and the devastation it brought saw the beginning of the rehabilitation movement, coinciding with the need for restoring function to those who were permanently disabled. One may ask why the rehabilitation field developed at that time and not in prior periods of recovery from war? The historical factors that led to the rehabilitation movement are outlined in Table 14–6. Until the 19th century, chronic illness and permanent disability in general were not always considered medical problems. Many people with chronic neurological and orthopedic disabilities were considered incurable and were either dependent upon family caregiving or institutionalized and mainly neglected. For instance, psychiatric illness and epilepsy were considered by the public as social problems rather than of medical concern. Treatment of psychiatric illness, if any, was stark, brutal, or radical. Before the rise of large institutions providing custodial care for psychiatric patients, the attitude toward chronic mental illness was at best benign neglect and at worst rejection and punishment. In a related area, birth injuries such as cerebral palsy were misunderstood by ancient cultures. Not until 1862, when W. T. Little, an English orthopedic surgeon, described the relationship between birth injury and neurological disorders, was there any dynamic understanding of this disability. Individuals with other chronic disabilities, such as arthritis, emphysema, stroke, cardiovascular disease, and spinal cord injuries, were left either to the family or worse were placed into the hands of charlatans who promised miraculous cures.

14.7.1 Social Welfare and Rehabilitation

The change from custodial care to therapeutic interventions and rehabilitation for individuals with chronic disabilities occurred at a period of time in history when social welfare had become a worldwide concern. The social welfare movement in general fostered women's rights, prison reform, child protection laws, health and safety protections for workers, and financial aid for the poor. Charitable agencies and government policies and laws fostered progressive changes. Social welfare policies were the forerunners in public health and medicine for the indigent with chronic disabilities. Germany, in 1883, and England, in 1897, were the first countries in Europe to enact legislation providing worker's compensation to cover disability and illness resulting from occupational accidents. The progress toward social and occupational health and safety is described in Figure 14–1. Governmental financial support, resulting from national policies on health and welfare, was necessary because of the enormous hospital resources and health personnel required in the rehabilitation of individuals with disabilities. In the United States, social security legislation, first enacted in 1935, has been a major impetus for the development of the rehabilitation movement. Change in societies' attitudes toward the individual with chronic disabilities, as evidenced in the social welfare movement, has encouraged the growth of the allied health professions.

14.7.2 The Development of Allied Health Professions—Phase I

Three major phases in the history of rehabilitation led directly to the growth of the allied health professions. The first phase occurred shortly after World War I. During this period, the need for the physical and social rehabilitation of individuals with disabilities was recognized by the medical community. Casualties from the First World War of 1914–1918 included individuals with lower extremity amputations, victims of poisonous

TABLE 14–6
HISTORICAL FACTORS LEADING TO THE REHABILITATION MOVEMENT
Incorporation of scientific methodology into clinical medicine
Industrialization and its impact on clinical procedures for diagnosis and treatment
Large population of veterans with disabilities from World War I
The availability of financial resources through Social Security and National Health Insurance schemes
Medical specialties and the development of allied health professions
Public acceptance that individuals with disabilities can be restored to independence through rehabilitation
Public acceptance of individuals with disabilities in social and work situations

ANTIQUITY	MEDIEVAL GUILDS	SOCIETY OF ARTIFICERS
➤ Manual labor and tradesmen neglected ➤ Occupational diseases ignored	➤ Voluntary associations formed for mutual aid protection of tradesman ➤ Assist worker with disabilities ➤ Assist in funeral expenses	➤ Established apprenticeship system ➤ Work day regulated 12–13 hours
PROTECTION OF MINERS (16th century) ➤ Ventilating machines for mines	OCCUPATIONAL MEDICINE (established 17th century) ➤ Relationship between occupation and disease investigated medically ➤ Prevention measures introduced—rest intervals, positioning, cleanliness, protective clothing	COMPILING OF VITAL STATISTICS ON OCCUPATIONAL DISEASE (18th century) ➤ Use of medical inspectors
PROTECTION OF VULNERABLE WORKERS IN DANGEROUS TRADES (19th century) ➤ Public health legislation to regulate child labor ➤ Work day reduced to 10 hours	WORKMEN'S COMPENSATION (1890–1910) ➤ Compensate workers for occupational accidents and diseases	NATIONAL WOMEN'S TRADE UNION (1920) ➤ Protection of women from dangerous industries WORKER HEALTH BUREAU (established 1927)
SOCIAL SECURITY LEGISLATION (1930s) ➤ Place safety and health activities within Labor Department	OCCUPATIONAL SAFETY AND HEALTH AGENCIES (OSHA; established 1970) ➤ Onsite inspections, regulations, and enforcement of laws relating to dangerous and unhealthy conditions in all industries	THE NATIONAL INSTITUTE FOR OCCUPATIONAL SAFETY AND HEALTH (NIOSH; Established 1970) ➤ Provide information through research, information, education and training to aid in improving safe and healthful working conditions
SCIENTIFIC INVESTIGATIONS OF PREVENTION AND TREATMENT OF OCCUPATIONAL INJURIES AND DISEASES (1980s) ➤ Application of ergonomics and rehabilitation of principles	FUTURE TRENDS IN OCCUPATIONAL MEDICINE ➤ Occupational health teams: ergonomist, occupational therapist, physician, industrial hygienist, physical therapist, safety officer, and nurse ➤ Investigation of physical, chemical, biological, and psychological factors in work environment that may cause or aggravate disease in individuals who are vulnerable ➤ Investigation of long-term effects of exposure to toxic chemicals, repetitive motion, vibration, excessive noise, extreme temperature, radiation, dust, bacteria ➤ Prevention of accidents or disease	

Figure 14–1 Progress toward social reform in occupational health and safety.

gas resulting in neurological disabilities and blindness, and soldiers with psychiatric disabilities that now would be labeled post-traumatic stress disorders. At that time, these veterans of the war with chronic disabilities needed assistance in readjusting to community living. Reconstruction workers mainly recruited from nursing staffs were the first health personnel in rehabilitation. These reconstruction workers became the first occupational therapists, and on March 15, 1917 the National Society for the Promotion of Occupational Therapy was established (see Box 14–1). Immediately after World War I, the goal of occupational therapy was primarily diversional and humane and adjunctive to the medical treatment. There was no direct effort by the occupational therapists to change the course of a disability or to make the individual with disabilities more functional. During the late 1920s, occupational therapy departments were established for the first time in hospitals. The health personnel recruited to work in these departments were, on the whole, dedicated people who applied caring support and activity to facilitate the patient's readjustment to the community. The purposes of rehabilitation and specific methods were formulated during these initial years.

Box 14-1. Selected International Landmarks in the History of Occupational Therapy

359 BCE (circa)   Idleness and lack of occupation tend—nay are dragged—towards evil. As to diseases make a habit of two things—to help, or at least, to do no harm. (Hippocrates)

172 CE   Employment is nature's best physician and is essential to human happiness. (Galen)

1752   Pennsylvania Hospital in Philadelphia established. Psychiatric patients were prescribed manual labor to counteract disease process.

1780   Clement-Joseph Tissot, a French physician in the cavalry, published a book prescribing the use of crafts and recreational activities for individuals with muscle and joint injuries.

BOX 14-1. SELECTED INTERNATIONAL LANDMARKS IN THE HISTORY OF OCCUPATIONAL THERAPY (CONTINUED)

1786   Philippe Pinel, a French psychiatrist in the Bicetre Asylum for the insane, prescribed humane treatment in the care of the mentally ill, including physical exercises, manual occupation, and music.

1803   Johanann Christian Reil, a German psychiatrist, advocated that activities such as swimming, dancing, gymnastics, arts and crafts, music, and theater be part of the everyday routine for patients.

1812   Benjamin Rush, the father of American psychiatry, prescribed work, leisure activities, chess and other board games, exercise, and theatre for treatment of mental illness.

1813   Samuel Tuke, an English Quaker, founded the Retreat Asylum for the Insane in York, England. Tuke introduced the term *moral treatment* which was the application of humane practices—including exercise, recreation, arts and crafts, gardening, and regular employment—in the maintenance of the hospital.

1833   Samuel Woodard, a physician at the Worcester State Lunatic Hospital in Massachusetts, introduced the term *occupational therapy* as a therapeutic method to keep inmates active in varied tasks and leisure activities in regular routines. The therapeutic program was observed to be clinically effective and produced a significant recovery rate.

1838   Jean Etienne Esquirol, a French psychiatrist, described the importance of corporal exercise, horseback riding, tennis, fencing, swimming, and travel for the treatment of depression.

1840   Francois Leuret, a French psychiatrist, advanced that moral treatment, including arts and crafts and work, are effective in treating individuals with mental illness and intellectual disabilities.

1843   Dorothea Dix, a social reformer, worked diligently in the United States for humanistic care for individuals with mental illness, which included the use of therapeutic activities.

1854   Thomas Kirkbride, one of the founders of the American Psychiatric Association advocated a highly structured regimen for patients that included exercise, lectures, music, arts and crafts, and entertainment.

1895   William Rush Dunton, a psychiatrist and innovator in applying occupational therapy, used arts-and-crafts activities at Sheppard and Pratt Asylum in Baltimore.

1895/1922   Adolph Meyer, a strong advocate of occupation, believed in a holistic approach to treatment centering on sleep habits, nutrition, work, play, and socialization.

1895   Mary Potter Meyer, a social worker and wife of Adolph Meyer, used arts and crafts activities in the State Hospital in Worcester, Massachusetts.

1904   Herbert Hall, a physician, prescribed occupation as a medicine to regulate the life and direct interests of the patient. He called this the "work cure."

1905   Susan Tracy, a nurse, applied occupational therapy activities in working with individuals with mental illness while she was director of the Training School for Nurses at the Adams Nervine Asylum in Boston.

1906   Herbert Hall was awarded a grant of $1,000 by Harvard University to study the application of activities and graded manual occupation in the treatment of psychiatric disorders.

1908   Training courses in occupations for hospital attendants were initiated at Chicago School of Civics and Philanthropy.

1909   Clifford Beers, founder of the National Committee for Mental Hygiene, described his emotional illness in the book, *A Mind that Found Itself* (1908). Beers reinforced the application of therapeutic activities in treating individuals with mental illness.

1910   Susan Tracy authored the first book on occupation studies, *Invalid Occupations: A Manual for Nurses and Attendants*.

1911   Susan Tracy initiated the first course on occupation at Massachusetts General Hospital in Boston.

1911   Eleanor Clark Slagle, a social worker, established an occupation department at Phipps Psychiatric Clinic at Johns Hopkins University in Baltimore.

1914   George Edward Barton, an architect who had contracted tuberculosis, introduced the term *occupational therapy* at a meeting in Boston of hospital workers.

(continued)

Box 14-1. Selected International Landmarks in the History of Occupational Therapy (continued)

1917   The National Society for the Promotion of Occupational Therapy was founded in Consolation House in Clifton Springs, New York. The charter members included George Barton, an architect; Eleanor Clark Slagle, a social worker at Hull House, Chicago; Thomas Kidner, vocational specialist from Canada; William Rush Dunton, a psychiatrist at Sheppard and Pratt Hospital in Baltimore; Susan Cox Johnson, an arts and crafts instructor from New York City; Isabel Newton; and Susan B. Tracy, a nurse at the Adams Nervine Asylum in Boston. This meeting led to the occupational therapy profession in the United States.

1917   Reconstruction aides were recruited to serve in US army hospitals during World War I, applying arts and crafts and exercises in the treatment of physical and mental disorders.

1918   Formal educational training programs in occupational therapy were established at the Henry B. Favil School in Chicago, Teachers College of Columbia University, and the Boston School of Occupational Therapy.

1919   Bird T. Baldwin authored the US *Army Manual on Occupational Therapy* that included information on evaluation and treatment procedures for the restoration of physical function.

1919   George Barton wrote the book *Teaching the Sick: A Manual of Occupational Therapy as Reeducation.*

1922   The *Archives of Occupational Therapy* was published and became the official journal of the American Association of Occupational Therapy.

1925   *Occupational Therapy and Rehabilitation* was first published

1928   Six programs available to prepare occupational therapists: Boston School; Philadelphia School; St. Louis School; Milwaukee-Downer College; University of Minnesota; and the University of Toronto

1931   National registry for the American Occupational Therapy Association was established.

1933   The American Medical Association (AMA) began the accreditation of occupational therapy educational programs.

1934   Essentials of an acceptable education curriculum in occupational therapy were adopted by the American Medical Education Council on Medical Education and Hospitals.

1939   Among all AMA-approved hospitals, 13% employed occupational therapists.

1943   The Barden-LaFollette Vocational Rehabilitation Act was passed by Congress providing coverage of medical services including occupational therapy for individuals in vocational rehabilitation programs.

1945   Eighteen approved programs in occupational therapy in the United States compared with five in 1940.

1947   First national registration examination for US occupational therapists was given.

1947   Advanced master's degree in occupational therapy was offered at the University of Southern California and New York University.

1947   Helen Willard and Clare S. Spackman, occupational therapy educators, authored the first textbook in occupational therapy.

1952   The World Federation of Occupational Therapists established. The ten founding member countries were Australia, Canada, Denmark, Great Britain, India, Israel, New Zealand, South Africa, Sweden, and the United States.

1958   Essentials and Guidelines for an approved Educational Program for Occupational Therapy Assistant in the US adopted.

1964   Certified occupational therapists assistants (COTAs) certified in the United States.

1964   The first entry-level master's program in occupational therapy established at the University of Southern California. Shortly thereafter, basic master's programs were begun at Boston University and Virginia Commonwealth University.

1965   The American Occupational Therapy Foundation (AOTF) established as a philanthropic organization for advancing the science of occupational therapy.

1973   The Rehabilitation Act passed by Congress protecting the rights of persons with disabilities. Section 504 of the Rehabilitation Act of 1973 prohibits discrimination based on disability in programs or activities receiving federal financial assistance. (See www.access.gpo.gov/nara/cfr/waisidx_99/34cfr104_99.html and www2.ed.gov/policy/speced/reg/narrative.html.)

(continued)

Box 14-1. Selected International Landmarks in the History of Occupational Therapy (continued)

1974   New York University developed the first doctoral program in occupational therapy.

1975   *Education for All Handicapped Children Act* (EHA; PL. 94–142) facilitated free appropriate public education services for students with disabilities at all levels and provided funding for these services. The concept of least restrictive environment, inherent in the law, specifies that students with disabilities are educated with typical students "to the maximum extent possible."

1976   Support was given to students for development of their organization on a national level, which was later named the American Student Occupational Therapy Alliance.

1979   "Uniform Terminology System for Reporting Occupational Therapy Services" developed and adopted by the Representative Assembly (RA).

1980   AOTF published the *Occupational Therapy Journal of Research*.

1981   Entry level role delineation for OTRs and COTAs adopted by RA.

1981   *Occupational Therapy Journal of Research* published.

1986   Medicare amendments expanded coverage for occupational therapy services under Part B in the United States.

1990   *The Americans with Disabilities Act* (ADA; PL 101–336; [42 USC 12101]) passed by Congress and signed by President Bush. The ADA guarantees equal opportunity for individuals with disabilities in employment, public accommodations, transportation, governmental services, and telecommunications (FCTD, 2010). (See also www.usdoj.gov/crt/ada/cguide.htm#anchor62335 and www.ada.gov.)

1990   PL 94–142 reauthorized and renamed the *Individuals with Disabilities Education Act* (IDEA). This law continued federal funding from 94–142, and increased services by adding related services, transition from school to work, and parental involvement. Under this act, occupational therapy is considered a related service in helping students with disabilities in public schools.

1991   The AOTA RA approved a physical agent modalities (PAMS) position paper that recommended the use of PAMS as an adjunct to purposeful activity to enhance occupational performance.

1994   *Occupational Therapy International* is founded as the first refereed journal publishing manuscripts by occupational therapists throughout the world.

1997   *The Balanced Budget Act* PL 105–33 (BBA) significantly changed the procedures for payment of services for rehabilitation personnel affecting the quality of care, especially in home health.

1999   The AOTA Representative Assembly passes a resolution to mandate that entry-level education in occupational therapy should be at the master's level.

1998   The *Assistive Technology Act* (PL105–394 [29 USC 2201]) passed. This legislation provides funds to the States to support the establishment of assistive technology (AT) demonstration centers, information centers, facilities, referral services, advocacy services to help people with disabilities to access AT services. The act also provides low interest loans to purchase AT (FCTD, 2010). (See also www.ataporg.org/atap/index.php and www.assistivetech.net/webresources/stateTechActProjects.php for information regarding state projects.)

1998   Carl D. Perkins Vocational and Technical Education Act Amendments of 1998 (PL105–332 Section 1 (b) [20 USC 2302]). This act requires schools to integrate academic, vocational, and technical training; increase technology use; provide professional development opportunities; develop, implement, and expand quality programs; and link secondary and post-secondary vocational education (FCTD, 2010). (See also www.ed.gov/offices/OVAE/CTE/legis.html.)

2001   *The International Classification of Functioning, Disability, and Health*, known more commonly as ICF, is a classification of health and health-related domains. These domains are classified from body, individual, and societal perspectives by means of two lists: a list of body functions and structure, and a list of domains of activity and participation. Since an individual's functioning and disability occurs in a context, the ICF also includes a list of environmental factors. The ICF is WHO's framework for measuring health and disability at both individual and population levels.

2002   *No Child Left Behind* (NCLB; PL 107–110; www2.ed.gov/policy/elsec/leg/esea02/index.html) enacted. As part of the need to improve education, the law focused on requiring each state to develop and implement a statewide accountability system that insured adequate yearly gain for all schools in reading and math. It is based on the concept that setting standards and measurable educational goals can improve academic performance in the classroom.

(continued)

Box 14-1. Selected International Landmarks in the History of Occupational Therapy (continued)

2002   The *Occupational Therapy Practice Framework: Domain and Process (Framework)* was developed in response to current practice needs, intended to "more clearly affirm and articulate occupational therapy's unique focus on occupation and daily life activities and the application of an intervention process that facilitates engagement in occupation to support participation in life" (AOTA, 2002, p. 609).

2004   The *Individuals with Disabilities Education Improvement Act of 2004* (IDEIA; PL108–556; http://idea.ed.gov/) is the reauthorization of PL 94–142 enacted in 1975. The law ensures services for more than 6.5 million eligible infants, toddlers, children, and youth with disabilities throughout the nation. With this reauthorization, IDEIA-2000 was aligned with NCLB. In addition to funding, IDEIA governs how states and public agencies provide early intervention, special education, and related services.

2005   The fourth edition of the *Canadian Occupational Performance Measure* (COPM; Law et al., 2005) is published. It is an individualized, client-centered measure designed for use by occupational therapists to detect change in a client's self-perception of occupational performance over time. It is designed to be used as an outcome measure. The COPM is designed for use with clients with a variety of disabilities and across all developmental stages. The COPM has been used in more than 35 countries and has been translated into over 20 languages.

2008   *Occupational Therapy Practice Framework (2nd edition) is published (AOTA, 2008; Roley et al., 2008).*

2009   New emerging areas of occupational therapy practice in the United States identified by AOTA: psychosocial needs of children and youth, health and wellness, driver rehabilitation, low vision services, ergonomics, community health, welfare to work and technology and assistive device development and consulting.

2009   Americans with Disabilities Act Amendment (PL 110–325; www.judiciary.state.nj.us/legis/110-325_Law.pdf) was signed on September 25, 2008 by President Bush and went into effect on January 1, 2009. Under the Amendment, millions more Americans qualify as "disabled" and fall under the Act's protections. Under the Amendment, the definition of disability has been modified to so that the individual is regarded as having an impairment, without regard to whether it substantially limits a major life activity. The Amendment also expands the term "major life activities" to "caring for oneself, performing manual tasks, seeing, hearing, eating, sleeping, walking, standing, lifting, bending, speaking, breathing, learning, reading, concentrating, thinking, communicating, and working." Another important change requires that impairments that are episodic or in remission qualify as a disability if they would qualify in their active stage.

2010   On March 23, President Obama signed the *Affordable Health Care for America Act* (PL 111–148; http://democrats.senate.gov/reform/patient-protection-affordable-care-act-as-passed.pdf). The general principle is to ensure that all Americans have access to quality, affordable health care. It is projected that the Bill will provide health care coverage to 95% of Americans. (See www.aota.org/Practitioners/Advocacy/Federal/Highlights/Reform.aspx, for the impact of the Act on occupational therapy.)

2010   *World Federation of Occupational Therapists (WFOT) meets in Santiago, Chile for its 15th Congress. There are 70 member countries of WFOT.*

2014   *The third edition of the Occupational Therapy Practice Framework Domain and Process is published by the AOTA.*

2014   *WFOT meets in Yokahoma, Japan for its 16th Congress.*

2016   AOTA attains the membership high milestone of 60,000 members; membership in 1917 was 40.

2017   *AOTA celebrates its 100th anniversary in Philadelphia during the Annual Conference.*

2018   *WFOT met in Cape Town, South Africa. There are now over 92 member organizations and approximately 400,000 occupational therapists internationally.*

2018   The capstone project as a requirement in receiving the occupational therapy doctorate (OTD) in the United States was introduced by the Accreditation Council for Occupational Therapy Education (ACOTE). There are now 217 educational programs that offer the OTD and require a capstone project for graduation.

2022   WFOT met in Paris, France for its 18th Congress.

2023   The WFOT consists of 107 Member Organizations and represents over 633,000 occupational therapists internationally.

2026   WFOT Congress plans to meet in Bangkok, Thailand.

TABLE 14–7

EARLY LANDMARKS IN REHABILITATION MOVEMENT—STAGE VI

REHABILITATION EVENTS	DATES	CONTRIBUTORS	SIGNIFICANCE
First comprehensive rehabilitation	1946	Howard Rusk	Served as model for physical medicine programs in a general hospital rehabilitation team approach
Physical therapy methods	1949	H.O. Kendall F.P. Kendall	Basis for physical therapy techniques for muscle testing and patient evaluation
Retraining methods of ADLs	1956	Edith Buchwald Lawton	Provided functional rehabilitation methods for increasing independence
Vocational rehabilitation	1957	Lloyd H. Lofquist	Established the role of the rehabilitation counselor
Aphasia rehabilitation	1955	Martha L. Taylor M. Marks	Provided rehabilitation techniques for speech therapy
Prosthetics	1959	M.H. Anderson C.O. Bechtol R.E. Sollars	Led to cooperative research by physicians, engineers, and prosthetists in the design of artificial limbs
Orthotics	1962	Muriel Zimmerman	Led to the development of self-help devices for the homemaker and worker with physical disabilities

14.7.3 The Education and Professionalization—Phase II

The second phase of rehabilitation, during the 1930s, 1940s, and 1950s, can be identified as the educational and professionalization phase. Table 14–7 lists the early landmarks in physical rehabilitation. During this time, programs in colleges and universities were initiated, professional associations grew, and rehabilitation services evolved. The training of allied health specialists who had a unique combination of knowledge in the application of activities and rehabilitation techniques, understanding of medical treatment, and a background in the social sciences were considered necessary preparation for working in a hospital setting. The concepts underlying rehabilitation at that time were taken from other clinical and applied disciplines such as anatomy, physiology, nutrition, language development, psychology, clinical medicine, and education.

14.7.4 Physical Medicine and Rehabilitation

The first rehabilitation medical service in a general hospital was created in 1946, in Bellevue Hospital, New York City (Rusk, 1971). This unit served as a model for the interdisciplinary rehabilitation team. In addition, the physiatry specialty in rehabilitation medicine was started. Conceptually, rehabilitation was defined as restoring the individual to the highest level of cognitive, physical, economic, social, and emotional independence. This process, involving a team evaluation of the patient's functions, establishment of treatment goals and priorities, and an interdisciplinary approach to treatment, became the model for rehabilitation. This process is listed in Figure 14–2.

CHRONIC DISABILITY	EVALUATION OF FUNCTION	TREATMENT
○ Amputee	○ Activities of daily living	○ Chemotherapy
○ Arthritis	○ Ambulation	○ Dietetics
○ Cardiovascular	○ Diet	○ Nursing care
○ Degenerative diseases of the CNS	○ Leisure activities	○ Occupational therapy
○ Emphysema and pulmonary disease	○ Muscular and joint function	○ Orthotics
○ Epilepsy	○ Neurological processes	○ Physical therapy
○ Spinal cord injury	○ Psychological factors	○ Prosthetics
○ Stroke	○ Speech and language	○ Psychological counseling
	○ Vocational adjustment	○ Social work
		○ Speech therapy
		○ Surgery
		○ Vocational rehabilitation

Figure 14–2 The process of physical medicine and rehabilitation. Rehabilitation is the process of restoring function in individuals with severe disabilities. Assessment of the physical, cognitive, psychosocial, and vocational factors are carried out before intervention is planned and implemented.

Parallel to the evolution of a medical rehabilitation team was the involvement of the federal and state governments in providing vocational rehabilitation services that resulted from the Vocational Rehabilitation Act of 1954. Sheltered workshops, such as Abilities, Inc. in New York City, Epi-Hab in Phoenix and Los Angeles, Community Workshops in Boston, and Goodwill Industries, provided the vocational training component and the specialized employment placement that helped re-employ individuals with disabilities.

14.7.5 Allied Health Treatment Technologies

As the training of allied health professionals developed during the 1940s and 1950s, a treatment technology emerged, especially in physical therapy. Methods for objectively assessing muscle function were established (Daniels, 1956; Kendall et al., 1971). Electrodiagnosis of muscle function, measurement of range of motion, and techniques for improving muscle and joint action through heat, ultraviolet rays, electrical stimulation, whirlpool, and cold packs were developed through trial and error and clinical practice. These techniques were a major part of the physical therapist's treatment procedures (Downer, 1988). The need for retraining patients in activities of daily living was recognized by therapists as an important area for intervention. Lawton (1956), working with Howard Rusk at the Institute of Physical Medicine and Rehabilitation, published a manual for therapists describing methods to retrain patients to become functionally independent in their everyday activities. The need to retrain patients with aphasia to regain their use of language as the result of a stroke or brain injury led to the development of sequentially programmed techniques (Taylor & Marks, 1955).

Another important component of rehabilitation was in the area of vocational rehabilitation. Lofquist (1957), McGowan (1967), and Patterson (1958) were some of the early workers who defined the role of the rehabilitation counselor in prevocational evaluation, special placement, and vocational training. Occupational therapy progressed as an integral part of the rehabilitation movement in a more general direction than physical therapy or speech therapy. The use of activities as treatment modalities in work, leisure, and activities of daily living was applied to a broader spectrum of disabilities. Occupational therapists worked mainly in rehabilitation departments, psychiatric state hospitals, Veteran Administration facilities, and state schools for those with physical and mental disabilities (Willard & Spackman, 1971). As the rehabilitation movement gained momentum in the 1950s, biomedical research in the replacement of limbs and joints led to the field of prosthetics. The design of component parts, fitting of the prosthesis, and gait training gave rise to another member of the physical rehabilitation team, the prosthetist (Anderson et al., 1959). Specialization in rehabilitation also occurred at a rapid rate within the fields of nutrition, social work, psychology, and nursing.

14.7.6 Psychiatric Rehabilitation

In comparison with physical rehabilitation techniques, psychiatric treatment has lagged behind in developing the technology to treat the individual with mental illness.

Scull (2015)

The initial optimism from 1930 to 1950 that was generated by biological interventions, such as electric convulsive therapy, insulin therapy, Metrazol treatment, and psychosurgery, has faded. From the 1960s to the 1990s psychiatric treatment remained in a state of disarray. The onset of neuroleptic drugs and the community mental health movement in the 1960s led to the dismantling of large psychiatric hospitals that had served as custodial "warehouses" for the patients who were chronically mentally ill.

Since the 1960s, the length of hospitalization for patients with psychiatric disorders has been drastically reduced, but the number of individuals with mental illness living in the community and homeless without treatment has increased dramatically. "The mean prevalence of any current mental disorder was estimated at 76.2% (95% CI 64.0% to 86.6%). The most common diagnostic categories were alcohol use disorders, at 36.7% (95% CI 27.7% to 46.2%), and drug use disorders, at 21.7% (95% CI 13.1% to 31.7%), followed by schizophrenia spectrum disorders (12.4% [95% CI 9.5% to 15.7%]) and major depression (12.6% [95% CI 8.0% to 18.2%])" (Gutwinski et al., 2021, p. e1003750).

Affiliations Expand

Current enlightened psychiatric treatment emphasizes early return to the community in combination with outpatient rehabilitation emphasizing teaching functional skills, providing housing support, and aiding in vocational placement. In the remaining state hospitals for those with mental illness, a large percentage of elderly patients form a residual population. This population is mainly rejected, untreated, and provided mainly with maintenance care. Other individuals with mental illness are in custodial care facilities, prisons or left untreated and mostly neglected in large cities as homeless populations.

Evaluation of psychiatric treatment still remains a fertile area for clinical researchers. Apart from descriptive observations, few comprehensive studies have analyzed intervention techniques in depth. Although many clinicians believe that what they are doing is beneficial, there is little evidence or hard data to support their claims.

Why has psychiatric rehabilitation lagged behind other areas of medical progress? First, there has been wide disagreement in identifying, diagnosing, and treating mental illness in spite of the attempt to classify it as exemplified in the *Diagnostic and Statistical Manual of Mental Disorders*, 5th edition (APA, 2013). Theorists have differed widely in their approaches in psychiatry, advocating specific treatment techniques for the broad spectrum of mental illness. Many clinical researchers have failed to recognize the individual needs of patients and the differential effects of specific interventions. A second reason for the lag in scientific progress in psychiatric rehabilitation is the lack of comprehensive studies. Psychiatric research has been fixed at the 19th century two-variable research stage model, which assumed a single-factor cause for mental illness. If progress in psychiatric rehabilitation is to occur, multidisciplinary efforts must investigate mental illness on a broad front, using a biopsychosocial model, rather than narrow, one-dimensional research. The promise in psychiatric rehabilitation lies in a holistic approach, the incorporation of a community mental health model relying on half-way houses, vocational programs, and support groups, with an individualized approach to evaluation, education, psychotherapy, counseling, and drug treatment.

14.7.7 Third Phase of Allied Health—1960 to Present

This development led to the present period of rehabilitation, which has been characterized by various treatment theories. Unfortunately, these theories have become so specialized that professionals in allied health fields can no longer change from one disability area to another without familiarizing themselves with a vast amount of knowledge and technology. For example, allied health professionals have advocated and applied various interventions such as constraint therapy, augmentative communication, driver rehabilitation, assistive technology, sensory integration therapy (SI), neurodevelopmental therapy, robotics, telemetry, cinematography, and biofeedback. These interventions are not unique to one profession. They are many times interdisciplinary in nature and incorporate theories and findings from the physical and social sciences.

Table 14–8 shows the rapid growth of the allied health professions from 1950 to 2014.

TABLE 14–8						
THE GROWTH OF HEALTH PROFESSION, 1950 TO 2022						
	POSTSECONDARY			ACTIVE PRACTITIONERS		
HEALTH SPECIALTY	TRAINING (YEARS)	1950	1972	1992	2014	2022
Audiologist[1]	6–8	—	—	—	13,200	14,400
Chiropractor	6–8	14,000	16,000	46,000	42,200	55,000
Dentist	8	75,300	105,000	183,000	151,500	155,000
Dietitian and nutritionists	4–5	15,000	33,000	50,000	66,700	78,600
Occupational therapist	5–6	2,300	7,500	40,000	114,000	139,600
Optometrist	7–8	17,000	18,700	31,000	40,000	43,400
Pharmacist	6–7	100,000	131,000	163,000	207,100	334,200
Physical therapist	6–7	4,500	18,000	90,000	210,900	246,800
Physician and surgeon[2]	8–16	200,000	316,500	556,000	708,300	816,900
Physician assistant[3]	4–6	—	303	22,305	94,400	148,000
Podiatrist	10–12	6,400	7,300	14,700	9,600	10,600
Psychologist	9–10	10,000	57,000	144,000	173,900	196,000
Registered nurse	3–5	300,500	750,000	1,835,000	2,751,000	3,172,500
Respiratory therapist	2–4	—	17,000	74,000	120,700	133,100
Speech-language pathologist	6	2,000	27,000	73,000	135,400	171,400
Social worker	4–8	100,000	185,000	484,000	649,300	728,600

[1] Audiologists were included with speech/language pathologists until 2008.

[2] Surgeons were added in 2008.

[3] Physician assistant programs were started in 1967.

Note. The information contained in this table is based on data from U.S. Department Labor, *Occupational Outlook Handbook.* Retrieved from http://stats.bls.gov/oco/

The extraordinary growth of the allied health professions since 1950 is apparent if one examines the percentage increase in the number of active practitioners and the number of professional schools. In comparison with the United States' population increase from 150 million in 1949 to 210 million in 1972, one would have expected the professions to increase about 40%. We find, however, that professions such as occupational therapy and physical therapy increased 300% during the same period. The number of radiologic technologists increased 685%, registered nurses increased 149%, and physicians increased 58% during this period. On the other hand, the smallest increases were in the numbers of chiropractic, osteopathy, optometry, and pharmacy professionals. The growth of the allied health professions has continued into the 1980s and 1990s with forecasts of continued growth far into the 21st century.

Another indication of the rapid expansion of the allied health professions is the emergence of new fields that did not exist 40 years ago. The *Occupational Outlook Handbook* (1951) did not include many allied health professions, which appeared in later editions, starting with 1972. (See Table 14–9.)

14.7.8 Rehabilitation Research Trends (1950–1975)

Goldberg (1974), in an analysis of rehabilitation research, identified ten areas at that time that were related to clinical practice.

- Program evaluation: the assessment of the effectiveness of a clinical program in reaching stated objectives or meeting a list of criteria
- Management: the study of factors related to health manpower, cost effectiveness, and comprehensive planning in providing health care to those in need of services
- Dissemination: the process of communicating research findings over a wide area, including to professional and lay persons
- Involvement of consumer groups: the identification of research problems
- Chronic severe disability: functional problems as a major focus of research in rehabilitation
- Social problems: alcoholism, adult crime, drug addiction, and juvenile delinquency as areas included under health-related problems instead of correctional problems
- Functional assessment methods: targeted to the individuals with severe disabilities who are in supported employment and working at home
- Need for follow-up and follow-along research: evaluation of the continuity of care
- Rehabilitation utilization: incorporation of rehabilitation research in clinical practices
- Rehabilitation engineering: interdisciplinary research in solving practical rehabilitation problems especially in the fields of prosthetics, orthotics, communication, mobility, and independent living.

These trends continue to have an impact on current rehabilitation research in the 21st century. From the initial emphasis on the physical restoration of the individual, researchers are now turning to the more complex chronic social problems that are associated with poverty, crime, homelessness, substandard housing, undernourishment, alienation, and addiction. Evidence shows that

TABLE 14–9					
GROWTH OF SELECTED HEALTH PROFESSIONS OF TECHNOLOGISTS AND ASSISTANTS, 1972–2022					
HEALTH FIELD	1972	1986	1996	2014	2022
Dental hygienist	17,000	87,000	133,000	200,500	219,400
Electrocardiograph (ECG) technician	10,000	18,000	15,000	112,000	142,800
Medical record technician	8,000	40,000	87,000	188,600	194,300
Nuclear medicine technologist	—	9,700	13,000	20,700	18,100
Occupational therapy assistant	6,000	9,000	16,000	41,900	49,000
Physical therapy assistant	10,000	12,000	84,000	128,700	145,100
Radiology and MRI technologist	55,000	1 15,000	174,000	230,000	264,100
Respiratory therapist	17,000	56,000	82,000	120,700	133,100
Surgical technician	25,000	37,000	49,000	99,800	128,900
Note. Data in this table are taken from the U.S. Department of Labor, *Occupational Outlook Handbook*, retrieved from www.bls.gov/ooh/.					

severe chronic disabilities on a global level, such as polio, tuberculosis, stroke, chronic obstructive pulmonary disease, and cardiovascular diseases, can be alleviated or reduced through public health immunization programs, healthy nutrition, exercise regimes, smoking cessation and self-monitoring of symptoms. The biopsychosocial holistic approach in occupational therapy is an important concept guiding rehabilitation. The cost of preventing chronic illnesses is much less than the cost of rehabilitation. Primary, secondary, and tertiary prevention have begun to make an impact in the work of allied health professionals. Research has an important part in justifying the efficacy of treatment interventions, either in restoring function or preventing chronic disability.

Key facts (WHO):

- Rehabilitation is an essential part of universal health coverage along with promotion of good health, prevention of disease, treatment and palliative care.
- Rehabilitation helps a child, adult, or older person to be as independent as possible in everyday activities and enables participation in education, work, recreation, and meaningful life roles such as taking care of family.
- Globally, an estimated 2.4 billion people are currently living with a health condition that benefits from rehabilitation.
- The need for rehabilitation worldwide is predicted to increase due to changes in the health and characteristics of the population. For example, people are living longer, but with more chronic disease and disability.
- Currently, the need for rehabilitation is largely unmet. In some low- and middle-income countries, more than 50% of people do not receive the rehabilitation services they require. Rehabilitation services are also amongst the health services most severely disrupted by the COVID-19 pandemic.

What Is Rehabilitation?

Rehabilitation is defined as "a set of interventions designed to optimize functioning and reduce disability in individuals with health conditions in interaction with their environment." (Nas, et al., 2015, p 8).

Put simply, rehabilitation helps a child, adult or older person to be as independent as possible in everyday activities and enables participation in education, work, recreation and meaningful life roles such as taking care of family. It does so by addressing underlying conditions (such as pain) and improving the way an individual functions in everyday life, supporting them to overcome difficulties with thinking, seeing, hearing, communicating, eating, or moving around.

Anybody may need rehabilitation at some point in their lives, following an injury, surgery, disease or illness, or because their functioning has declined with age.

Some examples of rehabilitation include:

- Exercises to improve a person's speech, language, and communication after a brain injury.
- Modifying an older person's home environment to improve their safety and independence at home and to reduce their risk of falls.
- Exercise training and education on healthy living for a person with a heart disease.
- Making, fitting, and educating an individual to use a prosthesis after a leg amputation.
- Positioning and splinting techniques to assist with skin healing, reduce swelling, and to regain movement after burn surgery.
- Prescribing medicine to reduce muscle stiffness for a child with cerebral palsy.
- Psychological support for a person with depression.
- Training in the use of a white cane, for a person with vision loss.

Rehabilitation is highly person-centered, meaning that the interventions and approach selected for each individual depends on their goals and preferences. Rehabilitation can be provided in many different settings, from inpatient or outpatient hospital settings, to private clinics, or community settings such as an individual's home.

The rehabilitation workforce is made up of different health workers, including but not limited to physiotherapists, occupational therapists, speech and language therapists and audiologists, orthotists and prosthetists, clinical psychologists, physical medicine and rehabilitation doctors, and rehabilitation nurses.

The Benefits of Rehabilitation

Rehabilitation can reduce the impact of a broad range of health conditions, including diseases (acute or chronic), illnesses or injuries. It can also complement other health interventions, such as medical and surgical interventions, helping to achieve the best outcome possible. For example, rehabilitation can help to reduce, manage or prevent complications associated with many health conditions, such as spinal cord injury, stroke, or a fracture.

Rehabilitation helps to minimize or slow down the disabling effects of chronic health conditions, such as cardiovascular disease, cancer and diabetes by equipping people with self-management strategies and the assistive products they require, or by addressing pain or other complications.

Rehabilitation is an investment, with cost benefits for both the individuals and society. It can help to avoid costly hospitalization, reduce hospital length of stay, and prevent readmissions. Rehabilitation also enables individuals to participate in education and gainful employment, remain independent at home, and minimize the need for financial or caregiver support.

Rehabilitation is an important part of universal health coverage and is a key strategy for achieving the UN's Sustainable Development Goal 3: "Ensure healthy lives and promote well-being for all at all ages."

Misconceptions About Rehabilitation

Rehabilitation is not only for people with long-term or physical impairments. Rather, rehabilitation is a core health service for anyone with an acute or chronic health condition, impairment or injury that limits functioning, and as such should be available for anyone who needs it.

Rehabilitation is not a luxury health service that is available only for those who can afford it. Nor is it an optional service to try only when other interventions to prevent or cure a health condition fail.

For the full extent of the social, economic, and health benefits of rehabilitation to be realized, timely, high-quality, and affordable rehabilitation interventions should be available to all. In many cases, this means starting rehabilitation as soon as a health condition is noted and continuing to deliver rehabilitation alongside other health interventions.

Unmet Global Need for Rehabilitation

Globally, about 2.4 billion people are currently living with a health condition that benefits from rehabilitation. With changes taking place in the health and characteristics of the population worldwide, this estimated need for rehabilitation is only going to increase in the coming years.

People are living longer, with the number of people over 60 years of age predicted to double by 2050, and more people are living with chronic diseases such as diabetes, stroke, and cancer. At the same time, there is an ongoing incidence of injury (such as a burn) and child developmental conditions (such as cerebral palsy). These health conditions can impact an individual's functioning and are linked to increased levels of disability, for which rehabilitation can be beneficial.

In many parts of the world, this increasing need for rehabilitation is going largely unmet. More than half of people living in some low- and middle-income countries who require rehabilitation services do not receive them.

Global rehabilitation needs continue to be unmet due to multiple factors, including:

- Lack of prioritization, funding, policies, and plans for rehabilitation at a national level.
- Lack of available rehabilitation services outside urban areas, and long waiting times.
- High out-of-pocket expenses and non-existent or inadequate means of funding.
- Lack of trained rehabilitation professionals, with less than ten skilled practitioners per 1 million population in many low- and middle-income settings.
- Lack of resources, including assistive technology, equipment, and consumables.
- The need for more research and data on rehabilitation.
- Ineffective and under-utilized referral pathways to rehabilitation.

Rehabilitation in Emergencies

Natural hazards such as earthquakes or disease outbreaks and human-induced hazards including conflict, terrorism, and industrial accidents can generate overwhelming rehabilitation needs as a result of injury or illness. They also simultaneously disrupt existing services and have the greatest impact on the most vulnerable populations and the weakest health systems.

While the important role of rehabilitation in emergencies is recognized in clinical and humanitarian guidelines, it is rarely considered as part of health system preparedness and early response. The result is that pre-existing limitations in rehabilitation services are magnified, health service delivery is less efficient, and people directly affected are at risk of increased impairment and disability.

WHO Response

For rehabilitation to reach its full potential, efforts should be directed towards strengthening the health system as a whole and making rehabilitation part of health care at all levels of the health system, and as part of universal health coverage.

In 2017, WHO launched the Rehabilitation 2030 initiative, which emphasizes the need for health system strengthening, and calls for all stakeholders worldwide to come together to work on different priority areas, including: improving leadership and governance; developing a strong multidisciplinary rehabilitation workforce; expanding financing for rehabilitation; and improving data collection and research on rehabilitation.

WHO is responding to the identified challenges and promoting health system strengthening for rehabilitation through:

- Providing technical support and building capacity at country level
- Increasing leadership, prioritization and resource mobilization
- Developing norms, standards and technical guidance
- Shaping the research agenda and monitoring progress.

(WHO, 2021)

14.8 HABILITATION AND SPECIAL EDUCATION—STAGE VII

The success of the rehabilitation movement led to the field of habilitation, which goes beyond the medical model. While the medical model traditionally relies on etiology, diagnosis, and treatment, habilitation includes the integration of psychological, sociological, and educational fields of knowledge emphasizing research in developmental theory and educational technology. Rehabilitation is

TABLE 14–10

THE PROCESS OF HABILITATION AND DEVELOPMENT OF FUNCTION

CHILDHOOD DISABILITIES RELATED TO GENETIC, EMBRYOLOGIC, OR TRAUMA INJURY	EVALUATION OF FUNCTION	EDUCATIONAL AND TREATMENT TECHNIQUES
• Attention-deficit/hyperactivity disorder (ADHD) • ASD • Cerebral palsy • Childhood amputee • Dyslexia • Epilepsy • Fetal alcohol spectrum disorders • Hearing impairment • Intellectual disabilities and developmental delay • Juvenile arthritis • Learning disabilities • Neuromotor impairments • Orthopedic impairments • Sensory integration disorder • Traumatic brain injury • Visual impairments	• Academic • ADLs • Cognitive • Leisure interests • Neuromuscular • Mental health • Memory • Neuropsychological • Prevocational • Psychosocial • Sensory	• Augmentative and alternative communication • Braille • Community-based instruction • Computer-assisted instruction • Explicit or direct instruction • Inclusive education • Individualized learning • Medical treatment • Motor therapy (occupational and physical therapy) • Orientation and mobility • Psychological counseling • Response to intervention • Self-care skills • Sensorimotor training • Sign language • Speech-language therapy • Strategic teaching • Vocational development
Children with special needs are evaluated and then taught using appropriate educational and treatment techniques.		

traditionally defined as the restoration of function and the maximization of abilities in individuals with chronic disabilities. In contrast, habilitation is defined as the development of functions and capabilities in individuals with disabilities occurring at birth, during childhood, or during a traumatic incident (e.g., traumatic brain injury, post-traumatic stress). The process of habilitation is presented in Table 14–10. The child with intellectual disability, the individual who is congenitally blind or deaf, the child born with a missing limb or with cerebral palsy, the child with autism, and the child who is extremely disadvantaged have needs that are different from adults who acquired a physical disability. Helping the child develop independence, coping skills, and physical and mental capabilities to adapt to societal demands requires specialized techniques. The child who is developmentally delayed, unlike the adult with a disability, has not lost a capacity or skill that requires remedial education, sensory retraining, or vocational readjustment. Instead, the child with a disability needs special education, sensorimotor or language training, occupational preparation, and training for activities of daily living basic to the habilitation process. Special education services, available for individuals with special needs, have been developed to provide training and instruction in functional skills necessary for independent living and self-support. What were the early historical precursors to the field of habilitation?

14.8.1 Initial Concern for Those with Disabilities

Although prior to the 20th century some services were available for individuals with disabilities, these services were minimal, generally no more than custodial care and assistance through the efforts of religious orders and voluntary charities. The earliest report of attempts to treat and educate the blind was the establishment of a hospital in 1260 (Special Education in Europe, 1981; Hallahan & Kauffman, 1993). Rousseau (1712–1779), a philosopher and theorist, petitioned in his treatise *Emile* for the study of children directly rather than using what was known about adults and applying that knowledge to children. "Nature intends that children shall be children before they are men… Treat your pupil as his age demands" (Rousseau, 1883, pp. 52–54).

During the mid-1800s, Jacob Rodreques Pereire (1715–1780), a Spanish medical doctor living in France, developed an oral method to teach individuals with severe hearing loss to read and speak. At the same time, a Frenchman, Abbé de l'Epée (1712–1789) developed a manual sign language for "deaf-mutes." "The natural language of the Deaf and Dumb is the language of signs; nature and their different wants are their only tutors in it: and they have no other language as long as they have no further instructors" (Epée, 1784/1820, as cited in Lane, 1976, p. 79).

Sicard (1742–1833), a French medical doctor influential in the education of the "deaf-mutes" expanded Epée's methods, producing a way to teach "deaf-mutes" to read and write:

> [Epée] saw that the deaf-mute expressed his physical needs without instruction; that one could, with the same signs, communicate to him the expression of the same needs and could indicate the things that one wanted to designate: these were the first words of a new language which this great man has enriched, to the astonishment of all of Europe.
>
> (Sicard, 1795, as cited in Lane, 1976, p. 79)

14.8.2 Itard's Influence

The earliest reported case of enlightened intervention with children identified of having intellectual disability was Jean-Marc Gaspard Itard's (1774–1838) work with Victor, "the wild boy of Aveyron" (Lane, 1976). Victor (ca. 1785–1828), who emerged from the forests of Aveyron between 1797 and 1800, was thought to have been abandoned by his parents as an infant or young child. Itard, a young physician, was assigned the responsibility to teach Victor. Itard applied methods developed earlier by Epée and Sicard. These methods included breaking up each task into small segments and using techniques that had been successful for "deaf-mutes." In this way, Itard believed that he could teach Victor to be social and use language (Lane, 1976; Winnie, 1912). After six years, even though Itard considered his work a failure, Victor had developed some social skills and could read a few words. On the other hand, Itard's work with Victor inspired him to further his methods for teaching "deaf-mutes":

> The child, who was called the wild boy of Aveyron, did not receive from my intensive care all the advantages that I had hoped. But the many observations that I could make and the techniques of instruction inspired by the inflexibility of his organs were not entirely fruitless, and I later found a more suitable application for them with some of our children whose mutism is the result of obstacles that are more easily overcome.
>
> (Itard, 1825, as cited in Lane, 1976, p. 185)

Several authors in education (Forness & Kavale, 1984; Hunt & Marshall, 2012; McDermott, 1994; Smith & Tyler, 2010) have recognized the significant contribution of Itard's work with Victor to present-day methods used in special education classes. In his effort to teach Victor, Itard developed methods that encompassed multiple senses (auditory, visual, kinesthetic) and demonstrated that individual instruction could be successful. Eduardo Séquin (1812–1880), a student of Itard, advanced these methods. He opened the first school for the "intellectually deficient" in 1837 and demonstrated that they could

be systematically trained and educated. Finally, as a physician involved in the education and treatment of individuals with disabilities, Itard played a significant part in the development of educational and treatment services for individuals with disabilities (Forness & Kavale, 1984). Initially, the emphasis of special education relied on a medical model using etiology, symptomology, differential diagnosis, and specialized treatment. This resulted in an educational system based on classification and segregation, rather than a system based on community participation and mainstreaming in general education. It is notable that Itard's work using a single case study has led to the development of general methods for teaching children with disabilities (Kirk et al., 2022).

14.8.3 Montessori's Contribution to Special Education

The following quote is from Marie Montessori who, as a physician and teacher, established the basis for special education in Italy at the end of the 19th century. "In this method the lesson corresponds to an experiment, the more fully the teacher is acquainted with the methods of experimental psychology, the better will she understand how to give the lesson" (Montessori, 1912, p. 107).

Montessori advocated that the special education teacher of individuals with intellectual disability should use observation and experimentation in sequencing pedagogical activities. Montessori, who acknowledges the influence of Itard and Séquin, was a forerunner in the movement to provide special education methods through perceptual-motor training to the child with disabilities. These materials and methods were based on concrete, three-dimensional manipulatives (hands-on activities) that allowed exploration and learning through discovery. Today these methods are used with populations of typical children and children with special needs (Shea & Bauer, 1994).

Theoretically, Montessori's method changed the direction of treatment from a medical model to a model based on education, psychology, and child development. This approach was not limited to the child with intellectual disability. For example, Louis Braille, who was blind, developed a system of reading for the blind over a period from 1825 to 1852 (Illingworth, 1910). This method of teaching was the basis of special education for the blind in the early 1900s. Analogous to Braille as a method for teaching the blind was sign language for the deaf, devised by Abbé de l'Epée around 1755 (Winnie, 1912). The oral method was later practiced in Germany by Heinicke and Hill, who felt that speech development in the deaf child should parallel normal speech development (Winnie, 1912). Because of the complexity in educating blind and deaf children, special schools that segregated them from the public schools were founded. The significance of the Montessori method for those with intellectual disability, of the Braille system for the blind, and of sign language for the deaf is that these methods compensate for the child's inability to learn in a typical classroom. They are specific, technological advances designed to help the child to learn. These methods have allowed special education to be effective for children who are blind, deaf, or intellectually disabled.

14.8.4 Early Services in the United States

Séquin's contribution to the education of individuals with disabilities extended to the United States. Through the efforts of Samuel Gridley Howe, Séquin immigrated to the United States in 1848 where he shared his knowledge of educational methods for teaching individuals with intellectual disability. He was later instrumental in founding the American Association on Intellectual and Developmental Disabilities (AAIDD), formerly known as the American Association on Mental Deficiency (AAMD). This association "promotes progressive policies, sound research, effective practices and universal human rights for people with intellectual and developmental disabilities."

(AAIDD, 2010, para 1)

In the United States, Reverend Thomas Gallaudet, Horace Mann, and Samuel Gridley Howe were pioneers in the early development of special schools for children with disabilities. In 1817, in Hartford, Connecticut, Gallaudet, assisted by Clerc, a "deaf-mute" trained by Sicard, founded the first residential school for the deaf (Lane, 1976). This outstanding school still exists. Gallaudet University, located in Washington, DC, is the only liberal arts college established for students with hearing impairments. The university was founded by Gallaudet's grandson in 1864 (Lane, 1976). In 1829, Howe opened the Perkins Institute at Watertown, Massachusetts, a residential school for students with visual impairments. This school is well known because Anne Sullivan, teacher of Helen Keller, was trained there. Fernald State School, the first institution for individuals with intellectual disability, was opened in 1848, with the Commonwealth of Massachusetts assuming full financial responsibility (Sigmon, 1987). In addition to Séquin and his work with intellectual disability, individuals such as Louis Braille and Alexander Graham Bell, who was instrumental in the amplification of sound for the hearing impaired, greatly influenced the teaching methods used in these early institutions (Kirk et al., 2022).

A major change in educational practices in the United States occurred when individual states mandated compulsory education between 1852 and 1918. Although some students with disabilities were taught in the general education program, the degree of severity in these individuals resulted in the creation of residential institutions, segregated day schools, and special classes. The first special education day school in the United States, the Horace Mann School, was opened in 1868 in Roxbury, Massachusetts. New Jersey, in 1911, was the first state to mandate programs for students with disabilities (Sigmon, 1987). Individuals confined to wheelchairs or with severe disabilities continued to be excluded from public schools until the 1960s and 1970s. The right for children with disabilities to be educated in a public school was mandated by court decisions such as Pennsylvania Association of Retarded Citizens (PARC) v. Pennsylvania (1971) and Mills v. Board of Education, Washington, DC (1971). Decisions from these judicial cases supported the position that individuals with disabilities were entitled to a free and appropriate public education (FAPE) regardless of the degree of severity or educational need (Turnbull III & Turnbull, 1998)

14.8.5 Special Education Assessment and Programming

In 1905, Alfred Binet (1857–1911), a French psychologist, was commissioned by the French government to provide a useful assessment tool that would identify those children who needed special techniques to learn. Binet began working to develop methods of assessing intelligence in 1886. His first book, published at that time, was entitled *Psychologie du Raissonnement* (*The Psychology of Reasoning*; 1899/1912). This was the beginning of intelligence testing as we know it today. In the United States, Lewis Terman (1877–1956) and Henry Herbert Goddard (1866–1957), strongly influenced by Binet, continued the development of intelligence tests. Both believed that intelligence was inherited, stable, and did not change over time. A student's failure in the general education curriculum was explained by their inadequate intellectual level, not by methods of teaching or environmental factors. As a result, in the first half of the 20th century, institutionalization and segregation of those individuals with severe intellectual deficits and physical disabilities became the norm. It was not until the 1960s when there was a major push toward normalization (Wolfensberger et al., 1972) and deinstitutionalization that individuals with intellectual disability and physical impairments were returned to the community and local school programs.

Historically, the habilitation of those with mild intellectual disability, blindness, and deafness has been more successful than the habilitation of individuals with brain damage, learning disabilities, autism, or social deprivation. One reason for these differences has been in the specialized educational curricula that have been developed to compensate for the child's disability. Methods for educating students with brain damage, learning disabilities, autism, or social deprivation were slower to develop.

During the latter half of the 19th century and the beginnings of the 20th century, physicians such as James

(Hinshelwood, 1917) and Samuel T. Orton (1879–1948) used adult models to understand reasons for learning difficulties in children who were not deaf, blind, or intellectually disabled. Both clinicians developed a multisensory method for teaching reading. Later, their ideas were expanded by special educators. The methods developed are still used today in many classrooms (Mercer et al., 2014)

The aftermath of World War I was another turning point in the development of educational programs for individuals with brain injuries. Kurt Goldstein (1878–1965), in his experimental work with soldiers who had sustained head injuries during battle, contributed much to the understanding of the consequences of brain damage. His work inspired Alfred Strauss and Heinz Werner (Strauss & Werner, 1941) to study children with brain damage during the 1930s and 1940s at Wayne County Training School in Michigan. Their findings led to the identification of a group of children with brain damage. Although these children appeared to be intellectually disabled, the cause of this was not genetic. Moreover, their behavioral characteristics were similar to the symptoms displayed by soldiers with brain injuries, such as perseveration, distractibility, inattention, and memory problems (Mercer 1983). In their classic book, *Psychopathology and Education of the Brain-Injured Child*, Strauss and Lehtinen (1947) described symptoms and behaviors of the child with brain injury and justified special education methods for teaching this group of children. Prior to the published works by Strauss and collaborators (Strauss & Kephart, 1940; Strauss & Werner, 1941; Strauss & Lehtinen, 1947) treatment for the child with brain damage was undifferentiated. Strauss and Lehtinen (1947) described the problem as follows: "The response of the brain-injured child to the school situation is frequently inadequate, conspicuously disturbing, and persistently troublesome" (p. 127).

Luria (1961) and Vygotsky (1934), Russian neuropsychologists were influential in the understanding of brain functioning and language development. Luria believed that the brain was made up of three functional units: the brainstem, involved with arousal and attention; the posterior portion, involved with taking in and processing of sensory information; and the anterior portion, implicated in planning, monitoring, and verifying one's performance. Luria and Vygotsky postulated that the development of language played an important part in one's ability to organize tasks involving planning, self-monitoring, and self-regulating. Individuals with brain damage who no longer use language for organization manifest extreme difficulties in self-regulatory and self-monitoring activities. Likewise, children who do not use language for organization do not develop self-regulation or planning skills. These ideas of Luria and Vygotsky have influenced the way we teach all students in developmentally appropriate early childhood classes.

Until recently, children with autism faced an even more uncertain future because of the lack of effective methods to compensate for their disability. For example Bettelheim (1967) described the initial reaction to the orthogenic school and the problems of communication in an 11-year-old girl with autism:

> At first what little speech she had consisted of very rare, simple, highly selective and only whispered echolalia. For example, when we asked her if she wanted some candy she would merely echo "candy." She would say "no" but never "yes…" It was not our language she used, but a private one of her own.
>
> (p. 162)

Currently, programs such as TEACCH (Treatment and Education of Autistic Children and Communication Handicapped Children) at the University of North Carolina in Chapel Hill provide expertise and technical assistance in diagnosis and treatment to teachers and parents of students with autism (Virues-Ortega et al., 2013).

As with the child with brain damage or autism, the child who is socially disadvantaged has been a challenge for special educators. Gordon (1968) characterized the child who is socially disadvantaged as unprepared for a normal educational experience. He wrote: "As a consequence, these children show in school disproportionately high rates of social maladjustment, behavioral disturbance, physical disability, academic retardation and mental subnormality [sic]" (p. 6). Many of the children formerly characterized as socially disadvantaged are now diagnosed with ADHD.

In 1963, at the first national meeting of what later became the Association for Children with Learning Disabilities (now named the Learning Disabilities Association of America), the term learning disabilities was identified by Samuel A. Kirk (1963):

> Recently I have used the term "Teaming disabilities" to describe a group of children who have disorders in development, in language, speech, reading, and associated communication skills needed for social interaction. In this group I do not include children who have sensory handicaps such as blindness or deafness, because we have methods of managing and training the deaf and the blind. I also exclude from this group children who have generalized mental retardation [sic].
>
> (p. 3)

Another impetus for the development of appropriate educational programs for individuals with disabilities was the formation of various organizations, such as the March of Dimes, National Easter Seal Society, and United Cerebral Palsy, designed to provide community-based services. Although these organizations originally provided resources for equipment and medical care for children with disabilities, parents of these children became politically proactive in obtaining rehabilitation hospitals and clinics, special education programs, community services, and barrier-free environments. These organizations have been instrumental in the development of support groups for families and in the publication and distribution of educational materials on prevention and treatment of disabilities.

Compared with children who have disabilities that cause severe problems in communication and learning; children with physical impairment who have normal language and sensory functions present different problems in habilitation. Physical barriers present problems in architectural design. Emotional and social adjustment is affected by the self-concept of children with disabilities, as well as by their feelings of competence. Other chronic disabilities of childhood such as juvenile arthritis, ulcerative colitis, childhood diabetes, heart defects, and epilepsy profoundly affect the child's development and require adaptive or specialized treatment methods.

14.8.6 Services for Individuals with Disabilities

Since the passing of Section 504 of the Rehabilitation Act in 1973, the Education for the Handicapped Act (EHA; Public Law 94–142) in 1974, the reauthorization and amendment of EHA as Public Law 99–457, the passing of the Americans with Disabilities Act (1990), the reauthorization and amendment of EHA as Public Law 101–456, also known as Individuals with Disabilities Education Act (IDEA) in 1990, the Individuals with Disabilities Education Act Amendments of 1997 (IDEA; PL. 105–117), No Child Left Behind in 2002 (NCLB, PL 107–110) and the reauthorization of IDEA through the Individuals with Disabilities Education Improvement Act (IDEIA; PL 108–446) in December, 2004, programs for students with special needs have grown by leaps and bounds. For example, in 1976–1977, approximately 3.5 million students, ages 6 to 18, were served in special education. By 1987–1988, this number had risen to 4.1 million, and by 1996–1997, there were 5.3 million students, ages 6 to 21, or approximately 8.5% of the population (United States Department of Education, 2000).

In 2020–2021, the number of students ages 3–21 who received special education services under the Individuals with Disabilities Education Act (IDEA) was 7.2 million, or 15 percent of all public school students. Among students receiving special education services, the most common category of disability was specific learning disabilities (33 percent).

Enacted in 1975, the Individuals with Disabilities Education Act (IDEA), formerly known as the Education for All Handicapped Children Act, mandates the provision of a free and appropriate public school education for eligible students ages 3–21. Eligible students are those identified by a team of professionals as having a disability that adversely affects academic performance and as being in need of special education and related services. Data collection activities to monitor compliance with IDEA began in 1976. From school year 2009–2010 through 2020–2021, the number of students ages 3–21 who received special education services under IDEA increased from 6.5 million, or 13 percent of total public school enrollment, to 7.2 million, or 15 percent of total public school enrollment. In fall 2020, after the beginning of the coronavirus pandemic, overall enrollment in public schools was 3 percent lower than in fall 2019 (see Public School Enrollment). Meanwhile, the number of students receiving IDEA services was about 1 percent lower in 2020–2021 than in 2019–202020. This was the first drop in the number of students receiving IDEA services since 2011–2012. However, the percentage of students who were served under IDEA was higher in 2020–2021 (15 percent) than in 2019–20 (14 percent), continuing the upward trend.

(NCES, 2022)

Approximately 16,000 occupational therapists were employed in educational and school settings during the 2020–2021 school year (Bureau of Labor Statistics, US Department of Labor, 2022). Treatment and educational services are provided by public schools for any student from birth to age 21 who is at risk or is disabled. In addition, a continuum of services are available that range from consulting with the general education teacher about a student's needs, to providing an intense, restrictive residential setting for a student. Augmentative communication, life-skills training, and assistive technology are provided to the student when needed (Meyen & Skrtic, 1988; Skrtic, 1991; Smith & Tyler, 2010).

During the 1950s, 1960s, and 1970s, services for students with special needs were available primarily in residential institutions, special day schools, or special classes that were often physically isolated and segregated from the mainstreamed students. The concept of least restrictive environment, delineated in EHA (PL. 94–142), states that each student will be educated in the program that allows him or her to be educated with their own peers to the maximum extent possible. Efficacy studies examining the effectiveness of special classes show mixed results. Earlier studies (Dunn, 1968; Epps & Tindal, 1987; Haynes & Jenkins, 1986) found special education to be ineffective; however more recent studies have suggested that students with learning disabilities and behavior disorders often show greater improvement in the special education classroom (Fuchs et al., 1993; Marston, 1987–1988). Madeline Will (1986), the Assistant Secretary of Education, strongly recommended that students with mild disabilities be returned to general education. She argued that general educators should take more responsibility for teaching these students. This position, originally called the Regular Education Initiative, is now known as the General Education Initiative. Although some individuals, such as Sailor (1991) and Stainback and Stainback (1992) proposed total inclusion, that is, placement of all students, regardless of their educational needs, into their home schools and into the regular classroom, others (Vergason & Anderegg, 1992) encouraged a range of inclusiveness, with each student's placement based on individual needs and related to specific long-term goals. This latter stance appears to be more in accord with the concept of least restrictive environment as stated in IDEA.

Two factors have influenced changes in how services are provided to students in special education. First, NCLB mandated that students with special needs have access to the general education curriculum. Second, following the passage of IDEIA (Congress, 2004), the Office of Special Education and Rehabilitation mandated the "implementation of a process known as response to intervention (RTI)" (Reynolds, 2008) be used with students with learning disabilities. As a result, the more than half of the students in special education are taught in the general education classroom with supports provided as needed (US Department of Education, Office of Special Education and Rehabilitative Services, Office of Special Education Programs, 2009). With the increase in inclusive classes, additional training in collaborative techniques has been provided for general educators, special educators, occupational therapists, physical therapists, speech-language pathologists, school psychologists, and audiologists. Students with severe disabilities may continue to receive educational services in special class placements, especially when the educational needs include self-care skills and independent living skills.

Although much has been achieved in the development of programs and services for those individuals with special needs, there is much more to accomplish. There continue to be a greater percentage of students from minority groups placed in special education than those from the majority population. We are only beginning to understand how to remediate and improve cognitive deficits with individuals diagnosed with Alzheimer's Disease. Augmentative communication, assistive technology, and the use of computer assisted instruction in education and training are still in the infancy stage of development. Although increased medical technology has made it possible to keep infants and patients with severe disabilities alive, we have only just begun to develop educational and training programs for these individuals so that they can live in home environments or supportive housing in the community. The age of "warehousing" individuals in large institutions with custodial care has been replaced with more humane care for individuals with severe disabilities.

14.9 Research and the Future of Health Care

What are the future directions and goals of health care? The physician, an individual educated in the arts and science of healing, historically has been the primary health practitioner. At first, education of the physician was "at the foot of a master;" later, formal training permitted one to legally practice medicine. It is only in the last 150 years that medicine has become a science with reliable and valid methods. The science of modern medicine began with Claude Bernard and Louis Pasteur, who provided the research methods and theory of disease that underlie clinical practice. Progress has been dramatic since the late 1800s, culminating with the elimination of many major diseases through vaccination, chemotherapy, surgery, and effective hospital care. Preventive medicine is now the cornerstone of health maintenance. Since the beginning of the 21st century, researchers are mobilizing their efforts to discover means to prevent premature deaths from heart disease, stroke, cancer, arthritis, emphysema, and AIDS. Ironically, chronic disabilities continue to persist as people live longer. As new diseases emerge (e.g., ebola virus, COVID), they present new challenges for medical researchers.

In 2023 a major trend in all aspects of society has been the application of artificial intelligence (AI). In 2019 Eric Topol published the book titled *Deep Medicine: How Artificial Intelligence Can Make Healthcare Human Again*. He describes how AI is being applied in diagnostics such as in breast cancer, mental health through Chatbots, and in personalized diets.

AI is also having an influence on occupational therapy practice:

With Artificial Intelligence, assistive technology (AT) has become more popular for Occupational Therapists (OT) to support the elderly and disabled people thanks to increased flexibility, efficiency, and productivity. If these technologies and tools are not improving the activity performance and do not match the abilities and skills of the client, the OTs change or adapt them, as he or she will use them. Hence, these assistive technology devices and services are important for occupational therapy intervention for supporting individuals in improving their performance and increasing their participation in their activities. AT plays an important role in self-care, play, leisure, and productivity. AT aids a person who has functional limitations due to some pathology. Some challenges, which have been observed in Occupational Therapy interventions, are the decreased use of emerging technologies such as augmented/virtual reality or smartphones, robotics, and multidisciplinary intervention in children and adolescents. The embracing of AT by OT will be braced by affordability, positive client–therapist relationships, time, education/training, increased awareness, and usability features of the assisted technology. To accomplish this, however, Occupational Therapists are required to equip with time, training, and education necessary to offer their clients ATs that are client-centered, usable, and affordable. This SI will present the most effective, innovative approaches to develop and use the next generation assisting technologies and tools to assist occupational therapists and occupational therapy assistants for better wellbeing.

(Yu et al., 2023)

Another trend in preventing and intervening in medical conditions is the rise of self-regulation of health care through education and monitoring of bodily symptoms through public health education and internet sites such as:

- Heart.org – www.heart.org/en. Information on heart disease and ways to prevent disease. From the American Heart Association.
- Diabetes.org – www.diabetes.org. Information on diabetes and ways to prevent, manage, and treat the disease. From the American Diabetes Association.
- Familydoctor.org. General health information for families. Produced by the American Academy of Family Physicians.
- Healthfinder.gov. General health information. Produced by the US Department of Health and Human Services.
- HealthyChildren.org – www.healthychildren.org/English/Pages/default.aspx. From the American Academy of Pediatrics.
- CDC – www.cdc.gov. Health information for all ages. From the Centers for Disease Control and Prevention.
- NIH Senior Health – www.nia.nih.gov/health. Health information for older adults. From the National Institutes of Health.

Educating the public toward an understanding of the relationship between mind and body is an example of the Wellness movement. The trend toward self-regulation in health will lead to more responsibility for one's own well-being in preventing illness through activities such as exercise, stress management, diet, tai chi, yoga, arts and crafts, and music. Scientific research will continue to explore the effectiveness of these methods. A holistic approach to health care has also generated changes in medicine through the specialties of integrative medicine and lifestyle physicians.

Another trend in health care is the growth of specialized health professions. Up until 1920, the doctor and the nurse were the main health care providers. More than 100 health-related professions now exist. These new positions, such as cardiovascular technologist, respiratory therapist, nuclear medicine technologist, cancer immunologist, sanitarian, and public health educator, are the result of progress made in medical technology and the advancement of public health methods. New professions will continue to emerge from advanced technology. As research refines the diagnosis and treatment of illness, there will be a parallel growth in specialized health professions.

The medical practice of the future may well be dominated by machines that monitor physiological changes; control the heart rate; stimulate nerves, muscle, and skin; replace bodily organs; and, in general, receive and transmit information to and from the body (Schmidt et al., 2019).

These medical machines will be designed to adapt to the internal organism of the body. Computers connected to the machines will be programmed to interpret accurately the information received. This relationship is shown in Table 14–11.

Another trend in rehabilitation medicine is the merging of technology in assisting individuals with disabilities. For many years, professionals in rehabilitation have recognized the need to develop devices and apparati to help individuals with disabilities maximize their independence and functional activities. The growth of the fields of robotics, orthotics (braces and splints), self-help devices, prosthetics (design of artificial limbs), and assistive technology is a direct result of this vision. Methodological research in health care is an example of interdisciplinary cooperation between scientists. Biomedical engineering,

TABLE 14–11

COMPUTER APPLICATION IN DIAGNOSIS AND TREATMENT

BODILY PROCESS	MACHINE MONITORING	COMPUTER DIAGNOSIS
• Circulatory • Gastrointestinal • Neurophysiological • Genitourinary • Skeletal-muscular • Respiration	• ECG • EEG • Respirator • MRI • CT Scan	• Aids in health professionals in diagnosis and prescription of treatment

which emerged as a complex multidisciplinary field incorporating medicine, engineering, psychology, economics, computer technology, law, sociology, and the environmental sciences, has grown rapidly in the last 80 years. Rushmer (1972), a researcher at the Center for Bioengineering, University of Washington, Seattle, was one of the first to describe the interaction of these multidisciplines. Table 14–12 is adapted from his early work.

The Defense Advanced Research Projects Agency (DARPA) launched an initiative to develop technologically sophisticated upper extremity prosthetic devices. The goals were to develop a prosthetic device that

TABLE 14–12

THE CURRENT SCOPE OF BIOMÉDICAL ENGINEERING: POTENTIAL AREAS OF INTERACTION BETWEEN LIFE SCIENCES AND ENGINEERING

APPLIED BIOENGINEERING

TECHNOLOGICAL DEVELOPMENT	THERAPEUTIC TECHNIQUES	HEALTH CARE SYSTEM	ENVIRONMENTAL ENGINEERING
Research Tools	*Therapies and Services*	*Components*	*Focus Areas*
• Physical measure • chemical composition • microscopy • isotope	• ssistive Technology • Occupational therapy • Physical therapy • Radiation therapy • Respiratory treatments • Special education • Speech-language therapy • Surgical interventions	• rganization • Medical economics • Long-range planning	• Pollution • air • water • noise • solid waste • food • Human fertility • Population control
Clinical Interventions	*Monitoring*	*Methods and Improvements*	*Aerospace*
• audiology • cardiology • gastrointestinal • genito-urinal • musculoskeletal • neurology • respiratory	• intensive care • surgical, postoperative • coronary care • ward supervision	• support functions • service functions • nursing • facilities design • medical care • community care • independent living	• environment control • closed ecological systems • physiological adaptation
Diagnostic data	*Artificial organs*	*Operations research*	*Underwater compression effects*
• automation • chemistry • microbiology • pathology • multiphasic screening	• sensory aids • heart-lung machine • artificial kidneys • artificial extremities: (e.g., myoelectric prostheses and mechanical arms, legs)	• optimization of laboratories • support functions • personnel • processing • scheduling	• Heat conservation • Communication
Computer applications	*Transplants*	*Cost benefit analysis*	
• data processing • analysis • retrieval • diagnosis	• liver • heart • blood vessels • kidneys	• cost accounting • evaluation of results • beneficial economy	

Source: Adapted from *Medical Engineering: Projections for Health Care Delivery*, (p. 13), by R. F. Rushmer, 1972, New York: Academic Press. Copyright 1994 by Academic Press.

could mimic the functioning of a normal healthy upper extremity including having five dexterous fingers, an articulating wrist with "normal" motion including flexion, extension, abduction, adduction, supination, and pronation. The limb is required to have an elbow strong enough to lift weight, and a shoulder with range of motion to allow flexion above the head and internal rotation to reach behind the back. Additionally, the device is required to have a power source to last an entire day, be waterproof, have "normal" looking skin, and weigh no more than 8 pounds (Beard, 2008).

> The LUKE Arm system was originally developed for DARPA by DEKA Research and Development Corporation. The modular, battery-powered arm enables dexterous arm and hand movement through a simple, intuitive control system that allows users to move multiple joints simultaneously. Years of testing and optimization in collaboration with the Department of Veterans Affairs led to clearance by the US Food and Drug Administration in May 2014 and creation of a commercial-scale manufacturer, Mobius Bionics, in July 2016. In June 2017, the first two LUKE Arm systems were prescribed to veterans.
>
> (DARPA, 2023)

The merging of medicine with the social sciences to find solutions to the complex problems of mental illness, alcoholism, drug addiction, and criminology is inevitable. Interdisciplinary approaches to prevention and rehabilitation will result in the merging of the physical and social sciences. The study of the relationship between psychology and physiology and the immune system has led to the field of psychoneuroimmuniology. The relationship of poverty, alienation, malaise, and hopelessness (which are social variables) to the onset of disease, self-destruction, and social aggression have attracted the attention of health researchers who work closely with social scientists.

The controversy in the United States during the 1990s and 2000s regarding the creation of a national health care system was influenced by the health consumer's concern about being denied the right to choose a health plan. The rise of health maintenance organizations and managed care in the 1990s brought attention to the issue of quality health care.

The Health Care Reform Bill of 2010 was signed into law by President Obama March 23, 2010 (Meckler & Hitt, 2010). This bill provides many substantial changes to the health care system in the United States. In 2010, subsidies were made available to small businesses to help offset the cost of providing health insurance coverage for their employees. A notable change during 2010 was that insurance companies were barred from denying health insurance coverage for children with pre-existing illnesses.

Additionally, children were allowed to stay on their parent's health insurance until the age of 26 years.

- During 2011 a long-term care program initiative began where people who pay premiums into the long-term care program will become eligible for long-term care support payments if they require assistance in daily living.
- In 2014 "exchanges" were created where individuals without employer health care insurance as well as small businesses could shop for health care coverage. Another significant change for 2014 was that insurance companies were barred from denying health insurance coverage to anyone with pre-existing conditions; 2014 also marked the year when Medicaid expanded (with State approval) to all Americans with income up to 133% of the federal poverty level. Additionally, grants were offered to small businesses to provide health insurance coverage (Meckler & Hitt, 2010).

The COVID-19 pandemic of 2019–2022 changed the nature of medical and health care. Telehealth and computer networks replaced in-person visits and interactions with the physician and health care professional. At the same time elective surgery dramatically decreased while patients sheltered in place. How will medicine and the allied health professions adopt to this new reality?

Currently, health care is still dominated by a biomedical model in which prescriptive drugs are foremost in medical treatment. It is estimated that there are more than 20,000 prescription drugs approved for marketing (FDA, 2019). Furthermore, it is estimated that approximately 66% of adults in the United States take prescription drugs (HPI, 2019).

It is hoped that research will resolve the conflict between the biomedical model and a holistic approach to health care. A delicate balance between governmental intervention and respect for the sanctity and privacy of the individual must be maintained. The right of every individual to the very best health care should be among the most important priorities for every nation. In evaluating and treating clients, occupational therapy and the allied health professions should be guided by the application of evidence-based research.

14.10 Summary

The growth of the profession of occupational therapy is a direct outcome of the progressive history of medicine into the 21st century. The previous chapters in this book highlight the impact that research has had on increasing the scope of clinical practice and its effectiveness.

In 2021 The American Occupational Therapy Association adopted the following description of the occupational therapy profession that has evolved in the last 100 years which is in part a result of research influencing evidence-based practice:

Definition of Occupational Therapy Practice for the AOTA Model Practice Act The practice of occupational therapy means the therapeutic use of everyday life occupations with persons, groups, or populations (clients) to support occupational performance and participation. Occupational therapy practice includes clinical reasoning and professional judgment to evaluate, analyze, and diagnose occupational challenges (e.g., issues with client factors, performance patterns, and performance skills) and provide occupation-based interventions to address them. Occupational therapy services include habilitation, rehabilitation, and the promotion of physical and mental health and wellness for clients with all levels of ability related needs. These services are provided for clients who have or are at risk for developing an illness, injury, disease, disorder, condition, impairment, disability, activity limitation, or participation restriction. Through the provision of skilled services and engagement in everyday activities, occupational therapy promotes physical and mental health and well-being by supporting occupational performance in people with, or at risk of experiencing, a range of developmental, physical, and mental health disorders. The practice of occupational therapy includes the following components:

A. Evaluation of factors affecting activities of daily living (ADLs), instrumental activities of daily living (IADLs), health management, rest and sleep, education, work, play, leisure, and social participation, including:

1. Context (environmental and personal factors) and occupational and activity demands that affect performance

2. Performance patterns including habits, routines, roles, and rituals

3. Performance skills, including motor skills (e.g., moving oneself or moving and interacting with objects), process skills (e.g., actions related to selecting, interacting with, and using tangible task objects), and social interaction skills (e.g., using verbal and non-verbal skills to communicate)

4. Client factors, including body functions (e.g., neuromuscular, sensory, visual, mental, psychosocial, cognitive, pain factors), body structures (e.g., cardiovascular, digestive, nervous, integumentary, genitourinary systems; structures related to movement), values, beliefs, and spirituality.

B. Methods or approaches to identify and select interventions, such as

1. Establishment, remediation, or restoration of a skill or ability that has not yet developed, is impaired, or is in decline

2. Compensation, modification, or adaptation of occupations, activities, and contexts to improve or enhance performance

3. Maintenance of capabilities to prevent decline in performance in everyday life occupations

4. Health promotion and wellness to enable or enhance performance in everyday life activities and quality of life

5. Prevention of occurrence or emergence of barriers to performance and participation, including injury and disability prevention

C. Interventions and procedures to promote or enhance safety and performance in ADLs, IADLs, health management, rest and sleep, education, work, play, leisure, and social participation, for example:

1. Therapeutic use of occupations and activities

2. Training in self-care, self-management, health management (e.g., medication management, health routines), home management, community/work integration, school activities, and work performance

3. Identification, development, remediation, or compensation of physical, neuromusculoskeletal, sensory–perceptual, emotional regulation, visual, mental, and cognitive functions; pain tolerance and management; praxis; developmental skills; and behavioral skills

4. Education and training of persons, including family members, caregivers, groups, populations, and others

5. Care coordination, case management, and transition services

6. Consultative services to persons, groups, populations, programs, organizations, and communities

7. Virtual interventions (e.g., simulated, real-time, and near-time technologies, including telehealth and mobile technology)

8. Modification of contexts (environmental and personal factors in settings such as home, work, school, and community) and adaptation of processes, including the application of ergonomic principles

9. Assessment, design, fabrication, application, fitting, and training in seating and positioning, assistive technology, adaptive devices, and orthotic devices, and training in the use of prosthetic devices

10. Assessment, recommendation, and training in techniques to enhance functional mobility, including fitting and management of wheelchairs and other mobility devices

11. Exercises, including tasks and methods to increase motion, strength, and endurance for occupational participation

12. Remediation of and compensation for visual deficits, including low vision rehabilitation

13. Driver rehabilitation and community mobility

14. Management of feeding, eating, and swallowing to enable eating and feeding performance

15. Application of physical agent and mechanical modalities and use of a range of specific therapeutic procedures (e.g., wound care management; techniques to enhance sensory, motor, perceptual, and cognitive processing; manual therapy techniques) to enhance performance skills

16. Facilitating the occupational participation of persons, groups, or populations through modification of contexts (environmental and personal) and adaptation of processes

17. Efforts directed toward promoting occupational justice and empowering clients to seek and obtain resources to fully participate in their everyday life occupations

18. Group interventions (e.g., use of dynamics of group and social interaction to facilitate learning and skill acquisition across the life course).

Adopted as part of the Occupational Therapy Scope of Practice document by the Representative Assembly Coordinating Council (RACC) for the Representative Assembly, 2021. (AOTA, 2023)

Occupational therapy as a health care profession has expanded dramatically worldwide in the last 50 years. Research has been a driving force in this expansion and will continue to be the engine for demonstrating the effectiveness of the profession in improving the health of the world's population. Research does not exist in a vacuum. There is a strong historical background for research that has led to progress in medicine, rehabilitation, and habilitation. Many occupational therapists are part of the behavioral medicine and humanistic tradition that applies non-surgical and non-pharmaceutical methods in the pursuit of better health. Occupational therapists employing techniques such as sensory integration therapy, task-oriented training, creative arts, relaxation therapy, and orthosis application can use the research methods described to strengthen the published evidence base of their practice in the 21st century. It is the authors' intention that the effort to develop and evaluate rigorous research protocols can be useful in the establishment of a scientific foundation for occupational therapy.

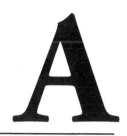

Commonly Used Abbreviations in Occupational Therapy

/d	per day	AT	assistive technology
a	of each	b.i.d.	twice a day
a.c.	before a meal	bal	balance
AAC	augmentative and alternative communication	BE	below elbow amputation
		bib.	drink
AAOx3	awake, alert, oriented to person, place	bilat	bilateral
AAROM	active assisted range of motion	BK	below knee amputation
ABI	acquired brain injury	BMI	body mass index
ACTH	adrenocorticotropic hormone	bol.	pill
ad lib.	freely	BP	blood pressure
ADA	Americans with Disabilities Act	BRP	bathroom privileges
ADD	attention deficit disorder	BSC	bedside commode
ADHD	attention-deficit hyperactivity disorder	c̄	with (usually written with a bar on top of the "c")
adm	admission		
admov.	apply	c/o	complains of
AFO	ankle foot orthosis	CA	cancer
AIDS	acquired immuno deficiency syndrome	CABG	coronary artery bypass graft
AK	above knee amputation	CBC	complete blood count
ALS	amyotrophic lateral sclerosis	Cc	cubic centimeters
alt.dieb	every other day	CHF	congestive heart failure
AMA	against medical advice	CMC	carpometacarpal joint
amb	ambulation or ambulate	CMV	cytomegalovirus
ap	before dinner	CNS	central nervous system
AROM	active range of motion	CP	cerebral palsy
as tol	as tolerated	CPR	cardio-pulmonary resuscitation
ASAP	as soon as possible	CRPS	complex regional pain syndrome

CSF	cerebrospinal fluid	ITP	Individualized Transition Plan
CT	computed tomography, also referred to as CAT (computer axial tomography)	IV	intravenous
		kg	kilogram
CTLSO	cervical thoracic lumbar sacral orthosis	KVO	keep vein open
CTS	carpal tunnel syndrome	lb	pound
CVA	cerebro vascular accident	LBP	low back pain
d	daily	LOB	loss of balance
D and C	dilatation and curettage	LOC	loss of consciousness
DIP	distal interphalangeal	LOS	length of stay
DM	diabetes mellitus	LP	lumbar puncture
DME	durable medical equipment	LTC	long-term care
DNR	do not resuscitate	MCA	middle cerebral artery
DO	Doctor of Osteopathic Medicine	MCP	metacarpophalangeal
DOB	date of birth	MD	muscular dystrophy
DOE	dyspnea on exertion	MED	minimum effective dose
DTR	deep tendon reflex	MET	metabolic equivalent
DUI	driving under the influence	MI	myocardial infarction
DV	domestic violence	MMR	measles-mumps-rubella vaccine
DVT	deep vein thrombosis	MP or MCP	metacarpophalangeal
Dx	diagnosis	MRI	magnetic resonance imaging
ECG	electrocardiogram	MRSA	methicillin resistant staphylococcum aureus
ED	emergency departure		
EEG	electroencephalogram	MS	multiple sclerosis
EMG	electromyogram	MVA	motor vehicle accident
EOB	edge of bed	MVR	mitral valve replacement
ER	emergency room	Nasogastric	a tube that leads from the nose or mouth into the stomach
FAE	fetal alcohol effects		
FAS	fetal alcohol syndrome	NG	nasogastric
FASD	fetal alcohol spectrum disorder	NICU	neonatal intensive care unit
FWB	full weight bearing	NKA	no known allergies
FWW	front wheeled walker	NP	nurse practitioner
fx	fracture	NPO	nothing by mouth; nothing to eat or drink usually within a defined time frame
GBS	Guillain-Barre syndrome		
GI	gastrointestinal		
H&P	history and physical	NSAID	non-steroidal anti-inflammatory drug
H/A	headache	NWB	non-weight bearing
H₂0	water	OA	osteoarthritis
Hct	hematocrit	OB/GYN	obstetrics and gynecology
Hgb	hemoglobin	OD	doctor of osteopathic medicine
HIV	human immunodeficiency virus	ODA	operating day admission
HR	heartrate	OOB	out of bed
HTN	hypertension	OR	operating room
Hx	history	ORIF	open reduction, internal fixation
ICU	intensive care unit	Ox3	oriented to person, place, time
IDEIA	Individuals with Disabilities Education Improvement Act of 2004 (Often referred to as IDEA-2004)	p	after
		p.c.	after meals
		p.o.	by mouth or orally
IEP	Individualized Education Plan	p.r.n.	as needed
IFSP	Individualized Family Service Plan	PA	physician's assistant
IM	intramuscular	PAC	premature atrial contraction
IP	interphalangeal	PDD	pervasive developmental disorder
IQ	intelligence quotient	PE	physical examination

per	by	**Rx**	prescription, treatment, or therapy
per os	by mouth	**S/P or s/p**	status post
PET	positron emission tomography	**SCI**	spinal cord injury
PICC Line	peripherally inserted central catheter for delivery of medication	**sine**	without
PIP	proximal interphalangeal	**SLP**	speech language pathologist
PROM	passive range of motion	**SNF**	skilled nursing facility
PTSD	post-traumatic stress disorder	**SOB**	shortness of breath
PVD	peripheral vascular disease	**STD**	sexually transmitted disease
PWB	partial weight bearing	**Strep**	streptococcus
q.h.	every hour	**Sx**	symptoms
q.i.d.	four times a day	**t.i.d.**	three times a day
q2h, q3h, …	every two hours, every three hours, etc.	**TBI**	traumatic brain injury
quotid	everyday	**THR or THA**	total hip replacement (arthroplasty)
R/O or r/o	rule out	**TIA**	transient ischemia attacks
R/R	respiratory rate	**TTWB**	toe-touch weight bearing
RA	rheumatoid arthritis	**USP**	United States Pharmacopoeia
RBC	red blood cells	**URI**	upper respiratory infection
RC	rotator cuff	**UTI**	urinary tract infection
REM	rapid eye movement	**VS**	vital signs
RESNA	Rehabilitation Engineering and Assistive Technology Society of North America	**VSD**	ventricular septal defect
ROM	range of motion	**w/**	with
RR	respiratory rate	**W/C**	wheelchair
RTW	return to work	**w/o**	without
		WB	weight bearing
		WBC	white blood cells
		WNL	within normal limits

B

Texas Woman's University Institutional Review Board (IRB)

GUIDE TO WRITING A CONSENT FORM

For studies that require written informed consent, these guidelines provide minimum standards for preparation of the written consent form. **When writing your consent document, make sure that all items on the consent form match the information provided to the IRB in the application form.**

REQUIRED ELEMENTS OF INFORMED CONSENT

1. The heading:

   TEXAS WOMAN'S UNIVERSITY
   CONSENT TO PARTICIPATE IN RESEARCH

2. The title of your study.

3. The names, degrees, TWU email addresses, and office phone numbers of the investigator(s) and faculty advisor (if investigator is a student). Note that the type of degree should be used as opposed to the prefix "Dr." and that the use of home phone numbers is not recommended.

4. A concise and focused presentation of <u>key information</u> that is organized and explained in a way that facilitates comprehension of the study.

   The purpose of this section is to assist a potential subject or legally authorized representative understand reasons why one might or might not want to participate in the research. Please note that the information presented in this section should be discussed in greater detail later in the consent form. Hence, it is important to keep this section brief and simple in language. The length of this section can vary from a paragraph to a maximum of one page depending upon the field/type of study. Possible key information includes, but is *not limited to,* a summary of the items below. Note that not all of these items may be key information for every study.

   - a statement that the study being conducted is for research (required),
   - the purpose of the research (required),
   - main study procedures or activities required of the subjects (required),
   - total time commitment,
   - major risks associated with participation in the study,
   - significant inclusion or exclusion criteria for participation,
   - setting of study,
   - benefits of the study, or
   - any other study-specific key information.

5. A description of the research study, which must include the following:

   - A description of the procedures to be used in the study, including details of the participant's involvement, and identification of any procedures that are experimental.
   - The total time commitment for the participant.
   - If audio or video recording will be used, an explanation of the purpose of the recording and who will have access to the recordings.

6. Potential risks

- A description of all potential risks to the participant and the steps that will be taken to minimize those risks.

  ➢ Include *loss of confidentiality* as a potential risk on the consent form as well as in the application since this can be a risk in every study involving human participants. Describe how the confidentiality of <u>identifiable private information</u> will be protected including where this information will be stored. If information will be destroyed as a protection of confidentiality, state how it will be destroyed and provide a timeframe such as "3 years from the end of the study." Note that if identifiable information will be kept indefinitely, this must be disclosed to the participant. The following statement must be included on all consent forms:

    Confidentiality will be protected to the extent that is allowed by law.

  ➢ If electronic transmission of information is used (i.e., email, internet, online meeting platforms, etc.), add the following statement:

    There is a potential risk of loss of confidentiality in all email, downloading, electronic meetings, and internet transactions.

7. Research collecting any <u>identifiable private information</u> and/or any <u>identifiable biospecimens</u> must inform the subjects in the study what will happen to their identifiable private information and/or biospecimens. Researchers must include the (1) or (2) below:

  (1) A statement that identifiers will be removed from the identifiable private information or identifiable biospecimens and that, after such removal, the information or biospecimens could be used for future research studies or distributed to another investigator for future research studies without additional informed consent from the subject or the legally authorized representative.

    If you would like to participate in the current study but not allow your de-identified data to be used for future research, please initial here_____

    _____.

  (2) A statement that the subject's information or biospecimens collected as part of the research, even if identifiers are removed, will not be used or distributed for future research studies.

8. TWU Disclaimer Statement (add verbatim)

  The researchers will try to prevent any problem that could happen because of this research. You should let the researchers know at once if there is a problem and they will help you. However, TWU does not provide medical services or financial

assistance for injuries that might happen because you are taking part in this research.

If using a Spanish consent form:

Los investigadores tratarán de prevenir cualquier problema que pudiera suceder a causa de este estudio de investigación. Usted deberá hacer del conocimiento de los investigadores tan pronto exista un problema, y ellos le ayudarán. Sin embargo, TWU no provee servicios médicos ni ayuda financiera para atender daños o heridas que pudieran suceder debido a su participación en este estudio.

9. A statement that participation is voluntary and participants may withdraw from the study at any time without penalty.

10. A description of any direct benefits or remuneration to the participant as a result of participation in the study. If there are no direct benefits, please state that there is none. If results will be available or provided to participants, include information on when and how the participant will be provided with results of the study, or how participants can ask for copies of the results.

11. Information for contacting TWU with questions

You will be given a copy of this signed and dated consent form to keep. If you have any questions about the research study you should ask the researchers; their contact information is at the top of this form. If you have questions about your rights as a participant in this research or the way this study has been conducted, you may contact the Texas Woman's University Office of Research and Sponsored Programs at 940-898-3378 or via e-mail at IRB@twu.edu.

If using a Spanish consent form:

Usted recibirá una copia firmada y fechada de esta forma de consentimiento. Si tuviera cualquier pregunta acerca de este estudio de investigación, favor de dirigir sus preguntas a los investigadores; sus números telefónicos se encuentran en la parte superior de esta forma. Si usted tuviera preguntas acerca de sus derechos como participante en este estudio o acerca de la forma en que este estudio se está llevando a cabo, puede ponerse en contacto con la Oficina de Investigación y de Proyectos Auspiciados por Fondos Externos de la Texas Woman's University al número 940-898-3378 o por correo electrónico a IRB@twu.edu

If obtaining consent online/electronically:

You may print a copy of this consent page to keep. If you have any questions about the research study you should ask the researcher; their contact information is at the top of this form. If you have questions about your rights as a participant in this research or the way this study has been conducted, you may contact the TWU Office of Research and Sponsored Programs at 940-898-3378 or via e-mail at IRB@twu.edu.

12. If the consent form is more than one page long, provide a line in the bottom right corner of each page except the signature page for the participant or parent/guardian to initial to indicate that they have read them. The pages of the consent form must be numbered using the following format: Page 1 of 3, Page 2 of 3, etc., under the line for participant initials.

13. Provide a signature line at the end of the consent form for the participant to sign and date the form. If the participant is a minor, provide a signature line for the parent/guardian to sign and date the form as well as an assent line for the minor if appropriate.

POTENTIAL ADDITIONAL ELEMENTS OF INFORMED CONSENT

When appropriate, the following elements(s) shall also be provided to each subject or the legally authorized representative:

1. A statement that the particular treatment or procedure may involve risks to the subject (or to the embryo or fetus, if the subject is or may become pregnant) that are currently unforeseeable;

2. Anticipated circumstances under which the subject's participation may be terminated by the investigator without regard to the subject's or the legally authorized representative's consent;

3. Any additional costs to the subject that may result from participation in the research;

4. The consequences of a subject's decision to withdraw from the research and procedures for orderly termination of participation by the subject;

5. A statement that significant new findings developed during the course of the research that may relate to the subject's willingness to continue participation will be provided to the subject;

6. The approximate number of subjects involved in the study;

7. A statement that the subject's biospecimens (even if identifiers are removed) may be used for commercial profit and whether the subject will or will not share in this commercial profit;

8. A statement regarding whether clinically relevant research results, including individual research results, will be disclosed to subjects, and if so, under what conditions; and

9. For research involving biospecimens, whether the research will (if known) or might include whole genome sequencing (i.e., sequencing of a human germline or somatic specimen with the intent to generate the genome or exome sequence of that specimen).

10. A section may be added at the end of the consent for the address where the results of the study may be sent.

Statistical Tables

TABLE C-1

RANDOM NUMBERS

427	8168	6022	1839	7551	7267	564	64	4222	1950
1885	7999	4901	722	5651	8026	4538	2708	7452	7185
5645	1859	5837	3022	7033	6079	9163	1294	4654	1751
7272	6252	8537	7784	4123	3723	7284	1009	7751	7957
6603	8698	9063	8612	7935	6835	4364	7568	171	359
1933	4688	8046	7018	5698	4972	4696	345	7031	3179
428	9076	7159	1140	8954	282	7156	3069	377	2840
5491	2932	7401	3914	9995	6403	9741	4253	5871	3239
7865	4053	6181	7053	9354	5612	4695	7449	3608	9309
1696	4956	3296	244	6718	5004	8328	1376	6646	420
6179	1046	3714	810	9147	2692	6401	6099	669	8070
4385	6107	2097	7800	9436	969	8948	215	7896	5162
3005	2849	1387	5231	9834	5303	6140	3450	4357	2246
1645	8446	6072	9321	6452	8687	6807	9294	9384	427
4352	5114	3458	557	4203	953	4706	9187	1881	4197
8097	6886	6117	3612	5835	6029	9914	2690	9935	4020
4319	9787	8537	442	5920	8919	6542	8858	3186	5251
534	422	2504	3190	5592	5344	9150	4082	869	6470
2699	234	82	924	9748	8198	8789	8730	7687	2632
8867	2771	1589	9630	5033	8720	9067	9478	8867	4530
2304	9779	9008	5321	5668	4491	7197	7064	9148	4923
888	6251	2110	506	9504	3517	2131	1564	2691	2627
2563	380	8805	6190	1595	7281	4167	5632	7715	2688
1786	3293	3752	7526	5646	6807	6694	9449	7124	5329
4712	3580	7627	4029	7676	7655	3567	1122	1874	3335
9882	9208	1618	5801	8704	7508	228	4341	5369	2478
8544	4571	7681	6847	2311	1801	1476	3521	8780	7339
6719	4638	8527	7588	551	6291	531	2090	1837	7324
8709	8569	9953	378	8475	905	9591	1728	9705	9611
8652	1830	505	9129	5314	4766	5920	2332	3008	4333

(continued)

TABLE C–1 (CONTINUED)

RANDOM NUMBERS

1595	143	5277	8354	9102	5071	8807	9340	9972	3130
8777	1096	7081	2112	712	8941	4650	742	9205	6917
8126	1021	1162	5014	8803	7157	8410	9875	7513	2531
4490	8445	9244	7937	1673	8441	7297	3349	5619	2608
5323	7144	5045	7122	4784	368	6908	7499	5399	4083
1107	5926	5966	2489	7955	5832	720	1504	932	8389
5241	2417	4227	4850	4047	4723	7251	9534	5538	253
1938	2683	4457	7591	7971	6626	4025	6117	8421	5663
9097	2967	6611	9832	5372	3222	833	5015	3778	5350
5499	4836	7250	5446	1007	1281	7239	6918	5068	3711

Source: The table was generated using Microsoft Office Excel 2013.

TABLE C–2

PROPORTION OF AREAS UNDER THE NORMAL CURVE (PERCENTILE RANK)

Z	0	0.01	0.02	0.03	0.04	0.05	0.06	0.07	0.08	0.09
0	.50000	.50399	.50798	.51197	.51595	.51994	.52392	.52790	.53188	.53586
0.1	.53983	.54380	.54776	.55172	.55567	.55962	.56356	.56749	.57142	.57535
0.2	.57926	.58317	.58706	.59095	.59483	.59871	.60257	.60642	.61026	.61409
0.3	.61791	.62172	.62552	.62930	.63307	.63683	.64058	.64431	.64803	.65173
0.4	.65542	.65910	.66276	.66640	.67003	.67364	.67724	.68082	.68439	.68793
0.5	.69146	.69497	.69847	.70194	.70540	.70884	.71226	.71566	.71904	.72240
0.6	.72575	.72907	.73237	.73565	.73891	.74215	.74537	.74857	.75175	.75490
0.7	.75804	.76115	.76424	.76730	.77035	.77337	.77637	.77935	.78230	.78524
0.8	.78814	.79103	.79389	.79673	.79955	.80234	.80511	.80785	.81057	.81327
0.9	.81594	.81859	.82121	.82381	.82639	.82894	.83147	.83398	.83646	.83891
1.0	.84134	.84375	.84614	.84849	.85083	.85314	.85543	.85769	.85993	.86214
1.1	.86433	.86650	.86864	.87076	.87286	.87493	.87698	.87900	.88100	.88298
1.2	.88493	.88686	.88877	.89065	.89251	.89435	.89617	.89796	.89973	.90147
1.3	.90320	.90490	.90658	.90824	.90988	.91149	.91309	.91466	.91621	.91774
1.4	.91924	.92073	.92220	.92364	.92507	.92647	.92785	.92922	.93056	.93189
1.5	.93319	.93448	.93574	.93699	.93822	.93943	.94062	.94179	.94295	.94408
1.6	.94520	.94630	.94738	.94845	.94950	.95053	.95154	.95254	.95352	.95449
1.7	.95543	.95637	.95728	.95818	.95907	.95994	.96080	.96164	.96246	.96327
1.8	.96407	.96485	.96562	.96638	.96712	.96784	.96856	.96926	.96995	.97062
1.9	.97128	.97193	.97257	.97320	.97381	.97441	.97500	.97558	.97615	.97670
2.0	.97725	.97778	.97831	.97882	.97932	.97982	.98030	.98077	.98124	.98169
2.1	.98214	.98257	.98300	.98341	.98382	.98422	.98461	.98500	.98537	.98574
2.2	.98610	.98645	.98679	.98713	.98745	.98778	.98809	.98840	.98870	.98899
2.3	.98928	.98956	.98983	.99010	.99036	.99061	.99086	.99111	.99134	.99158
2.4	.99180	.99202	.99224	.99245	.99266	.99286	.99305	.99324	.99343	.99361
2.5	.99379	.99396	.99413	.99430	.99446	.99461	.99477	.99492	.99506	.99520
2.6	.99534	.99547	.99560	.99573	.99585	.99598	.99609	.99621	.99632	.99643
2.7	.99653	.99664	.99674	.99683	.99693	.99702	.99711	.99720	.99728	.99736
2.8	.99744	.99752	.99760	.99767	.99774	.99781	.99788	.99795	.99801	.99807
2.9	.99813	.99819	.99825	.99831	.99836	.99841	.99846	.99851	.99856	.99861
3.0	.99865	.99869	.99874	.99878	.99882	.99886	.99889	.99893	.99896	.99900
3.1	.99903	.99906	.99910	.99913	.99916	.99918	.99921	.99924	.99926	.99929
3.2	.99931	.99934	.99936	.99938	.99940	.99942	.99944	.99946	.99948	.99950
3.3	.99952	.99953	.99955	.99957	.99958	.99960	.99961	.99962	.99964	.99965
3.4	.99966	.99968	.99969	.99970	.99971	.99972	.99973	.99974	.99975	.99976
3.5	.99977	.99978	.99978	.99979	.99980	.99981	.99981	.99982	.99983	.99983
3.6	.99984	.99985	.99985	.99986	.99986	.99987	.99987	.99988	.99988	.99989

(continued)

TABLE C–2 (CONTINUED)

PROPORTION OF AREAS UNDER THE NORMAL CURVE (PERCENTILE RANK)

Z	0	0.01	0.02	0.03	0.04	0.05	0.06	0.07	0.08	0.09
3.7	.99989	.99990	.99990	.99990	.99991	.99991	.99992	.99992	.99992	.99992
3.8	.99993	.99993	.99993	.99994	.99994	.99994	.99994	.99995	.99995	.99995
3.9	.99995	.99995	.99996	.99996	.99996	.99996	.99996	.99996	.99997	.99997
4.0	.99997	.99997	.99997	.99997	.99997	.99997	.99998	.99998	.99998	.99998
4.1	.99998	.99998	.99998	.99998	.99998	.99998	.99998	.99998	.99999	.99999
4.2	.99999	.99999	.99999	.99999	.99999	.99999	.99999	.99999	.99999	.99999
4.3	.99999	.99999	.99999	.99999	.99999	.99999	.99999	.99999	.99999	.99999
4.4	.99999	.99999	>.99999	>.99999	>.99999	>.99999	>.99999	>.99999	>.99999	>.99999

Note: z-score values are provided at two decimal places. For example, a z-score of 1.27 represents .89796 proportion of the normal curve or percentile rank.

Source: The table was generated using Microsoft Office Excel 2013.

TABLE C–3

CRITICAL VALUES FOR *T*-TEST

LEVEL OF SIGNIFICANCE FOR ONE-TAILED TEST

	0.1	0.05	0.025	0.01	0.005	0.0005

LEVEL OF SIGNIFICANCE FOR TWO-TAILED TEST

DF	0.2	0.1	0.05	0.02	0.01	0.001
1	3.0777	6.3138	12.7062	31.8205	63.6567	636.6192
2	1.8856	2.9200	4.3027	6.9646	9.9248	31.5991
3	1.6377	2.3534	3.1824	4.5407	5.8409	12.9240
4	1.5332	2.1318	2.7764	3.7469	4.6041	8.6103
5	1.4759	2.0150	2.5706	3.3649	4.0321	6.8688
6	1.4398	1.9432	2.4469	3.1427	3.7074	5.9588
7	1.4149	1.8946	2.3646	2.9980	3.4995	5.4079
8	1.3968	1.8595	2.3060	2.8965	3.3554	5.0413
9	1.3830	1.8331	2.2622	2.8214	3.2498	4.7809
10	1.3722	1.8125	2.2281	2.7638	3.1693	4.5869
11	1.3634	1.7959	2.2010	2.7181	3.1058	4.4370
12	1.3562	1.7823	2.1788	2.6810	3.0545	4.3178
13	1.3502	1.7709	2.1604	2.6503	3.0123	4.2208
14	1.3450	1.7613	2.1448	2.6245	2.9768	4.1405
15	1.3406	1.7531	2.1314	2.6025	2.9467	4.0728
16	1.3368	1.7459	2.1199	2.5835	2.9208	4.0150
17	1.3334	1.7396	2.1098	2.5669	2.8982	3.9651
18	1.3304	1.7341	2.1009	2.5524	2.8784	3.9216
19	1.3277	1.7291	2.0930	2.5395	2.8609	3.8834
20	1.3253	1.7247	2.0860	2.5280	2.8453	3.8495
21	1.3232	1.7207	2.0796	2.5176	2.8314	3.8193
22	1.3212	1.7171	2.0739	2.5083	2.8188	3.7921
23	1.3195	1.7139	2.0687	2.4999	2.8073	3.7676
24	1.3178	1.7109	2.0639	2.4922	2.7969	3.7454
25	1.3163	1.7081	2.0595	2.4851	2.7874	3.7251
26	1.3150	1.7056	2.0555	2.4786	2.7787	3.7066
27	1.3137	1.7033	2.0518	2.4727	2.7707	3.6896
28	1.3125	1.7011	2.0484	2.4671	2.7633	3.6739
29	1.3114	1.6991	2.0452	2.4620	2.7564	3.6594
30	1.3104	1.6973	2.0423	2.4573	2.7500	3.6460

(continued)

TABLE C–3 (CONTINUED)

CRITICAL VALUES FOR *T*-TEST

LEVEL OF SIGNIFICANCE FOR ONE-TAILED TEST

	0.1	0.05	0.025	0.01	0.005	0.0005

LEVEL OF SIGNIFICANCE FOR TWO-TAILED TEST

DF	0.2	0.1	0.05	0.02	0.01	0.001
31	1.3095	1.6955	2.0395	2.4528	2.7440	3.6335
32	1.3086	1.6939	2.0369	2.4487	2.7385	3.6218
33	1.3077	1.6924	2.0345	2.4448	2.7333	3.6109
34	1.3070	1.6909	2.0322	2.4411	2.7284	3.6007
35	1.3062	1.6896	2.0301	2.4377	2.7238	3.5911
36	1.3055	1.6883	2.0281	2.4345	2.7195	3.5821
37	1.3049	1.6871	2.0262	2.4314	2.7154	3.5737
38	1.3042	1.6860	2.0244	2.4286	2.7116	3.5657
39	1.3036	1.6849	2.0227	2.4258	2.7079	3.5581
40	1.3031	1.6839	2.0211	2.4233	2.7045	3.5510
41	1.3025	1.6829	2.0195	2.4208	2.7012	3.5442
42	1.3020	1.6820	2.0181	2.4185	2.6981	3.5377
43	1.3016	1.6811	2.0167	2.4163	2.6951	3.5316
44	1.3011	1.6802	2.0154	2.4141	2.6923	3.5258
45	1.3006	1.6794	2.0141	2.4121	2.6896	3.5203
46	1.3002	1.6787	2.0129	2.4102	2.6870	3.5150
47	1.2998	1.6779	2.0117	2.4083	2.6846	3.5099
48	1.2994	1.6772	2.0106	2.4066	2.6822	3.5051
49	1.2991	1.6766	2.0096	2.4049	2.6800	3.5004
50	1.2987	1.6759	2.0086	2.4033	2.6778	3.4960
51	1.2984	1.6753	2.0076	2.4017	2.6757	3.4918
52	1.2980	1.6747	2.0066	2.4002	2.6737	3.4877
53	1.2977	1.6741	2.0057	2.3988	2.6718	3.4838
54	1.2974	1.6736	2.0049	2.3974	2.6700	3.4800
55	1.2971	1.6730	2.0040	2.3961	2.6682	3.4764
56	1.2969	1.6725	2.0032	2.3948	2.6665	3.4729
57	1.2966	1.6720	2.0025	2.3936	2.6649	3.4696
58	1.2963	1.6716	2.0017	2.3924	2.6633	3.4663
59	1.2961	1.6711	2.0010	2.3912	2.6618	3.4632
60	1.2958	1.6706	2.0003	2.3901	2.6603	3.4602

(continued)

TABLE C–3 (CONTINUED)

CRITICAL VALUES FOR *t*-TEST

LEVEL OF SIGNIFICANCE FOR ONE-TAILED TEST

	0.1	0.05	0.025	0.01	0.005	0.0005

LEVEL OF SIGNIFICANCE FOR TWO-TAILED TEST

DF	0.2	0.1	0.05	0.02	0.01	0.001
61	1.2956	1.6702	1.9996	2.3890	2.6589	3.4573
62	1.2954	1.6698	1.9990	2.3880	2.6575	3.4545
63	1.2951	1.6694	1.9983	2.3870	2.6561	3.4518
64	1.2949	1.6690	1.9977	2.3860	2.6549	3.4491
65	1.2947	1.6686	1.9971	2.3851	2.6536	3.4466
66	1.2945	1.6683	1.9966	2.3842	2.6524	3.4441
67	1.2943	1.6679	1.9960	2.3833	2.6512	3.4417
68	1.2941	1.6676	1.9955	2.3824	2.6501	3.4394
69	1.2939	1.6672	1.9949	2.3816	2.6490	3.4372
70	1.2938	1.6669	1.9944	2.3808	2.6479	3.4350
71	1.2936	1.6666	1.9939	2.3800	2.6469	3.4329
72	1.2934	1.6663	1.9935	2.3793	2.6459	3.4308
73	1.2933	1.6660	1.9930	2.3785	2.6449	3.4289
74	1.2931	1.6657	1.9925	2.3778	2.6439	3.4269
75	1.2929	1.6654	1.9921	2.3771	2.6430	3.4250
76	1.2928	1.6652	1.9917	2.3764	2.6421	3.4232
77	1.2926	1.6649	1.9913	2.3758	2.6412	3.4214
78	1.2925	1.6646	1.9908	2.3751	2.6403	3.4197
79	1.2924	1.6644	1.9905	2.3745	2.6395	3.4180
80	1.2922	1.6641	1.9901	2.3739	2.6387	3.4163
81	1.2921	1.6639	1.9897	2.3733	2.6379	3.4147
82	1.2920	1.6636	1.9893	2.3727	2.6371	3.4132
83	1.2918	1.6634	1.9890	2.3721	2.6364	3.4116
84	1.2917	1.6632	1.9886	2.3716	2.6356	3.4102
85	1.2916	1.6630	1.9883	2.3710	2.6349	3.4087
86	1.2915	1.6628	1.9879	2.3705	2.6342	3.4073
87	1.2914	1.6626	1.9876	2.3700	2.6335	3.4059
88	1.2912	1.6624	1.9873	2.3695	2.6329	3.4045
89	1.2911	1.6622	1.9870	2.3690	2.6322	3.4032
90	1.2910	1.6620	1.9867	2.3685	2.6316	3.4019

(continued)

TABLE C–3 (CONTINUED)

CRITICAL VALUES FOR *T*-TEST

	LEVEL OF SIGNIFICANCE FOR ONE-TAILED TEST					
	0.1	*0.05*	*0.025*	*0.01*	*0.005*	*0.0005*
	LEVEL OF SIGNIFICANCE FOR TWO-TAILED TEST					
DF	*0.2*	*0.1*	*0.05*	*0.02*	*0.01*	*0.001*
91	1.2909	1.6618	1.9864	2.3680	2.6309	3.4007
92	1.2908	1.6616	1.9861	2.3676	2.6303	3.3994
93	1.2907	1.6614	1.9858	2.3671	2.6297	3.3982
94	1.2906	1.6612	1.9855	2.3667	2.6291	3.3971
95	1.2905	1.6611	1.9853	2.3662	2.6286	3.3959
96	1.2904	1.6609	1.9850	2.3658	2.6280	3.3948
97	1.2903	1.6607	1.9847	2.3654	2.6275	3.3937
98	1.2902	1.6606	1.9845	2.3650	2.6269	3.3926
99	1.2902	1.6604	1.9842	2.3646	2.6264	3.3915
100	1.2901	1.6602	1.9840	2.3642	2.6259	3.3905
101	1.2900	1.6601	1.9837	2.3638	2.6254	3.3895
102	1.2899	1.6599	1.9835	2.3635	2.6249	3.3885
103	1.2898	1.6598	1.9833	2.3631	2.6244	3.3875
104	1.2897	1.6596	1.9830	2.3627	2.6239	3.3865
105	1.2897	1.6595	1.9828	2.3624	2.6235	3.3856
106	1.2896	1.6594	1.9826	2.3620	2.6230	3.3847
107	1.2895	1.6592	1.9824	2.3617	2.6226	3.3838
108	1.2894	1.6591	1.9822	2.3614	2.6221	3.3829
109	1.2894	1.6590	1.9820	2.3610	2.6217	3.3820
110	1.2893	1.6588	1.9818	2.3607	2.6213	3.3812
111	1.2892	1.6587	1.9816	2.3604	2.6208	3.3803
112	1.2892	1.6586	1.9814	2.3601	2.6204	3.3795
113	1.2891	1.6585	1.9812	2.3598	2.6200	3.3787
114	1.2890	1.6583	1.9810	2.3595	2.6196	3.3779
115	1.2890	1.6582	1.9808	2.3592	2.6193	3.3771
116	1.2889	1.6581	1.9806	2.3589	2.6189	3.3764
117	1.2888	1.6580	1.9804	2.3586	2.6185	3.3756
118	1.2888	1.6579	1.9803	2.3584	2.6181	3.3749
119	1.2887	1.6578	1.9801	2.3581	2.6178	3.3742
120	1.2886	1.6577	1.9799	2.3578	2.6174	3.3735

(continued)

TABLE C–3 (CONTINUED)

CRITICAL VALUES FOR *T*-TEST

LEVEL OF SIGNIFICANCE FOR ONE-TAILED TEST

	0.1	0.05	0.025	0.01	0.005	0.0005

LEVEL OF SIGNIFICANCE FOR TWO-TAILED TEST

DF	0.2	0.1	0.05	0.02	0.01	0.001
121	1.2886	1.6575	1.9798	2.3576	2.6171	3.3728
122	1.2885	1.6574	1.9796	2.3573	2.6167	3.3721
123	1.2885	1.6573	1.9794	2.3570	2.6164	3.3714
124	1.2884	1.6572	1.9793	2.3568	2.6161	3.3707
125	1.2884	1.6571	1.9791	2.3565	2.6157	3.3701
126	1.2883	1.6570	1.9790	2.3563	2.6154	3.3694
127	1.2883	1.6569	1.9788	2.3561	2.6151	3.3688
128	1.2882	1.6568	1.9787	2.3558	2.6148	3.3682
129	1.2881	1.6568	1.9785	2.3556	2.6145	3.3675
130	1.2881	1.6567	1.9784	2.3554	2.6142	3.3669
131	1.2880	1.6566	1.9782	2.3552	2.6139	3.3663
132	1.2880	1.6565	1.9781	2.3549	2.6136	3.3658
133	1.2879	1.6564	1.9780	2.3547	2.6133	3.3652
134	1.2879	1.6563	1.9778	2.3545	2.6130	3.3646
135	1.2879	1.6562	1.9777	2.3543	2.6127	3.3641
136	1.2878	1.6561	1.9776	2.3541	2.6125	3.3635
137	1.2878	1.6561	1.9774	2.3539	2.6122	3.3630
138	1.2877	1.6560	1.9773	2.3537	2.6119	3.3624
139	1.2877	1.6559	1.9772	2.3535	2.6117	3.3619
140	1.2876	1.6558	1.9771	2.3533	2.6114	3.3614
141	1.2876	1.6557	1.9769	2.3531	2.6111	3.3609
142	1.2875	1.6557	1.9768	2.3529	2.6109	3.3604
143	1.2875	1.6556	1.9767	2.3527	2.6106	3.3599

(continued)

TABLE C–3 (CONTINUED)

CRITICAL VALUES FOR *T*-TEST

LEVEL OF SIGNIFICANCE FOR ONE-TAILED TEST

	0.1	0.05	0.025	0.01	0.005	0.0005

LEVEL OF SIGNIFICANCE FOR TWO-TAILED TEST

DF	0.2	0.1	0.05	0.02	0.01	0.001
144	1.2875	1.6555	1.9766	2.3525	2.6104	3.3594
145	1.2874	1.6554	1.9765	2.3523	2.6102	3.3589
146	1.2874	1.6554	1.9763	2.3522	2.6099	3.3584
147	1.2873	1.6553	1.9762	2.3520	2.6097	3.3579
148	1.2873	1.6552	1.9761	2.3518	2.6095	3.3575
149	1.2873	1.6551	1.9760	2.3516	2.6092	3.3570
150	1.2872	1.6551	1.9759	2.3515	2.6090	3.3566

STEPS IN DETERMINING CRITICAL VALUES FOR T FOR TABLE C–3.

1. Calculate the degrees of freedom (*df*):
   - In one-sample *t*-test it is number of cases of the sample minus 1
   - In paired-data of correlated *t*-test it is number of pairs minus 1
   - In independent *t*-test it is number of cases in $N_1 + N_2$ minus 2
2. Determine if hypothesis is one-tailed or two-tailed test.
3. Establish level of significance (.05 or.01)
4. Locate *t* critical (crit) value:

   e.g., 10 *df*, two-tailed test, .05 level
   t_{crit} = 2.2281

5. Note that these critical values are the same for negative or positive numbers.
6. Calculate *t* observed (obs) using an appropriate *t*-test formula (e.g., one-sample, paired, or independent *t*-test).
7. Decision rule:
   - If t_{obs} is equal to or above t_{crit} then reject the null hypothesis.
   - If t_{obs} is below t_{crit} then accept the null hypothesis.

Source: The table was generated using Microsoft Office Excel 2013.

TABLE C–4

CRITICAL VALUES FOR F (ANALYSIS OF VARIANCE, ANOVA)

DENOMINATOR df	A	NUMERATOR df 1	2	3	4	5	6	7	8	9	10
1	0.01	4052	4999	5403	5625	5764	5859	5928	5981	6022	6056
	0.05	161.4	199.5	215.7	224.6	230.2	234.0	236.8	238.9	240.5	241.9
2	0.01	98.50	99.00	99.17	99.25	99.30	99.33	99.36	99.37	99.39	99.40
	0.05	18.513	19.000	19.164	19.247	19.296	19.330	19.353	19.371	19.385	19.396
3	0.01	34.116	30.817	29.457	28.710	28.237	27.911	27.672	27.489	27.345	27.229
	0.05	10.1280	9.5521	9.2766	9.1172	9.0135	8.9406	8.8867	8.8452	8.8123	8.7855
4	0.01	21.198	18.000	16.694	15.977	15.522	15.207	14.976	14.799	14.659	14.546
	0.05	7.7086	6.9443	6.5914	6.3882	6.2561	6.1631	6.0942	6.0410	5.9988	5.9644
5	0.01	16.258	13.274	12.060	11.392	10.967	10.672	10.456	10.289	10.158	10.051
	0.05	6.6079	5.7861	5.4095	5.1922	5.0503	4.9503	4.8759	4.8183	4.7725	4.7351
6	0.01	13.7450	10.9248	9.7795	9.1483	8.7459	8.4661	8.2600	8.1017	7.9761	7.8741
	0.05	5.9874	5.1433	4.7571	4.5337	4.3874	4.2839	4.2067	4.1468	4.0990	4.0600
7	0.01	12.2464	9.5466	8.4513	7.8466	7.4604	7.1914	6.9928	6.8400	6.7188	6.6201
	0.05	5.5914	4.7374	4.3468	4.1203	3.9715	3.8660	3.7870	3.7257	3.6767	3.6365
8	0.01	11.2586	8.6491	7.5910	7.0061	6.6318	6.3707	6.1776	6.0289	5.9106	5.8143
	0.05	5.3177	4.4590	4.0662	3.8379	3.6875	3.5806	3.5005	3.4381	3.3881	3.3472
9	0.01	10.5614	8.0215	6.9919	6.4221	6.0569	5.8018	5.6129	5.4671	5.3511	5.2565
	0.05	5.1174	4.2565	3.8625	3.6331	3.4817	3.3738	3.2927	3.2296	3.1789	3.1373
10	0.01	10.0443	7.5594	6.5523	5.9943	5.6363	5.3858	5.2001	5.0567	4.9424	4.8491
	0.05	4.9646	4.1028	3.7083	3.4780	3.3258	3.2172	3.1355	3.0717	3.0204	2.9782
11	0.01	9.6460	7.2057	6.2167	5.6683	5.3160	5.0692	4.8861	4.7445	4.6315	4.5393
	0.05	4.8443	3.9823	3.5874	3.3567	3.2039	3.0946	3.0123	2.9480	2.8962	2.8536
12	0.01	9.3302	6.9266	5.9525	5.4120	5.0643	4.8206	4.6395	4.4994	4.3375	4.2961
	0.05	4.7472	3.8853	3.4903	3.2592	3.1059	2.9961	2.9134	2.8486	2.7964	2.7534

13	0.01	9.0738	6.7010	5.7394	5.2053	4.8616	4.6204	4.4410	4.3021	4.1911	4.1003
	0.05	4.6672	3.8056	3.4105	3.1791	3.0254	2.9153	2.8321	2.7669	2.7144	2.6710
14	0.01	8.8616	6.5149	5.5639	5.0354	4.6950	4.4558	4.2779	4.1399	4.0297	3.9394
	0.05	4.6001	3.7389	3.3439	3.1122	2.9582	2.8477	2.7642	2.6987	2.6458	2.6022
15	0.01	8.6831	6.3589	5.4170	4.8932	4.5556	4.3183	4.1415	4.0045	3.8948	3.8049
	0.05	4.5431	3.6823	3.2874	3.0556	2.9013	2.7905	2.7066	2.6408	2.5876	2.5437
16	0.01	8.5310	6.2262	5.2922	4.7726	4.4374	4.2016	4.0259	3.8896	3.7804	3.6909
	0.05	4.4940	3.6337	3.2389	3.0069	2.8524	2.7413	2.6572	2.5911	2.5377	2.4935
17	0.01	8.3997	6.1121	5.1850	4.6690	4.3359	4.1015	3.9267	3.7910	3.6822	3.5931
	0.05	4.4513	3.5915	3.1968	2.9647	2.8100	2.6987	2.6143	2.5480	2.4943	2.4499
18	0.01	8.2854	6.0129	5.0919	4.5790	4.2479	4.0146	3.8406	3.7054	3.5971	3.5082
	0.05	4.4139	3.5546	3.1599	2.9277	2.7729	2.6613	2.5767	2.5102	2.4563	2.4117
19	0.01	8.1849	5.9259	5.0103	4.5003	4.1708	3.9386	3.7653	3.6305	3.5225	3.4338
	0.05	4.3807	3.5219	3.1274	2.8951	2.7401	2.6283	2.5435	2.4768	2.4227	2.3779
20	0.01	8.0960	5.8489	4.9382	4.4307	4.1027	3.8714	3.6987	3.5644	3.4567	3.3682
	0.05	4.3512	3.4928	3.0984	2.8661	2.7109	2.5990	2.5140	2.4471	2.3928	2.3479
21	0.01	8.0166	5.7804	4.8740	4.3688	4.0421	3.8117	3.6396	3.5056	3.3981	3.3098
	0.05	4.3248	3.4668	3.0725	2.8401	2.6848	2.5727	2.4876	2.4205	2.3660	2.3210
22	0.01	7.9454	5.7190	4.8166	4.3134	3.9880	3.7583	3.5867	3.4530	3.3458	3.2576
	0.05	4.3009	3.4434	3.0491	2.8167	2.6613	2.5491	2.4638	2.3965	2.3419	2.2967
23	0.01	7.8811	5.6637	4.7649	4.2636	3.9392	3.7102	3.5390	3.4057	3.2986	3.2106
	0.05	4.2793	3.4221	3.0280	2.7955	2.6400	2.5277	2.4422	2.3748	2.3201	2.2747
24	0.01	7.8229	5.6136	4.7181	4.2184	3.8951	3.6667	3.4959	3.3629	3.2560	3.1681
	0.05	4.2597	3.4028	3.0088	2.7763	2.6207	2.5082	2.4226	2.3551	2.3002	2.2547
25	0.01	7.7698	5.5680	4.6755	4.1774	3.8550	3.6272	3.4568	3.3239	3.2172	3.1294
	0.05	4.2417	3.3852	2.9912	2.7587	2.6030	2.4904	2.4047	2.3371	2.2821	2.2365
26	0.01	7.7213	5.5263	4.6366	4.1400	3.8183	3.5911	3.4210	3.2884	3.1818	3.0941
	0.05	4.2252	3.3690	2.9752	2.7426	2.5868	2.4741	2.3883	2.3205	2.2655	2.2197

(continued)

Table C-4 (Continued)
Critical Values for F (Analysis of Variance, ANOVA)

DENOMINATOR df	A	NUMERATOR df									
		1	2	3	4	5	6	7	8	9	10
27	0.01	7.6767	5.4881	4.6009	4.1056	3.7848	3.5580	3.3882	3.2558	3.1494	3.0618
	0.05	4.2100	3.3541	2.9604	2.7278	2.5719	2.4591	2.3732	2.3053	2.2501	2.2043
28	0.01	7.6356	5.4529	4.5681	4.0740	3.7539	3.5276	3.3581	3.2259	3.1195	3.0320
	0.05	4.1960	3.3404	2.9467	2.7141	2.5581	2.4453	2.3593	2.2913	2.2360	2.1900
29	0.01	7.5977	5.4204	4.5378	4.0449	3.7254	3.4995	3.3303	3.1982	3.0920	3.0045
	0.05	4.1830	3.3277	2.9340	2.7014	2.5454	2.4324	2.3463	2.2783	2.2229	2.1768
30	0.01	7.5625	5.3903	4.5097	4.0179	3.6990	3.4735	3.3045	3.1726	3.0665	2.9791
	0.05	4.1709	3.3158	2.9223	2.6896	2.5336	2.4205	2.3343	2.2662	2.2107	2.1646
35	0.01	7.4191	5.2679	4.3957	3.9082	3.5919	3.3679	3.2000	3.0687	2.9630	2.8758
	0.05	4.1213	3.2674	2.8742	2.6415	2.4851	2.3718	2.2852	2.2167	2.1608	2.1143
40	0.01	7.3141	5.1785	4.3126	3.8283	3.5138	3.2910	3.1238	2.9930	2.8876	2.8005
	0.05	4.0847	3.2317	2.8387	2.6060	2.4495	2.3359	2.2490	2.1802	2.1240	2.0772
45	0.01	7.2339	5.1103	4.2492	3.7674	3.4544	3.2325	3.0658	2.9353	2.8301	2.7432
	0.05	4.0566	3.2043	2.8115	2.5787	2.4221	2.3083	2.2212	2.1521	2.0958	2.0487
50	0.01	7.1706	5.0566	4.1993	3.7195	3.4077	3.1864	3.0202	2.8900	2.7850	2.6981
	0.05	4.0343	3.1826	2.7900	2.5572	2.4004	2.2864	2.1992	2.1299	2.0734	2.0261
55	0.01	7.1194	5.0132	4.1591	3.6809	3.3700	3.1493	2.9834	2.8534	2.7485	2.6617
	0.05	4.0162	3.1650	2.7725	2.5397	2.3828	2.2687	2.1813	2.1119	2.0552	2.0078
60	0.01	7.0771	4.9774	4.1259	3.6490	3.3389	3.1187	2.9530	2.8233	2.7185	2.6318
	0.05	4.0012	3.1504	2.7581	2.5252	2.3683	2.2541	2.1665	2.0970	2.0401	1.9926

80	0.01	6.9627	4.8807	4.0363	3.5631	3.2550	3.0361	2.8713	2.7420	2.6374	2.5508
	0.05	3.9604	3.1108	2.7188	2.4859	2.3287	2.2142	2.1263	2.0564	1.9991	1.9512
100	0.01	6.8953	4.8239	3.9837	3.5127	3.2059	2.9877	2.8233	2.6943	2.5898	2.5033
	0.05	3.9361	3.0873	2.6955	2.4626	2.3053	2.1906	2.1025	2.0323	1.9748	1.9267
120	0.01	6.8509	4.7865	3.9491	3.4795	3.1735	2.9559	2.7918	2.6629	2.5586	2.4721
	0.05	3.9201	3.0718	2.6802	2.4472	2.2899	2.1750	2.0868	2.0164	1.9588	1.9105

STEPS IN DETERMINING CRITICAL VALUES FOR F FOR TABLE C–4.

1. Calculate the degrees of freedom (df) for numerator and denominator:
   - The df for numerator is derived from the number of groups in the study minus 1. For example, if three treatment methods are being compared, then df equals 3 minus 1, or 2 df for numerator.
   - The df for denominator is derived from the total number of subjects in all groups being compared minus the number of groups. For example for three treatment methods with 6 subjects in each group the df for the denominator will equal 18 minus 3, or 15 df.
2. Apply the level of significance, such as .05 or .01.
3. Locate critical value of F.
4. e.g., df equals 2 / 15 at .05 level then F_{crit} = 6.3589.
5. Calculate F_{obs} for data.
6. Decision rule:
   - If F_{obs} is equal to or above F_{crit} then reject the null hypothesis.
   - If F_{obs} is below F_{crit} accept the null hypothesis.

Source: The table was generated using Microsoft Office Excel 2013.

TABLE C–5

CRITICAL VALUES FOR THE PEARSON PRODUCT-MOMENT CORRELATION COEFFICIENT (R)

LEVEL OF SIGNIFICANCE FOR ONE-TAILED TEST

	0.1	0.05	0.025	0.01	0.005	0.0005
	LEVEL OF SIGNIFICANCE FOR TWO-TAILED TEST					
DF	0.2	0.1	0.05	0.02	0.01	0.001
1	0.951057	0.987688	0.996917	0.999507	0.999877	0.999999
2	0.8	0.9	0.95	0.98	0.99	0.999
3	0.687049	0.805384	0.878339	0.934333	0.958735	0.991139
4	0.6084	0.729299	0.811401	0.882194	0.9172	0.974068
5	0.550863	0.669439	0.754492	0.832874	0.874526	0.950883
6	0.506727	0.621489	0.706734	0.78872	0.834342	0.924904
7	0.471589	0.582206	0.666384	0.749776	0.797681	0.89826
8	0.442796	0.549357	0.631897	0.715459	0.764592	0.872115
9	0.418662	0.521404	0.602069	0.685095	0.734786	0.847047
10	0.398062	0.497265	0.575983	0.65807	0.707888	0.823305
11	0.380216	0.476156	0.552943	0.633863	0.683528	0.800962
12	0.364562	0.4575	0.532413	0.612047	0.661376	0.779998
13	0.350688	0.440861	0.513977	0.59227	0.641145	0.760351
14	0.338282	0.425902	0.497309	0.574245	0.622591	0.741934
15	0.327101	0.41236	0.482146	0.557737	0.605506	0.724657
16	0.316958	0.400027	0.468277	0.542548	0.589714	0.708429
17	0.307702	0.388733	0.455531	0.528517	0.575067	0.693163
18	0.29921	0.378341	0.443763	0.515505	0.561435	0.678781
19	0.291384	0.368737	0.432858	0.503397	0.548711	0.665208
20	0.28414	0.359827	0.422714	0.492094	0.5368	0.652378
21	0.277411	0.351531	0.413247	0.481512	0.52562	0.64023
22	0.271137	0.343783	0.404386	0.471579	0.515101	0.62871
23	0.26527	0.336524	0.39607	0.462231	0.505182	0.617768
24	0.259768	0.329705	0.388244	0.453413	0.495808	0.60736
25	0.254594	0.323283	0.380863	0.445078	0.486932	0.597446
26	0.249717	0.317223	0.373886	0.437184	0.478511	0.587988
27	0.24511	0.31149	0.367278	0.429693	0.470509	0.578956
28	0.240749	0.306057	0.361007	0.422572	0.462892	0.570317
29	0.236612	0.300898	0.355046	0.415792	0.455631	0.562047
30	0.232681	0.295991	0.34937	0.409327	0.448699	0.554119

(continued)

| TABLE C–5 (CONTINUED) |

CRITICAL VALUES FOR THE PEARSON PRODUCT-MOMENT CORRELATION COEFFICIENT (*R*)

	LEVEL OF SIGNIFICANCE FOR ONE-TAILED TEST					
	0.1	*0.05*	*0.025*	*0.01*	*0.005*	*0.0005*
	LEVEL OF SIGNIFICANCE FOR TWO-TAILED TEST					
DF	*0.2*	*0.1*	*0.05*	*0.02*	*0.01*	*0.001*
35	0.215598	0.274611	0.324573	0.380976	0.418211	0.518898
40	0.201796	0.257278	0.304396	0.357787	0.393174	0.48957
45	0.190345	0.242859	0.287563	0.338367	0.372142	0.464673
50	0.180644	0.23062	0.273243	0.321796	0.354153	0.443201
60	0.164997	0.210832	0.250035	0.294846	0.324818	0.407865
65	0.158558	0.202673	0.240447	0.283682	0.31264	0.393085
70	0.152818	0.195394	0.231883	0.273695	0.301734	0.379799
75	0.147659	0.188847	0.224174	0.264694	0.291895	0.367771
80	0.14299	0.182916	0.217185	0.256525	0.282958	0.356816
85	0.138738	0.177511	0.210811	0.249069	0.274794	0.346782
90	0.134844	0.172558	0.204968	0.242227	0.267298	0.337549
95	0.13126	0.167998	0.199584	0.235919	0.260383	0.329014
100	0.127947	0.163782	0.194604	0.230079	0.253979	0.321095

STEPS IN DETERMINING CRITICAL VALUES FOR PEARSON R FOR TABLE C–5.

1. Determine the number of variables being correlated. For example if $x = 20$ and $y = 20$, then $n = 20$.
2. Determine if hypothesis calls for a one-tailed or two-tailed test. Usually a null hypothesis indicates a one-tailed test and a directional hypothesis indicates a two-tailed test of significance.
3. Apply level of significance, for example, .05 or .01.
4. Locate critical value of *r* from statistical table. For example, with $n = 20$, two-tailed test, .05 level, then $r_{crit} = .4438$ $df = 18$.
5. Calculate r_{ohs} from data.
6. Decision Rule:
   ○ If r_{obs} is equal to or greater then r_{crit}, then reject null hypothesis.
   ○ If r_{obs} is below r_{crit} then accept null hypothesis.

Source: The table was generated using Microsoft Office Excel 2013.

TABLE C–6

SPEARMAN RANK ORDER CORRELATION COEFFICIENT (r)

LEVEL OF SIGNIFICANCE FOR ONE-TAILED TEST

	.05	.025	.01	.005

LEVEL OF SIGNIFICANCE FOR TWO-TAILED TEST

N*	.10	.05	.02	.01
5	.900	1.000	1.000	—
6	.829	.886	.943	1.000
7	.714	.786	.893	.929
8	.643	.738	.833	.881
9	.600	.683	.783	.833
10	.564	.648	.746	.794
12	.506	.591	.712	.777
14	.456	.544	.645	.715
16	.425	.506	.601	.665
18	.399	.475	.564	.625
20	.377	.450	.534	.591
22	.359	.428	.508	.562
24	.343	.409	.485	.537
26	.329	.392	.465	.515
28	.317	.377	.448	.496
30	.306	.364	.432	.478

STEPS IN DETERMINING CRITICAL VALUES FOR SPEARMAN R_S (FORMERLY RHO) FOR TABLE C–6.

1. Determine the number of pairs of variables being correlated.
2. Determine if hypothesis calls for a one-tailed or two-tailed test.
3. Apply level of significance, .05 or.01.
4. Locate critical value of r_S from statistical table. For example, with $n = 12$, two-tailed test, .05 level, then $r_{S\text{-critl}} = .591$.
5. Calculate $r_{S\text{-obs}}$ from data.
6. Decision Rule:
   ○ If $r_{S\text{-obs}}$ is equal to or greater then $r_{S\text{-crit}}$, then reject the null hypothesis.
   ○ If $r_{S\text{-obs}}$ is below $r_{S\text{-crit}}$ then accept the null hypothesis.

*n = number of pairs

Source: Adapted from Olds (1938, 1949) and Runyon and Haber (1967). Reprinted with permission of the publishers.

TABLE C–7A

CRITICAL VALUES FOR THE MANN-WHITNEY *U* TEST* (ONE-TAILED TEST AT .025 OR A TWO-TAILED TEST AT .05)

NA

NB	1	2	3	4	5	6	7	8	9	10	11	12	13	14	15	16	17	18	19	20	21	22	23	24	25
1																									
1																									
2								16	18	20	22	23	25	27	29	31	32	34	36	38	39	41	43	45	47
2								0	0	0	0	1	1	1	1	1	2	2	2	2	3	3	3	3	3
3					15	17	20	22	25	27	30	32	35	37	40	42	45	47	50	52	55	57	60	62	65
3					0	1	1	2	2	3	3	4	4	5	5	6	6	7	7	8	8	9	9	10	10
4				16	19	22	25	28	32	35	38	41	44	47	50	53	57	60	63	66	69	72	75	79	82
4				0	1	2	3	4	4	5	6	7	8	9	10	11	11	12	13	14	15	16	17	17	18
5			15	19	23	27	30	34	38	42	46	49	53	57	61	65	68	72	76	80	83	87	91	95	98
5			0	1	2	3	5	6	7	8	9	11	12	13	14	15	17	18	19	20	22	23	24	25	27
6			17	22	27	31	36	40	44	49	53	58	62	67	71	75	80	84	89	93	97	102	106	111	115
6			1	2	3	5	6	8	10	11	13	14	16	17	19	21	22	24	25	27	29	30	32	33	35
7			20	25	30	36	41	46	51	56	61	66	71	76	81	86	91	96	101	106	111	116	121	126	131
7			1	3	5	6	8	10	12	14	16	18	20	22	24	26	28	30	32	34	36	38	40	42	44
8		16	22	28	34	40	46	51	57	63	69	74	80	86	91	97	102	108	114	119	125	131	136	142	147
8		0	2	4	6	8	10	13	15	17	19	22	24	26	29	31	34	36	38	41	43	45	48	50	53
9		18	25	32	38	44	51	57	64	70	76	82	89	95	101	107	114	120	126	132	139	145	151	157	163
9		0	2	4	7	10	12	15	17	20	23	26	28	31	34	37	39	42	45	48	50	53	56	59	62
10		20	27	35	42	49	56	63	70	77	84	91	97	104	111	118	125	132	138	145	152	159	166	173	179
10		0	3	5	8	11	14	17	20	23	26	29	33	36	39	42	45	48	52	55	58	61	64	67	71

(continued)

TABLE C–7A (CONTINUED)

CRITICAL VALUES FOR THE MANN-WHITNEY U TEST* (ONE-TAILED TEST AT .025 OR A TWO-TAILED TEST AT .05)

NB											NA														
	1	2	3	4	5	6	7	8	9	10	11	12	13	14	15	16	17	18	19	20	21	22	23	24	25
11		0	3	6	9	13	16	19	23	26	30	33	37	40	44	47	51	55	58	62	65	69	73	76	80
11			22	38	46	53	61	69	76	84	91	99	106	114	121	129	136	143	151	158	166	173	180	188	195
12		1	4	7	11	14	18	22	26	29	33	37	41	45	49	53	57	61	65	69	73	77	81	85	89
12			23	41	49	58	66	74	82	91	99	107	115	123	131	139	147	155	163	171	179	187	195	203	211
13		1	4	8	12	16	20	24	28	33	37	41	45	50	54	59	63	67	72	76	80	85	89	94	98
13			25	44	53	62	71	80	89	97	106	115	124	132	141	149	158	167	175	184	193	201	210	218	227
14		1	5	9	13	17	22	26	31	36	40	45	50	55	59	64	69	74	78	83	88	93	98	102	107
14			27	47	57	67	76	86	95	104	114	123	132	141	151	160	169	178	188	197	206	215	224	234	243
15		1	5	10	14	19	24	29	34	39	44	49	54	59	64	70	75	80	85	90	96	101	106	111	117
15			29	50	61	71	81	91	101	111	121	131	141	151	161	170	180	190	200	210	219	229	239	249	258
16		1	6	11	15	21	26	31	37	42	47	53	59	64	70	75	81	86	92	98	103	109	115	120	126
16			31	53	65	75	86	97	107	118	129	139	149	160	170	181	191	202	212	222	233	243	253	264	274
17		2	6	11	17	22	28	34	39	45	51	57	63	69	75	81	87	93	99	105	111	117	123	129	135
17			32	57	68	80	91	102	114	125	136	147	158	169	180	191	202	213	224	235	246	257	268	279	290
18		2	7	12	18	24	30	36	42	48	55	61	67	74	80	86	93	99	106	112	119	125	132	138	145
18			34	60	72	84	96	108	120	132	143	155	167	178	190	202	213	225	236	248	259	271	282	294	305

n_A	2	3	4	5	6	7	8	9	10	11	12	13	14	15	16	17	18	19	20	21	22	23	24	25
19	2	7	13	19	25	32	38	45	52	58	65	72	78	85	92	99	106	113	119	126	133	140	147	154
19	36	50	63	76	89	101	114	126	138	151	163	175	188	200	212	224	236	248	261	273	285	297	309	321
20	2	8	14	20	27	34	41	48	55	62	69	76	83	90	98	105	112	119	127	134	141	149	156	163
20	38	52	66	80	93	106	119	132	145	158	171	184	197	210	222	235	248	261	273	286	299	311	324	337
21	3	8	15	22	29	36	43	50	58	65	73	80	88	96	103	111	119	126	134	142	150	157	165	173
21	39	55	69	83	97	111	125	139	152	166	179	193	206	219	233	246	259	273	286	299	312	326	339	352
22	3	9	16	23	30	38	45	53	61	69	77	85	93	101	109	117	125	133	141	150	158	166	174	182
22	41	57	72	87	102	116	131	145	159	173	187	201	215	229	243	257	271	285	299	312	326	340	354	368
23	3	9	17	24	32	40	48	56	64	73	81	89	98	106	115	123	132	140	149	157	166	175	183	192
23	43	60	75	91	106	121	136	151	166	180	195	210	224	239	253	268	282	297	311	326	340	354	369	383
24	3	10	17	25	33	42	50	59	67	76	85	94	102	111	120	129	138	147	156	165	174	183	192	201
24	45	62	79	95	111	126	142	157	173	188	203	218	234	249	264	279	294	309	324	339	354	369	384	399
25	3	10	18	27	35	44	53	62	71	80	89	98	107	117	126	135	145	154	163	173	182	192	201	211
25	47	65	82	98	115	131	147	163	179	195	211	227	243	258	274	290	305	321	337	352	368	383	399	414

*Test for a one-tailed test at .025 or a two-tailed test at .05. If the U_{obs} value falls within the two values in the table for n_A and n_B, do not reject the null hypothesis. If the U_{obs} is less than or equal to the lower value in the table or greater than or equal to the larger value in the table then reject the null hypothesis.

TABLE C-7B

CRITICAL VALUES FOR THE MANN-WHITNEY U TEST* (ONE-TAILED TEST AT .05 OR A TWO-TAILED TEST AT .10)

na (columns). In each n_b pair the first row is the lower critical value and the second (underlined) row is the upper critical value.

nb	1	2	3	4	5	6	7	8	9	10	11	12	13	14	15	16	17	18	19	20	21	22	23	24	25
1																				0	0	0	0	0	0
1																				20	21	22	23	24	25
2					0	0	0	1	1	1	1	2	2	3	3	3	3	4	4	4	5	5	5	6	6
2					10	12	14	15	17	19	21	22	24	25	27	29	31	32	34	36	37	39	41	42	44
3			0	0	1	2	2	3	4	4	5	5	6	7	7	8	9	9	10	11	11	12	13	13	14
3			9	12	14	16	19	21	23	26	28	31	33	35	38	40	42	45	47	49	52	54	56	59	61
4			0	1	2	3	4	5	6	7	8	9	10	11	12	14	15	16	17	18	19	20	21	22	23
4			12	15	18	21	24	27	30	33	36	39	42	45	48	50	53	56	59	62	65	68	71	74	77
5		0	1	2	4	5	6	8	9	11	12	13	15	16	18	19	20	22	23	25	26	28	29	30	32
5		10	14	18	21	25	29	32	36	39	43	47	50	54	57	61	65	68	72	75	79	82	86	90	93
6		0	2	3	5	7	8	10	12	14	16	17	19	21	23	25	26	28	30	32	34	36	37	39	41
6		12	16	21	25	29	34	38	42	46	50	55	59	63	67	71	76	80	84	88	92	96	101	105	109
7		0	2	4	6	8	11	13	15	17	19	21	24	26	28	30	33	35	37	39	41	44	46	48	50
7		14	19	24	29	34	38	43	48	53	58	63	67	72	77	82	86	91	96	101	106	110	115	120	125
8		1	3	5	8	10	13	15	18	20	23	26	28	31	33	36	39	41	44	47	49	52	54	57	60
8		15	21	27	32	38	43	49	54	60	65	70	76	81	87	92	97	103	108	113	119	124	130	135	140
9		1	4	6	9	12	15	18	21	24	27	30	33	36	39	42	45	48	51	54	57	60	63	66	69
9		17	23	30	36	42	48	54	60	66	72	78	84	90	96	102	108	114	120	126	132	138	144	150	156

10	1	4	7	11	14	17	20	24	27	31	34	37	41	44	48	51	55	58	62	65	68	72	75	79
10	19	26	33	39	46	53	60	66	73	79	86	93	99	106	112	119	125	132	138	145	152	158	165	171
11	1	5	8	12	16	19	23	27	31	34	38	42	46	50	54	57	61	65	69	73	77	81	85	89
11	21	28	36	43	50	58	65	72	79	87	94	101	108	115	122	130	137	144	151	158	165	172	179	186
12	2	5	9	13	17	21	26	30	34	38	42	47	51	55	60	64	68	72	77	81	85	90	94	98
12	22	31	39	47	55	63	70	78	86	94	102	109	117	125	132	140	148	156	163	171	179	186	194	202
13	2	6	10	15	19	24	28	33	37	42	47	51	56	61	65	70	75	80	84	89	94	98	103	108
13	24	33	42	50	59	67	76	84	93	101	109	118	126	134	143	151	159	167	176	184	192	201	209	217
14	2	7	11	16	21	26	31	36	41	46	51	56	61	66	71	77	82	87	92	97	102	107	113	118
14	25	35	45	54	63	72	81	90	99	108	117	126	135	144	153	161	170	179	188	197	206	215	223	232
15	3	7	12	18	23	28	33	39	44	50	55	61	66	72	77	83	88	94	100	105	111	116	122	128
15	27	38	48	57	67	77	87	96	106	115	125	134	144	153	163	172	182	191	200	210	219	229	238	247
16	3	8	14	19	25	30	36	42	48	54	60	65	71	77	83	89	95	101	107	113	119	125	131	137
16	29	40	50	61	71	82	92	102	112	122	132	143	153	163	173	183	193	203	213	223	233	243	253	263
17	3	9	15	20	26	33	39	45	51	57	64	70	77	83	89	96	102	109	115	121	128	134	141	147
17	31	42	53	65	76	86	97	108	119	130	140	151	161	172	183	193	204	214	225	236	246	257	267	278
18	4	9	16	22	28	35	41	48	55	61	68	75	82	88	95	102	109	116	123	130	136	143	150	157
18	32	45	56	68	80	91	103	114	125	137	148	159	170	182	193	204	215	226	237	248	260	271	282	293

(continued)

TABLE C-7B (CONTINUED)

CRITICAL VALUES FOR THE MANN-WHITNEY U TEST* (ONE-TAILED TEST AT .05 OR A TWO-TAILED TEST AT .10)

na

nb	1	2	3	4	5	6	7	8	9	10	11	12	13	14	15	16	17	18	19	20	21	22	23	24	25
19		4	10	17	23	30	37	44	51	58	65	72	80	87	94	101	109	116	123	130	138	145	152	160	167
		34	47	59	72	84	96	108	120	132	144	156	167	179	191	203	214	226	238	250	261	273	285	296	308
20	0	4	11	18	25	32	39	47	54	62	69	77	84	92	100	107	115	123	130	138	146	154	161	169	177
	20	36	49	62	75	88	101	113	126	138	151	163	176	188	200	213	225	237	250	262	274	286	299	311	323
21	0	5	11	19	26	34	41	49	57	65	73	81	89	97	105	113	121	130	138	146	154	162	170	179	187
	21	37	52	65	79	92	106	119	132	145	158	171	184	197	210	223	236	248	261	274	287	300	313	325	338
22	0	5	12	20	28	36	44	52	60	68	77	85	94	102	111	119	128	136	145	154	162	171	179	188	197
	22	39	54	68	82	96	110	124	138	152	165	179	192	206	219	233	246	260	273	286	300	313	327	340	353
23	0	5	13	21	29	37	46	54	63	72	81	90	98	107	116	125	134	143	152	161	170	179	189	198	207
	23	41	56	71	86	101	115	130	144	158	172	186	201	215	229	243	257	271	285	299	313	327	340	354	368
24	0	6	13	22	30	39	48	57	66	75	85	94	103	113	122	131	141	150	160	169	179	188	198	207	217
	24	42	59	74	90	105	120	135	150	165	179	194	209	223	238	253	267	282	296	311	325	340	354	369	383
25	0	6	14	23	32	41	50	60	69	79	89	98	108	118	128	137	147	157	167	177	187	197	207	217	227
	25	44	61	77	93	109	125	140	156	171	186	202	217	232	247	263	278	293	308	323	338	353	368	383	398

*Test for a one-tailed test at .05 or a two-tailed test at .10. If the U_{obs} value falls within the two values in the table for n_A and n_B, do not reject the null hypothesis. If the U_{obs} value is less than or equal to the lower value in the table or greater than or equal to the larger value in the table then reject the null hypothesis.

TABLE C-7C
CRITICAL VALUES FOR THE MANN-WHITNEY U TEST* (ONE-TAILED TEST AT .01 OR A TWO-TAILED TEST AT .02)

| | | | | | | | | | | | | | na | | | | | | | | | | | | |
nb	1	2	3	4	5	6	7	8	9	10	11	12	13	14	15	16	17	18	19	20	21	22	23	24	25
1																									
1																									
2													0	0	0	0	0	0	1	1	1	1	1	1	1
2													26	28	30	32	34	36	37	39	41	43	45	47	49
3							0	0	1	1	1	2	2	2	3	3	4	4	4	5	5	5	6	6	7
3							21	24	26	29	32	34	37	40	42	45	47	50	53	55	58	60	63	66	68
4					0	1	1	2	3	3	4	5	5	6	7	7	8	9	9	10	11	11	12	13	13
4					20	23	27	30	33	37	40	43	47	50	53	57	60	63	67	70	73	77	80	83	87
5				0	1	2	3	4	5	6	7	8	9	10	11	12	13	14	15	16	17	18	19	20	21
5				20	24	28	32	36	40	44	48	52	56	60	64	68	72	76	80	84	88	92	96	100	104
6				1	2	3	4	6	7	8	9	11	12	13	15	16	18	19	20	22	23	24	26	27	29
6				23	28	33	38	42	47	52	57	61	66	71	75	80	84	89	94	98	103	108	112	117	121
7			0	1	3	4	6	7	9	11	12	14	16	17	19	21	23	24	26	28	30	31	33	35	36
7			21	27	32	38	43	49	54	59	65	70	75	81	86	91	96	102	107	112	117	123	128	133	139
8			0	2	4	6	7	9	11	13	15	17	20	22	24	26	28	30	32	34	36	38	40	42	45
8			24	30	36	42	49	55	61	67	73	79	84	90	96	102	108	114	120	126	132	138	144	150	155
9			1	3	5	7	9	11	14	16	18	21	23	26	28	31	33	36	38	40	43	45	48	50	53
9			26	33	40	47	54	61	67	74	81	87	94	100	107	113	120	126	133	140	146	153	159	166	172
10			1	3	6	8	11	13	16	19	22	24	27	30	33	36	38	41	44	47	50	53	55	58	61
10			29	37	44	52	59	67	74	81	88	96	103	110	117	124	132	139	146	153	160	167	175	182	189

(continued)

Table C-7C (Continued)

Critical Values for the Mann-Whitney U Test* (One-Tailed Test at .01 or a Two-Tailed Test at .02)

nb	1	2	3	4	5	6	7	8	9	10	11	12	13	14	15	16	17	18	19	20	21	22	23	24	25
11			32	40	48	57	65	73	81	88	96	104	112	120	128	135	143	151	159	167	174	182	190	198	205
11			1	4	7	9	12	15	18	22	25	28	31	34	37	41	44	47	50	53	57	60	63	66	70
12			34	43	52	61	70	79	87	96	104	113	121	130	138	146	155	163	172	180	188	197	205	213	222
12			2	5	8	11	14	17	21	24	28	31	35	38	42	46	49	53	56	60	64	67	71	75	78
13		26	37	47	56	66	75	84	94	103	112	121	130	139	148	157	166	175	184	193	202	211	220	229	238
13		0	2	5	9	12	16	20	23	27	31	35	39	43	47	51	55	59	63	67	71	75	79	83	87
14		28	40	50	60	71	81	90	100	110	120	130	139	149	159	168	178	187	197	207	216	226	235	245	255
14		0	2	6	10	13	17	22	26	30	34	38	43	47	51	56	60	65	69	73	78	82	87	91	95
15		30	42	53	64	75	86	96	107	117	128	138	148	159	169	179	189	200	210	220	230	240	251	261	271
15		0	3	7	11	15	19	24	28	33	37	42	47	51	56	61	66	70	75	80	85	90	94	99	104
16		32	45	57	68	80	91	102	113	124	135	146	157	168	179	190	201	212	222	233	244	255	266	276	287
16		0	3	7	12	16	21	26	31	36	41	46	51	56	61	66	71	76	82	87	92	97	102	108	113
17		34	47	60	72	84	96	108	120	132	143	155	166	178	189	201	212	224	235	247	258	269	281	292	303
17		0	4	8	13	18	23	28	33	38	44	49	55	60	66	71	77	82	88	93	99	105	110	116	122
18		36	50	63	76	89	102	114	126	139	151	163	175	187	200	212	224	236	248	260	272	284	296	308	320
18		0	4	9	14	19	24	30	36	41	47	53	59	65	70	76	82	88	94	100	106	112	118	124	130

na

n_A	2	3	4	5	6	7	8	9	10	11	12	13	14	15	16	17	18	19	20	21	22	23	24	25
19	1	4	9	15	20	26	32	38	44	50	56	63	69	75	82	88	94	101	107	113	120	126	133	139
19	37	53	67	80	94	107	120	133	146	159	172	184	197	210	222	235	248	260	273	286	298	311	323	336
20	1	5	10	16	22	28	34	40	47	53	60	67	73	80	87	93	100	107	114	121	127	134	141	148
20	39	55	70	84	98	112	126	140	153	167	180	193	207	220	233	247	260	273	286	299	313	326	339	352
21	1	5	11	17	23	30	36	43	50	57	64	71	78	85	92	99	106	113	121	128	135	142	150	157
21	41	58	73	88	103	117	132	146	160	174	188	202	216	230	244	258	272	286	299	313	327	341	354	368
22	1	5	11	18	24	31	38	45	53	60	67	75	82	90	97	105	112	120	127	135	143	150	158	166
22	43	60	77	92	108	123	138	153	167	182	197	211	226	240	255	269	284	298	313	327	341	356	370	384
23	1	6	12	19	26	33	40	48	55	63	71	79	87	94	102	110	118	126	134	142	150	158	167	175
23	45	63	80	96	112	128	144	159	175	190	205	220	235	251	266	281	296	311	326	341	356	371	385	400
24	1	6	13	20	27	35	42	50	58	66	75	83	91	99	108	116	124	133	141	150	158	167	175	184
24	47	66	83	100	117	133	150	166	182	198	213	229	245	261	276	292	308	323	339	354	370	385	401	416
25	1	7	13	21	29	36	45	53	61	70	78	87	95	104	113	122	130	139	148	157	166	175	184	192
25	49	68	87	104	121	139	155	172	189	205	222	238	255	271	287	303	320	336	352	368	384	400	416	433

*Test for a one-tailed test at .01 or a two-tailed test at .02. If the U_{obs} value falls within the two values in the table for n_A and n_B, do not reject the null hypothesis. If the U_{obs} is less than or equal to the lower value in the table or greater than or equal to the larger value in the table then reject the null hypothesis.

Source: The table was generated using R, version 3.43.

TABLE C–8

CRITICAL VALUES OF *T* FOR THE WILCOX SIGNED RANKS TEST

SIGNIFICANCE LEVELS FOR ONE-TAILED TEST				SIGNIFICANCE LEVELS FOR ONE-TAILED TEST				
	0.05	0.025	0.01	0.005		0.05	0.025	0.01	0.005
SIGNIFICANCE LEVELS FOR TWO-TAILED TEST				SIGNIFICANCE LEVELS FOR TWO-TAILED TEST				
N	0.1	0.05	0.02	0.01	N	0.1	0.05	0.02	0.01
5	0				33	187	170	151	138
6	2	0			34	200	182	162	148
7	3	2	0		35	213	195	173	159
8	5	3	1	0	36	227	208	185	171
9	8	5	3	1	37	241	221	198	182
10	10	8	5	3	38	256	235	211	194
11	13	10	7	5	39	271	249	224	207
12	17	13	9	7	40	286	264	238	220
13	21	17	12	9	41	302	279	252	233
14	25	21	15	12	42	319	294	266	247
15	30	25	19	15	43	336	310	281	261
16	35	29	23	19	44	353	327	296	276
17	41	34	27	23	45	371	343	312	291
18	47	40	32	27	46	389	361	328	307
19	53	46	37	32	47	407	378	345	322
20	60	52	43	37	48	426	396	362	339
21	67	58	49	42	49	446	415	379	355
22	75	65	55	48	50	466	434	397	373
23	83	73	62	54	51	486	453	416	390
24	91	81	69	61	52	507	473	434	408
25	100	89	76	68	53	529	494	454	427
26	110	98	84	75	54	550	514	473	445
27	119	107	92	83	55	573	536	493	465
28	130	116	101	91	56	595	557	514	484
29	140	126	110	100	57	618	579	535	504
30	151	137	120	109	58	642	602	556	525
31	163	147	130	118	59	666	625	578	546
32	175	159	140	128	60	690	648	600	567

Note: The T_{crit} value indicates the smaller sum of ranks associated with differences that are all of the same sign. For any given N (number of ranked differences), the T_{obs} is significant at a given level if it is equal to or less than the critical value in the table.

Source: The table was generated using R, version 3.43.

TABLE C–9

STUDENT RANGE STATISTIC FOR TUKEY'S HONESTLY SIGNIFICANTLY DIFFERENCE TEST (HSD)

k = NUMBER OF TREATMENTS

df FOR ERROR TERM	2	3	4	5	6	7	8	9	10	11	12
4	**3.927**	**5.040**	**5.757**	**6.287**	**6.706**	**7.053**	**7.347**	**7.602**	**7.826**	**8.027**	**8.208**
4	6.511	8.120	9.173	9.958	10.583	11.101	11.542	11.925	12.263	12.565	12.839
5	**3.635**	**4.602**	**5.218**	**5.673**	**6.033**	**6.330**	**6.582**	**6.801**	**6.995**	**7.167**	**7.323**
5	5.702	6.976	7.804	8.421	8.913	9.321	9.669	9.971	10.239	10.479	10.696
6	**3.460**	**4.339**	**4.896**	**5.305**	**5.628**	**5.895**	**6.122**	**6.319**	**6.493**	**6.649**	**6.789**
6	5.243	6.331	7.033	7.556	7.972	8.318	8.612	8.869	9.097	9.300	9.485
7	**3.344**	**4.165**	**4.681**	**5.060**	**5.359**	**5.606**	**5.815**	**5.997**	**6.158**	**6.302**	**6.431**
7	4.949	5.919	6.542	7.005	7.373	7.678	7.939	8.166	8.367	8.548	8.711
8	**3.261**	**4.041**	**4.529**	**4.886**	**5.167**	**5.399**	**5.596**	**5.767**	**5.918**	**6.053**	**6.175**
8	4.745	5.635	6.204	6.625	6.959	7.237	7.474	7.680	7.863	8.027	8.176
9	**3.199**	**3.948**	**4.415**	**4.755**	**5.024**	**5.244**	**5.432**	**5.595**	**5.738**	**5.867**	**5.983**
9	4.596	5.428	5.957	6.347	6.657	6.915	7.134	7.325	7.494	7.646	7.784
10	**3.151**	**3.877**	**4.327**	**4.654**	**4.912**	**5.124**	**5.304**	**5.460**	**5.598**	**5.722**	**5.833**
10	4.482	5.270	5.769	6.136	6.428	6.669	6.875	7.054	7.213	7.356	7.485
11	**3.113**	**3.820**	**4.256**	**4.574**	**4.823**	**5.028**	**5.202**	**5.353**	**5.486**	**5.605**	**5.713**
11	4.392	5.146	5.621	5.970	6.247	6.476	6.671	6.841	6.992	7.127	7.250
12	**3.081**	**3.773**	**4.199**	**4.508**	**4.750**	**4.950**	**5.119**	**5.265**	**5.395**	**5.510**	**5.615**
12	4.320	5.046	5.502	5.836	6.101	6.320	6.507	6.670	6.814	6.943	7.060
13	**3.055**	**3.734**	**4.151**	**4.453**	**4.690**	**4.884**	**5.049**	**5.192**	**5.318**	**5.431**	**5.533**
13	4.260	4.964	5.404	5.726	5.981	6.192	6.372	6.528	6.666	6.791	6.903
14	**3.033**	**3.701**	**4.111**	**4.407**	**4.639**	**4.829**	**4.990**	**5.130**	**5.253**	**5.364**	**5.463**
14	4.210	4.895	5.322	5.634	5.881	6.085	6.258	6.409	6.543	6.663	6.772
15	**3.014**	**3.673**	**4.076**	**4.367**	**4.595**	**4.782**	**4.940**	**5.077**	**5.198**	**5.306**	**5.403**
15	4.167	4.836	5.252	5.556	5.796	5.994	6.162	6.309	6.438	6.555	6.660
16	**2.998**	**3.649**	**4.046**	**4.333**	**4.557**	**4.741**	**4.896**	**5.031**	**5.150**	**5.256**	**5.352**
16	4.131	4.786	5.192	5.489	5.722	5.915	6.079	6.222	6.348	6.461	6.564
17	**2.984**	**3.628**	**4.020**	**4.303**	**4.524**	**4.705**	**4.858**	**4.991**	**5.108**	**5.212**	**5.306**
17	4.099	4.742	5.140	5.430	5.659	5.847	6.007	6.147	6.270	6.380	6.480
18	**2.971**	**3.609**	**3.997**	**4.276**	**4.494**	**4.673**	**4.824**	**4.955**	**5.071**	**5.173**	**5.266**
18	4.071	4.703	5.094	5.379	5.603	5.787	5.944	6.081	6.201	6.309	6.407
19	**2.960**	**3.593**	**3.977**	**4.253**	**4.468**	**4.645**	**4.794**	**4.924**	**5.037**	**5.139**	**5.231**
19	4.046	4.669	5.054	5.334	5.553	5.735	5.889	6.022	6.141	6.246	6.342

(continued)

TABLE C-9 (CONTINUED)

STUDENT RANGE STATISTIC FOR TUKEY'S HONESTLY SIGNIFICANTLY DIFFERENCE TEST (HSD)

k = NUMBER OF TREATMENTS

df FOR ERROR TERM	2	3	4	5	6	7	8	9	10	11	12
20	**2.950**	**3.578**	**3.958**	**4.232**	**4.445**	**4.620**	**4.768**	**4.895**	**5.008**	**5.108**	**5.199**
20	4.024	4.639	5.018	5.293	5.510	5.688	5.839	5.970	6.086	6.190	6.285
25	**2.913**	**3.523**	**3.890**	**4.153**	**4.358**	**4.526**	**4.667**	**4.789**	**4.897**	**4.993**	**5.079**
25	3.942	4.527	4.885	5.144	5.347	5.513	5.655	5.778	5.886	5.983	6.070
30	**2.888**	**3.486**	**3.845**	**4.102**	**4.301**	**4.464**	**4.601**	**4.720**	**4.824**	**4.917**	**5.001**
30	3.889	4.455	4.799	5.048	5.242	5.401	5.536	5.653	5.756	5.848	5.932
35	**2.871**	**3.461**	**3.814**	**4.066**	**4.261**	**4.421**	**4.555**	**4.606**	**4.773**	**4.863**	**4.945**
35	3.852	4.404	4.739	4.980	5.169	5.323	5.453	5.566	5.666	5.755	5.835
40	**2.858**	**3.442**	**3.791**	**4.039**	**4.232**	**4.388**	**4.521**	**4.634**	**4.735**	**4.824**	**4.904**
40	3.825	4.367	4.695	4.931	5.114	5.265	5.392	5.502	5.599	5.685	5.764
50	**2.841**	**3.416**	**3.758**	**4.002**	**4.190**	**4.344**	**4.473**	**4.584**	**4.681**	**4.768**	**4.846**
50	3.787	4.316	4.634	4.863	5.040	5.185	5.308	5.414	5.507	5.590	5.665
60	**2.829**	**3.399**	**3.737**	**3.977**	**4.163**	**4.314**	**4.441**	**4.550**	**4.646**	**4.732**	**4.808**
60	3.762	4.282	4.594	4.818	4.991	5.133	5.253	5.356	5.447	5.528	5.601
80	**2.814**	**3.377**	**3.711**	**3.947**	**4.129**	**4.277**	**4.402**	**4.509**	**4.603**	**4.686**	**4.761**
80	3.732	4.241	4.545	4.763	4.931	5.069	5.185	5.284	5.372	5.451	5.521
100	**2.806**	**3.365**	**3.695**	**3.929**	**4.109**	**4.256**	**4.379**	**4.484**	**4.577**	**4.659**	**4.733**
100	3.714	4.216	4.516	4.730	4.896	5.031	5.144	5.242	5.328	5.405	5.474
150	**2.794**	**3.348**	**3.674**	**3.905**	**4.083**	**4.227**	**4.348**	**4.451**	**4.542**	**4.623**	**4.696**
150	3.690	4.184	4.478	4.687	4.849	4.980	5.091	5.187	5.270	5.345	5.412
200	**2.789**	**3.339**	**3.664**	**3.893**	**4.069**	**4.212**	**4.332**	**4.435**	**4.525**	**4.605**	**4.677**
200	3.678	4.168	4.459	4.666	4.826	4.956	5.065	5.159	5.242	5.315	5.381

Note: Bolded critical Q-values are at p =.05. Non-bolded critical Q-values are at p =.01.

Source: The table was generated using R, version 2.13.0.

TABLE C-10

CRITICAL VALUES FOR THE CHI-SQUARE DISTRIBUTION (X^2)

df	α						
	0.25	0.1	0.05	0.025	0.01	0.005	0.001
1	1.3233	2.7055	3.8415	5.0239	6.6349	7.8794	10.8276
2	2.7726	4.6052	5.9915	7.3778	9.2103	10.5966	13.8155
3	4.1083	6.2514	7.8147	9.3484	11.3449	12.8382	16.2662
4	5.3853	7.7794	9.4877	11.1433	13.2767	14.8603	18.4668
5	6.6257	9.2364	11.0705	12.8325	15.0863	16.7496	20.5150
6	7.8408	10.6446	12.5916	14.4494	16.8119	18.5476	22.4577
7	9.0371	12.0170	14.0671	16.0128	18.4753	20.2777	24.3219
8	10.2189	13.3616	15.5073	17.5345	20.0902	21.9550	26.1245
9	11.3888	14.6837	16.9190	19.0228	21.6660	23.5894	27.8772
10	12.5489	15.9872	18.3070	20.4832	23.2093	25.1882	29.5883
11	13.7007	17.2750	19.6751	21.9200	24.7250	26.7568	31.2641
12	14.8454	18.5493	21.0261	23.3367	26.2170	28.2995	32.9095
13	15.9839	19.8119	22.3620	24.7356	27.6882	29.8195	34.5282
14	17.1169	21.0641	23.6848	26.1189	29.1412	31.3193	36.1233
15	18.2451	22.3071	24.9958	27.4884	30.5779	32.8013	37.6973
16	19.3689	23.5418	26.2962	28.8454	31.9999	34.2672	39.2524
17	20.4887	24.7690	27.5871	30.1910	33.4087	35.7185	40.7902
18	21.6049	25.9894	28.8693	31.5264	34.8053	37.1565	42.3124
19	22.7178	27.2036	30.1435	32.8523	36.1909	38.5823	43.8202
20	23.8277	28.4120	31.4104	34.1696	37.5662	39.9968	45.3147
21	24.9348	29.6151	32.6706	35.4789	38.9322	41.4011	46.7970
22	26.0393	30.8133	33.9244	36.7807	40.2894	42.7957	48.2679
23	27.1413	32.0069	35.1725	38.0756	41.6384	44.1813	49.7282
24	28.2412	33.1962	36.4150	39.3641	42.9798	45.5585	51.1786
25	29.3389	34.3816	37.6525	40.6465	44.3141	46.9279	52.6197
26	30.4346	35.5632	38.8851	41.9232	45.6417	48.2899	54.0520
27	31.5284	36.7412	40.1133	43.1945	46.9629	49.6449	55.4760
28	32.6205	37.9159	41.3371	44.4608	48.2782	50.9934	56.8923
29	33.7109	39.0875	42.5570	45.7223	49.5879	52.3356	58.3012
30	34.7997	40.2560	43.7730	46.9792	50.8922	53.6720	59.7031
31	35.8871	41.4217	44.9853	48.2319	52.1914	55.0027	61.0983
32	36.9730	42.5847	46.1943	49.4804	53.4858	56.3281	62.4872
33	38.0575	43.7452	47.3999	50.7251	54.7755	57.6484	63.8701
34	39.1408	44.9032	48.6024	51.9660	56.0609	58.9639	65.2472
35	40.2228	46.0588	49.8018	53.2033	57.3421	60.2748	66.6188

(continued)

TABLE C–10 (CONTINUED)

CRITICAL VALUES FOR THE CHI-SQUARE DISTRIBUTION (X^2)

df	α 0.25	0.1	0.05	0.025	0.01	0.005	0.001
36	41.3036	47.2122	50.9985	54.4373	58.6192	61.5812	67.9852
37	42.3833	48.3634	52.1923	55.6680	59.8925	62.8833	69.3465
38	43.4619	49.5126	53.3835	56.8955	61.1621	64.1814	70.7029
39	44.5395	50.6598	54.5722	58.1201	62.4281	65.4756	72.0547
40	45.6160	51.8051	55.7585	59.3417	63.6907	66.7660	73.4020
41	46.6916	52.9485	56.9424	60.5606	64.9501	68.0527	74.7449
42	47.7663	54.0902	58.1240	61.7768	66.2062	69.3360	76.0838
43	48.8400	55.2302	59.3035	62.9904	67.4593	70.6159	77.4186
44	49.9129	56.3685	60.4809	64.2015	68.7095	71.8926	78.7495
45	50.9849	57.5053	61.6562	65.4102	69.9568	73.1661	80.0767
46	52.0562	58.6405	62.8296	66.6165	71.2014	74.4365	81.4003
47	53.1267	59.7743	64.0011	67.8206	72.4433	75.7041	82.7204
48	54.1964	60.9066	65.1708	69.0226	73.6826	76.9688	84.0371
49	55.2653	62.0375	66.3386	70.2224	74.9195	78.2307	85.3506
50	56.3336	63.1671	67.5048	71.4202	76.1539	79.4900	86.6608

Source: The table was generated using Microsoft Office Excel 2013.

STEPS IN DETERMINING CRITICAL VALUES FOR CHI-SQUARE FOR TABLE C–10

1. Calculate the degrees of freedom (*df*). The formula is df = (*r* − 1) (*c* − 1), where

    r = number of rows in the matrix
    c = number of columns in the matrix.
    For example, in a 2 × 3 matrix, 2 rows and 3 columns, $df = (2 − 1) (3 − 1) = 2$ *df*.

2. Apply level of significance such as .05 or .01.

3. Locate critical value for chi-square from statistical table. For example, *df* = 2, .05 level, chi-square$_{crit}$ = 5.9915.

4. Calculate chi-square$_{obs}$ from data.

5. Decision rule:

    - If chi-square$_{obs}$ is equal to or above chi-square$_{crit}$ reject the null hypothesis.
    - If chi-square$_{obs}$ is below chi-square$_{crit}$ accept the null hypothesis.

TABLE C–11

BINOMIAL PROBABILITIES DISTRIBUTION

							p						
x	*n*	*0.01*	*0.05*	*0.1*	*0.15*	*0.2*	*0.25*	*0.3*	*0.35*	*0.4*	*0.45*	*0.5*	*n-x*
0	1	0.990	0.950	0.900	0.850	0.800	0.750	0.700	0.650	0.600	0.550	0.500	1
1	1	0.010	0.050	0.100	0.150	0.200	0.250	0.300	0.350	0.400	0.450	0.500	0
0	2	0.980	0.903	0.810	0.723	0.640	0.563	0.490	0.423	0.360	0.303	0.250	2
1	2	0.020	0.095	0.180	0.255	0.320	0.375	0.420	0.455	0.480	0.495	0.500	1
2	2	0.000	0.003	0.010	0.023	0.040	0.063	0.090	0.123	0.160	0.203	0.250	0
0	3	0.970	0.857	0.729	0.614	0.512	0.422	0.343	0.275	0.216	0.166	0.125	3
1	3	0.029	0.135	0.243	0.325	0.384	0.422	0.441	0.444	0.432	0.408	0.375	2
2	3	0.000	0.007	0.027	0.057	0.096	0.141	0.189	0.239	0.288	0.334	0.375	1
3	3	0.000	0.000	0.001	0.003	0.008	0.016	0.027	0.043	0.064	0.091	0.125	0
0	4	0.961	0.815	0.656	0.522	0.410	0.316	0.240	0.179	0.130	0.092	0.063	4
1	4	0.039	0.171	0.292	0.368	0.410	0.422	0.412	0.384	0.346	0.299	0.250	3
2	4	0.001	0.014	0.049	0.098	0.154	0.211	0.265	0.311	0.346	0.368	0.375	2
3	4	0.000	0.000	0.004	0.011	0.026	0.047	0.076	0.111	0.154	0.200	0.250	1
4	4	0.000	0.000	0.000	0.001	0.002	0.004	0.008	0.015	0.026	0.041	0.063	0
0	5	0.951	0.774	0.590	0.444	0.328	0.237	0.168	0.116	0.078	0.050	0.031	5
1	5	0.048	0.204	0.328	0.392	0.410	0.396	0.360	0.312	0.259	0.206	0.156	4
2	5	0.001	0.021	0.073	0.138	0.205	0.264	0.309	0.336	0.346	0.337	0.313	3
3	5	0.000	0.001	0.008	0.024	0.051	0.088	0.132	0.181	0.230	0.276	0.313	2
4	5	0.000	0.000	0.000	0.002	0.006	0.015	0.028	0.049	0.077	0.113	0.156	1
5	5	0.000	0.000	0.000	0.000	0.000	0.001	0.002	0.005	0.010	0.018	0.031	0
0	6	0.941	0.735	0.531	0.377	0.262	0.178	0.118	0.075	0.047	0.028	0.016	6
1	6	0.057	0.232	0.354	0.399	0.393	0.356	0.303	0.244	0.187	0.136	0.094	5
2	6	0.001	0.031	0.098	0.176	0.246	0.297	0.324	0.328	0.311	0.278	0.234	4
3	6	0.000	0.002	0.015	0.041	0.082	0.132	0.185	0.235	0.276	0.303	0.313	3
4	6	0.000	0.000	0.001	0.005	0.015	0.033	0.060	0.095	0.138	0.186	0.234	2
5	6	0.000	0.000	0.000	0.000	0.002	0.004	0.010	0.020	0.037	0.061	0.094	1
6	6	0.000	0.000	0.000	0.000	0.000	0.000	0.001	0.002	0.004	0.008	0.016	0
0	7	0.932	0.698	0.478	0.321	0.210	0.133	0.082	0.049	0.028	0.015	0.008	7
1	7	0.066	0.257	0.372	0.396	0.367	0.311	0.247	0.185	0.131	0.087	0.055	6

(continued)

TABLE C–11 (CONTINUED)

BINOMIAL PROBABILITIES DISTRIBUTION

x	n	0.01	0.05	0.1	0.15	0.2	0.25	0.3	0.35	0.4	0.45	0.5	n-x
2	7	0.002	0.041	0.124	0.210	0.275	0.311	0.318	0.298	0.261	0.214	0.164	5
3	7	0.000	0.004	0.023	0.062	0.115	0.173	0.227	0.268	0.290	0.292	0.273	4
4	7	0.000	0.000	0.003	0.011	0.029	0.058	0.097	0.144	0.194	0.239	0.273	3
5	7	0.000	0.000	0.000	0.001	0.004	0.012	0.025	0.047	0.077	0.117	0.164	2
6	7	0.000	0.000	0.000	0.000	0.000	0.001	0.004	0.008	0.017	0.032	0.055	1
7	7	0.000	0.000	0.000	0.000	0.000	0.000	0.000	0.001	0.002	0.004	0.008	0
0	8	0.923	0.663	0.430	0.272	0.168	0.100	0.058	0.032	0.017	0.008	0.004	8
1	8	0.075	0.279	0.383	0.385	0.336	0.267	0.198	0.137	0.090	0.055	0.031	7
2	8	0.003	0.051	0.149	0.238	0.294	0.311	0.296	0.259	0.209	0.157	0.109	6
3	8	0.000	0.005	0.033	0.084	0.147	0.208	0.254	0.279	0.279	0.257	0.219	5
4	8	0.000	0.000	0.005	0.018	0.046	0.087	0.136	0.188	0.232	0.263	0.273	4
5	8	0.000	0.000	0.000	0.003	0.009	0.023	0.047	0.081	0.124	0.172	0.219	3
6	8	0.000	0.000	0.000	0.000	0.001	0.004	0.010	0.022	0.041	0.070	0.109	2
7	8	0.000	0.000	0.000	0.000	0.000	0.000	0.001	0.003	0.008	0.016	0.031	1
8	8	0.000	0.000	0.000	0.000	0.000	0.000	0.000	0.000	0.001	0.002	0.004	0
0	9	0.914	0.630	0.387	0.232	0.134	0.075	0.040	0.021	0.010	0.005	0.002	9
1	9	0.083	0.299	0.387	0.368	0.302	0.225	0.156	0.100	0.060	0.034	0.018	8
2	9	0.003	0.063	0.172	0.260	0.302	0.300	0.267	0.216	0.161	0.111	0.070	7
3	9	0.000	0.008	0.045	0.107	0.176	0.234	0.267	0.272	0.251	0.212	0.164	6
4	9	0.000	0.001	0.007	0.028	0.066	0.117	0.172	0.219	0.251	0.260	0.246	5
5	9	0.000	0.000	0.001	0.005	0.017	0.039	0.074	0.118	0.167	0.213	0.246	4
6	9	0.000	0.000	0.000	0.001	0.003	0.009	0.021	0.042	0.074	0.116	0.164	3
7	9	0.000	0.000	0.000	0.000	0.000	0.001	0.004	0.010	0.021	0.041	0.070	2
8	9	0.000	0.000	0.000	0.000	0.000	0.000	0.000	0.001	0.004	0.008	0.018	1
9	9	0.000	0.000	0.000	0.000	0.000	0.000	0.000	0.000	0.000	0.001	0.002	0
0	10	0.904	0.599	0.349	0.197	0.107	0.056	0.028	0.013	0.006	0.003	0.001	10
1	10	0.091	0.315	0.387	0.347	0.268	0.188	0.121	0.072	0.040	0.021	0.010	9
2	10	0.004	0.075	0.194	0.276	0.302	0.282	0.233	0.176	0.121	0.076	0.044	8
3	10	0.000	0.010	0.057	0.130	0.201	0.250	0.267	0.252	0.215	0.166	0.117	7
4	10	0.000	0.001	0.011	0.040	0.088	0.146	0.200	0.238	0.251	0.238	0.205	6
5	10	0.000	0.000	0.001	0.008	0.026	0.058	0.103	0.154	0.201	0.234	0.246	5

(continued)

Table C–11 (Continued)

Binomial Probabilities Distribution

x	n	0.01	0.05	0.1	0.15	0.2	0.25	0.3	0.35	0.4	0.45	0.5	n-x
6	10	0.000	0.000	0.000	0.001	0.006	0.016	0.037	0.069	0.111	0.160	0.205	4
7	10	0.000	0.000	0.000	0.000	0.001	0.003	0.009	0.021	0.042	0.075	0.117	3
8	10	0.000	0.000	0.000	0.000	0.000	0.000	0.001	0.004	0.011	0.023	0.044	2
9	10	0.000	0.000	0.000	0.000	0.000	0.000	0.000	0.001	0.002	0.004	0.010	1
10	10	0.000	0.000	0.000	0.000	0.000	0.000	0.000	0.000	0.000	0.000	0.001	0
0	11	0.895	0.569	0.314	0.167	0.086	0.042	0.020	0.009	0.004	0.001	0.000	11
1	11	0.099	0.329	0.384	0.325	0.236	0.155	0.093	0.052	0.027	0.013	0.005	10
2	11	0.005	0.087	0.213	0.287	0.295	0.258	0.200	0.140	0.089	0.051	0.027	9
3	11	0.000	0.014	0.071	0.152	0.221	0.258	0.257	0.225	0.177	0.126	0.081	8
4	11	0.000	0.001	0.016	0.054	0.111	0.172	0.220	0.243	0.236	0.206	0.161	7
5	11	0.000	0.000	0.002	0.013	0.039	0.080	0.132	0.183	0.221	0.236	0.226	6
6	11	0.000	0.000	0.000	0.002	0.010	0.027	0.057	0.099	0.147	0.193	0.226	5
7	11	0.000	0.000	0.000	0.000	0.002	0.006	0.017	0.038	0.070	0.113	0.161	4
8	11	0.000	0.000	0.000	0.000	0.000	0.001	0.004	0.010	0.023	0.046	0.081	3
9	11	0.000	0.000	0.000	0.000	0.000	0.000	0.001	0.002	0.005	0.013	0.027	2
10	11	0.000	0.000	0.000	0.000	0.000	0.000	0.000	0.000	0.001	0.002	0.005	1
11	11	0.000	0.000	0.000	0.000	0.000	0.000	0.000	0.000	0.000	0.000	0.000	0
0	12	0.886	0.540	0.282	0.142	0.069	0.032	0.014	0.006	0.002	0.001	0.000	12
1	12	0.107	0.341	0.377	0.301	0.206	0.127	0.071	0.037	0.017	0.008	0.003	11
2	12	0.006	0.099	0.230	0.292	0.283	0.232	0.168	0.109	0.064	0.034	0.016	10
3	12	0.000	0.017	0.085	0.172	0.236	0.258	0.240	0.195	0.142	0.092	0.054	9
4	12	0.000	0.002	0.021	0.068	0.133	0.194	0.231	0.237	0.213	0.170	0.121	8
5	12	0.000	0.000	0.004	0.019	0.053	0.103	0.158	0.204	0.227	0.222	0.193	7
6	12	0.000	0.000	0.000	0.004	0.016	0.040	0.079	0.128	0.177	0.212	0.226	6
7	12	0.000	0.000	0.000	0.001	0.003	0.011	0.029	0.059	0.101	0.149	0.193	5
8	12	0.000	0.000	0.000	0.000	0.001	0.002	0.008	0.020	0.042	0.076	0.121	4
9	12	0.000	0.000	0.000	0.000	0.000	0.000	0.001	0.005	0.012	0.028	0.054	3
10	12	0.000	0.000	0.000	0.000	0.000	0.000	0.000	0.001	0.002	0.007	0.016	2
11	12	0.000	0.000	0.000	0.000	0.000	0.000	0.000	0.000	0.000	0.001	0.003	1
12	12	0.000	0.000	0.000	0.000	0.000	0.000	0.000	0.000	0.000	0.000	0.000	0
0	13	0.878	0.513	0.254	0.121	0.055	0.024	0.010	0.004	0.001	0.000	0.000	13
1	13	0.115	0.351	0.367	0.277	0.179	0.103	0.054	0.026	0.011	0.004	0.002	12

(continued)

TABLE C–11 (CONTINUED)

BINOMIAL PROBABILITIES DISTRIBUTION

x	n	0.01	0.05	0.1	0.15	0.2	0.25	0.3	0.35	0.4	0.45	0.5	n-x
2	13	0.007	0.111	0.245	0.294	0.268	0.200	0.139	0.084	0.045	0.022	0.010	11
3	13	0.000	0.021	0.100	0.190	0.246	0.252	0.218	0.165	0.111	0.066	0.035	10
4	13	0.000	0.003	0.028	0.084	0.154	0.210	0.234	0.222	0.184	0.135	0.087	9
5	13	0.000	0.000	0.006	0.027	0.069	0.126	0.180	0.215	0.221	0.199	0.157	8
6	13	0.000	0.000	0.001	0.006	0.023	0.056	0.103	0.155	0.197	0.217	0.209	7
7	13	0.000	0.000	0.000	0.001	0.006	0.019	0.044	0.083	0.131	0.177	0.209	6
8	13	0.000	0.000	0.000	0.000	0.001	0.005	0.014	0.034	0.066	0.109	0.157	5
9	13	0.000	0.000	0.000	0.000	0.000	0.001	0.003	0.010	0.024	0.050	0.087	4
10	13	0.000	0.000	0.000	0.000	0.000	0.000	0.001	0.002	0.006	0.016	0.035	3
11	13	0.000	0.000	0.000	0.000	0.000	0.000	0.000	0.000	0.001	0.004	0.010	2
12	13	0.000	0.000	0.000	0.000	0.000	0.000	0.000	0.000	0.000	0.000	0.002	1
13	13	0.000	0.000	0.000	0.000	0.000	0.000	0.000	0.000	0.000	0.000	0.000	0
0	14	0.869	0.488	0.229	0.103	0.044	0.018	0.007	0.002	0.001	0.000	0.000	14
1	14	0.123	0.359	0.356	0.254	0.154	0.083	0.041	0.018	0.007	0.003	0.001	13
2	14	0.008	0.123	0.257	0.291	0.250	0.180	0.113	0.063	0.032	0.014	0.006	12
3	14	0.000	0.026	0.114	0.206	0.250	0.240	0.194	0.137	0.085	0.046	0.022	11
4	14	0.000	0.004	0.035	0.100	0.172	0.220	0.229	0.202	0.155	0.104	0.061	10
5	14	0.000	0.000	0.008	0.035	0.086	0.147	0.196	0.218	0.207	0.170	0.122	9
6	14	0.000	0.000	0.001	0.009	0.032	0.073	0.126	0.176	0.207	0.209	0.183	8
7	14	0.000	0.000	0.000	0.002	0.009	0.028	0.062	0.108	0.157	0.195	0.209	7
8	14	0.000	0.000	0.000	0.000	0.002	0.008	0.023	0.051	0.092	0.140	0.183	6
9	14	0.000	0.000	0.000	0.000	0.000	0.002	0.007	0.018	0.041	0.076	0.122	5
10	14	0.000	0.000	0.000	0.000	0.000	0.000	0.001	0.005	0.014	0.031	0.061	4
11	14	0.000	0.000	0.000	0.000	0.000	0.000	0.000	0.001	0.003	0.009	0.022	3
12	14	0.000	0.000	0.000	0.000	0.000	0.000	0.000	0.000	0.001	0.002	0.006	2
13	14	0.000	0.000	0.000	0.000	0.000	0.000	0.000	0.000	0.000	0.000	0.001	1
14	14	0.000	0.000	0.000	0.000	0.000	0.000	0.000	0.000	0.000	0.000	0.000	0
0	15	0.860	0.463	0.206	0.087	0.035	0.013	0.005	0.002	0.000	0.000	0.000	15
1	15	0.130	0.366	0.343	0.231	0.132	0.067	0.031	0.013	0.005	0.002	0.000	14
2	15	0.009	0.135	0.267	0.286	0.231	0.156	0.092	0.048	0.022	0.009	0.003	13
3	15	0.000	0.031	0.129	0.218	0.250	0.225	0.170	0.111	0.063	0.032	0.014	12
4	15	0.000	0.005	0.043	0.116	0.188	0.225	0.219	0.179	0.127	0.078	0.042	11
5	15	0.000	0.001	0.010	0.045	0.103	0.165	0.206	0.212	0.186	0.140	0.092	10

(continued)

Table C–11 (Continued)

Binomial Probabilities Distribution

| | | p | | | | | | | | | | | |
x	n	0.01	0.05	0.1	0.15	0.2	0.25	0.3	0.35	0.4	0.45	0.5	n-x
6	15	0.000	0.000	0.002	0.013	0.043	0.092	0.147	0.191	0.207	0.191	0.153	9
7	15	0.000	0.000	0.000	0.003	0.014	0.039	0.081	0.132	0.177	0.201	0.196	8
8	15	0.000	0.000	0.000	0.001	0.003	0.013	0.035	0.071	0.118	0.165	0.196	7
9	15	0.000	0.000	0.000	0.000	0.001	0.003	0.012	0.030	0.061	0.105	0.153	6
10	15	0.000	0.000	0.000	0.000	0.000	0.001	0.003	0.010	0.024	0.051	0.092	5
11	15	0.000	0.000	0.000	0.000	0.000	0.000	0.001	0.002	0.007	0.019	0.042	4
12	15	0.000	0.000	0.000	0.000	0.000	0.000	0.000	0.000	0.002	0.005	0.014	3
13	15	0.000	0.000	0.000	0.000	0.000	0.000	0.000	0.000	0.000	0.001	0.003	2
14	15	0.000	0.000	0.000	0.000	0.000	0.000	0.000	0.000	0.000	0.000	0.000	1
15	15	0.000	0.000	0.000	0.000	0.000	0.000	0.000	0.000	0.000	0.000	0.000	0
0	16	0.851	0.440	0.185	0.074	0.028	0.010	0.003	0.001	0.000	0.000	0.000	16
1	16	0.138	0.371	0.329	0.210	0.113	0.053	0.023	0.009	0.003	0.001	0.000	15
2	16	0.010	0.146	0.275	0.277	0.211	0.134	0.073	0.035	0.015	0.006	0.002	14
3	16	0.000	0.036	0.142	0.229	0.246	0.208	0.146	0.089	0.047	0.022	0.009	13
4	16	0.000	0.006	0.051	0.131	0.200	0.225	0.204	0.155	0.101	0.057	0.028	12
5	16	0.000	0.001	0.014	0.056	0.120	0.180	0.210	0.201	0.162	0.112	0.067	11
6	16	0.000	0.000	0.003	0.018	0.055	0.110	0.165	0.198	0.198	0.168	0.122	10
7	16	0.000	0.000	0.000	0.005	0.020	0.052	0.101	0.152	0.189	0.197	0.175	9
8	16	0.000	0.000	0.000	0.001	0.006	0.020	0.049	0.092	0.142	0.181	0.196	8
9	16	0.000	0.000	0.000	0.000	0.001	0.006	0.019	0.044	0.084	0.132	0.175	7
10	16	0.000	0.000	0.000	0.000	0.000	0.001	0.006	0.017	0.039	0.075	0.122	6
11	16	0.000	0.000	0.000	0.000	0.000	0.000	0.001	0.005	0.014	0.034	0.067	5
12	16	0.000	0.000	0.000	0.000	0.000	0.000	0.000	0.001	0.004	0.011	0.028	4
13	16	0.000	0.000	0.000	0.000	0.000	0.000	0.000	0.000	0.001	0.003	0.009	3
14	16	0.000	0.000	0.000	0.000	0.000	0.000	0.000	0.000	0.000	0.001	0.002	2
15	16	0.000	0.000	0.000	0.000	0.000	0.000	0.000	0.000	0.000	0.000	0.000	1
16	16	0.000	0.000	0.000	0.000	0.000	0.000	0.000	0.000	0.000	0.000	0.000	0
0	17	0.843	0.418	0.167	0.063	0.023	0.008	0.002	0.001	0.000	0.000	0.000	17
1	17	0.145	0.374	0.315	0.189	0.096	0.043	0.017	0.006	0.002	0.001	0.000	16
2	17	0.012	0.158	0.280	0.267	0.191	0.114	0.058	0.026	0.010	0.004	0.001	15
3	17	0.001	0.041	0.156	0.236	0.239	0.189	0.125	0.070	0.034	0.014	0.005	14
4	17	0.000	0.008	0.060	0.146	0.209	0.221	0.187	0.132	0.080	0.041	0.018	13
5	17	0.000	0.001	0.017	0.067	0.136	0.191	0.208	0.185	0.138	0.087	0.047	12

(continued)

TABLE C–11 (CONTINUED)

BINOMIAL PROBABILITIES DISTRIBUTION

x	n	0.01	0.05	0.1	0.15	0.2	0.25	0.3	0.35	0.4	0.45	0.5	n-x
6	17	0.000	0.000	0.004	0.024	0.068	0.128	0.178	0.199	0.184	0.143	0.094	11
7	17	0.000	0.000	0.001	0.007	0.027	0.067	0.120	0.168	0.193	0.184	0.148	10
8	17	0.000	0.000	0.000	0.001	0.008	0.028	0.064	0.113	0.161	0.188	0.185	9
9	17	0.000	0.000	0.000	0.000	0.002	0.009	0.028	0.061	0.107	0.154	0.185	8
10	17	0.000	0.000	0.000	0.000	0.000	0.002	0.009	0.026	0.057	0.101	0.148	7
11	17	0.000	0.000	0.000	0.000	0.000	0.001	0.003	0.009	0.024	0.052	0.094	6
12	17	0.000	0.000	0.000	0.000	0.000	0.000	0.001	0.002	0.008	0.021	0.047	5
13	17	0.000	0.000	0.000	0.000	0.000	0.000	0.000	0.001	0.002	0.007	0.018	4
14	17	0.000	0.000	0.000	0.000	0.000	0.000	0.000	0.000	0.000	0.002	0.005	3
15	17	0.000	0.000	0.000	0.000	0.000	0.000	0.000	0.000	0.000	0.000	0.001	2
16	17	0.000	0.000	0.000	0.000	0.000	0.000	0.000	0.000	0.000	0.000	0.000	1
17	17	0.000	0.000	0.000	0.000	0.000	0.000	0.000	0.000	0.000	0.000	0.000	0
0	18	0.835	0.397	0.150	0.054	0.018	0.006	0.002	0.000	0.000	0.000	0.000	18
1	18	0.152	0.376	0.300	0.170	0.081	0.034	0.013	0.004	0.001	0.000	0.000	17
2	18	0.013	0.168	0.284	0.256	0.172	0.096	0.046	0.019	0.007	0.002	0.001	16
3	18	0.001	0.047	0.168	0.241	0.230	0.170	0.105	0.055	0.025	0.009	0.003	15
4	18	0.000	0.009	0.070	0.159	0.215	0.213	0.168	0.110	0.061	0.029	0.012	14
5	18	0.000	0.001	0.022	0.079	0.151	0.199	0.202	0.166	0.115	0.067	0.033	13
6	18	0.000	0.000	0.005	0.030	0.082	0.144	0.187	0.194	0.166	0.118	0.071	12
7	18	0.000	0.000	0.001	0.009	0.035	0.082	0.138	0.179	0.189	0.166	0.121	11
8	18	0.000	0.000	0.000	0.002	0.012	0.038	0.081	0.133	0.173	0.186	0.167	10
9	18	0.000	0.000	0.000	0.000	0.003	0.014	0.039	0.079	0.128	0.169	0.185	9
10	18	0.000	0.000	0.000	0.000	0.001	0.004	0.015	0.038	0.077	0.125	0.167	8
11	18	0.000	0.000	0.000	0.000	0.000	0.001	0.005	0.015	0.037	0.074	0.121	7
12	18	0.000	0.000	0.000	0.000	0.000	0.000	0.001	0.005	0.015	0.035	0.071	6
13	18	0.000	0.000	0.000	0.000	0.000	0.000	0.000	0.001	0.004	0.013	0.033	5
14	18	0.000	0.000	0.000	0.000	0.000	0.000	0.000	0.000	0.001	0.004	0.012	4
15	18	0.000	0.000	0.000	0.000	0.000	0.000	0.000	0.000	0.000	0.001	0.003	3
16	18	0.000	0.000	0.000	0.000	0.000	0.000	0.000	0.000	0.000	0.000	0.001	2
17	18	0.000	0.000	0.000	0.000	0.000	0.000	0.000	0.000	0.000	0.000	0.000	1
18	18	0.000	0.000	0.000	0.000	0.000	0.000	0.000	0.000	0.000	0.000	0.000	0
0	19	0.826	0.377	0.135	0.046	0.014	0.004	0.001	0.000	0.000	0.000	0.000	19
1	19	0.159	0.377	0.285	0.153	0.068	0.027	0.009	0.003	0.001	0.000	0.000	18

(continued)

TABLE C–11 (Continued)

BINOMIAL PROBABILITIES DISTRIBUTION

x	n	0.01	0.05	0.1	0.15	0.2	0.25	0.3	0.35	0.4	0.45	0.5	n-x
							p						
2	19	0.014	0.179	0.285	0.243	0.154	0.080	0.036	0.014	0.005	0.001	0.000	17
3	19	0.001	0.053	0.180	0.243	0.218	0.152	0.087	0.042	0.017	0.006	0.002	16
4	19	0.000	0.011	0.080	0.171	0.218	0.202	0.149	0.091	0.047	0.020	0.007	15
5	19	0.000	0.002	0.027	0.091	0.164	0.202	0.192	0.147	0.093	0.050	0.022	14
6	19	0.000	0.000	0.007	0.037	0.095	0.157	0.192	0.184	0.145	0.095	0.052	13
7	19	0.000	0.000	0.001	0.012	0.044	0.097	0.153	0.184	0.180	0.144	0.096	12
8	19	0.000	0.000	0.000	0.003	0.017	0.049	0.098	0.149	0.180	0.177	0.144	11
9	19	0.000	0.000	0.000	0.001	0.005	0.020	0.051	0.098	0.146	0.177	0.176	10
10	19	0.000	0.000	0.000	0.000	0.001	0.007	0.022	0.053	0.098	0.145	0.176	9
11	19	0.000	0.000	0.000	0.000	0.000	0.002	0.008	0.023	0.053	0.097	0.144	8
12	19	0.000	0.000	0.000	0.000	0.000	0.000	0.002	0.008	0.024	0.053	0.096	7
13	19	0.000	0.000	0.000	0.000	0.000	0.001	0.002	0.008	0.023	0.052	6	
14	19	0.000	0.000	0.000	0.000	0.000	0.000	0.000	0.001	0.002	0.008	0.022	5
15	19	0.000	0.000	0.000	0.000	0.000	0.000	0.000	0.000	0.001	0.002	0.007	4
16	19	0.000	0.000	0.000	0.000	0.000	0.000	0.000	0.000	0.000	0.000	0.002	3
17	19	0.000	0.000	0.000	0.000	0.000	0.000	0.000	0.000	0.000	0.000	0.000	2
18	19	0.000	0.000	0.000	0.000	0.000	0.000	0.000	0.000	0.000	0.000	0.000	1
19	19	0.000	0.000	0.000	0.000	0.000	0.000	0.000	0.000	0.000	0.000	0.000	0
0	20	0.818	0.358	0.122	0.039	0.012	0.003	0.001	0.000	0.000	0.000	0.000	20
1	20	0.165	0.377	0.270	0.137	0.058	0.021	0.007	0.002	0.000	0.000	0.000	19
2	20	0.016	0.189	0.285	0.229	0.137	0.067	0.028	0.010	0.003	0.001	0.000	18
3	20	0.001	0.060	0.190	0.243	0.205	0.134	0.072	0.032	0.012	0.004	0.001	17
4	20	0.000	0.013	0.090	0.182	0.218	0.190	0.130	0.074	0.035	0.014	0.005	16
5	20	0.000	0.002	0.032	0.103	0.175	0.202	0.179	0.127	0.075	0.036	0.015	15
6	20	0.000	0.000	0.009	0.045	0.109	0.169	0.192	0.171	0.124	0.075	0.037	14
7	20	0.000	0.000	0.002	0.016	0.055	0.112	0.164	0.184	0.166	0.122	0.074	13
8	20	0.000	0.000	0.000	0.005	0.022	0.061	0.114	0.161	0.180	0.162	0.120	12
9	20	0.000	0.000	0.000	0.001	0.007	0.027	0.065	0.116	0.160	0.177	0.160	11
10	20	0.000	0.000	0.000	0.000	0.002	0.010	0.031	0.069	0.117	0.159	0.176	10
11	20	0.000	0.000	0.000	0.000	0.000	0.003	0.012	0.034	0.071	0.119	0.160	9
12	20	0.000	0.000	0.000	0.000	0.000	0.001	0.004	0.014	0.035	0.073	0.120	8
13	20	0.000	0.000	0.000	0.000	0.000	0.000	0.001	0.004	0.015	0.037	0.074	7
14	20	0.000	0.000	0.000	0.000	0.000	0.000	0.000	0.001	0.005	0.015	0.037	6
15	20	0.000	0.000	0.000	0.000	0.000	0.000	0.000	0.000	0.001	0.005	0.015	5

(continued)

TABLE C–11 (CONTINUED)

BINOMIAL PROBABILITIES DISTRIBUTION

| | | p | | | | | | | | | | | |
x	n	0.01	0.05	0.1	0.15	0.2	0.25	0.3	0.35	0.4	0.45	0.5	n-x
16	20	0.000	0.000	0.000	0.000	0.000	0.000	0.000	0.000	0.000	0.001	0.005	4
17	20	0.000	0.000	0.000	0.000	0.000	0.000	0.000	0.000	0.000	0.000	0.001	3
18	20	0.000	0.000	0.000	0.000	0.000	0.000	0.000	0.000	0.000	0.000	0.000	2
19	20	0.000	0.000	0.000	0.000	0.000	0.000	0.000	0.000	0.000	0.000	0.000	1
20	20	0.000	0.000	0.000	0.000	0.000	0.000	0.000	0.000	0.000	0.000	0.000	0

Note: x = number of successes, n = number of opportunities, p = probability level.

Source: The table was generated using Microsoft Office Excel 2013.

This binomial distribution table is applicable to determine the probabilities of "yes/no" questions being answered one way or the other. The values in the row at the top that goes from .01 to .5 are probabilities, where the .01 is a 1% chance that something is occurring and .5 is a 50% chance that something is occurring. For instance, in the first two rows where n = 1, at the p =.5 the binomial distribution says that there is an equal chance of success with each (x = 0 and x = 1) equaling 50%. That is, the exact probability at finding either success or failure is.5. Conceptually, using smaller ps may make more sense when considering more possibilities. For example, for n = 6 possibilities, if the .01 column is chosen (which means that it is virtually impossible with only 1% chance of success) and where x = 0 and n = 6 (meaning that given 6 chances, 0 successes occurred, the probability of this being true is.941. In this example, let's take a coin toss. Someone says "I bet you that you can't get six heads in a row out of six tries" the probability is over 94% that the person who predicted no success in the heads coming up 6 times in a row would win the bet.

Glossary

A

a priori: Reasoning from cause to effect. A priori criteria are criteria that an investigator states before collecting data.

AB research design: Single subject research where the A phase represents the collection of baseline data and the B phase represents the intervention phase. Variations of this include ABA, ABAB, and other related research designs. *See also* case study.

abscissa: The horizontal coordinate, or x-axis, in a distribution.

abstract: A summary of a published article (150 to 300 words) that contains the important points of each section, including purpose of study, literature review, methodology, results, limitations of research design, and recommendations for further research.

action research: Application of research to a site-specific environment using a problem-solving approach. It is an outgrowth of both qualitative and quantitative research. For example, an occupational therapist is interested in finding the best splint to use with a client who has a cumulative trauma injury. The methodology may be replicated in another setting to test of generalizability of the results.

alpha (α): The probability of a Type I error predetermined to be acceptable in research. It is usually set at .05 or .01 in the social sciences. It is also referred to as *significance level*. The p-value of a particular comparison is compared to the alpha level in order to decide to reject the null hypothesis or not.

alternative hypothesis (H): The hypothesis that is the opposite of the stated hypothesis and is not predicted to be true.

analysis of covariance (ANCOVA): A statistical test arising from an analysis of variance that adjusts for a priori differences in comparison groups.

analysis of variance (ANOVA): An inferential statistical test that is applied to data when comparing two or more independent group means. An F score is derived. The formula for F in a one-way ANOVA is:

$$F = \frac{variance\ among\ group\ means}{variance\ within\ groups}$$

annotated bibliography: Includes the bibliographical citation and the abstract, perhaps with critical commentary.

ANOVA: *See also* analysis of variance.

a posteriori: A Latin phrase that refers to reasoning backwards from effect to causes. It sometimes can lead to false conclusions. For example earthquakes being the result of immoral behavior.

applied research: The direct application of research to improving the quality of life in areas such as reduction of work injuries, prevention of alcoholism, and evaluation of clinical treatment methods. *See also* problem-oriented research.

aptitude: Inherent, natural ability of an individual; underlying capacity to learn or perform in a specific area.

artifact: An unexplained result in an experiment not caused by the independent variable.

associational relationship: Degree of correlation between two variables.

attitude scale: A measure of an individual's feeling, belief, or opinion toward a subject or topic.

Average: There are three different types of average:
1. **Mean**: What one often thinks of as average—add all the values and divide by the number of values added together.
2. **Median (or midpoint)**: The value in the exact center of the list of responses.
3. **Mode**: The most commonly appearing value.

B

bar graph: A histogram with unattached bars.

baseline data: The results of initial testing of a subject before intervention.

basic research: Investigations in areas related to processes, functions, and attributes that can lead to applied research. An example of basic research is examining how serotonin, a neurochemical transmitter, operates in the brain. The results of basic research often have important significance for clinical researchers.

before-and-after design: An experimental research design in which performance or characteristics are measured before and after an intervention. Often referred to as a *pre- and post-test repeated measures design*.

beta (β): The probability of a Type 2 error in research. *See also* power.

bias: Any prejudicial factor in the researcher or methodology that may distort results.

biased sample: A sample that is not representative of a target population from which it is drawn. As it does not reflect the major characteristics of the target population, the results from a biased sample cannot be confidently generalized.

bibliographical citation: The exact reference for a journal, book, or article referred to in the research paper or manuscript. The citation includes the author; title of article, journal, or book; volume and page numbers; and in books, the place of publication and the publisher.

bimodal: A frequency distribution showing the two highest points.

binomial distribution: Probability distribution used to describe dichotomous outcomes in a population.

bivariate analysis: Statistical analysis in which there is one dependent variable and one independent variable.

box-and-whisker plots, box plots, box graphs: Type of exploratory data analysis that produces descriptive figures which display the maximum and minimum scores and the median and quartiles in a rectangular box. Useful in demonstrating graphically the degree of skewness of data.

C

case study: Intensive study of an individual or a defined entity through a comprehensive extraction of data from many sources, including observation, interview, and document analysis.

central tendency: A summary measure of a distribution indicated by the mean, median, or mode. Frequently referred to as *measures of central tendency*.

chi-square: A nonparametric statistical technique that tests the probability between observed and expected frequencies derived from nominal (categorical) level measurement.

clinical observation research: The systematic and objective investigation of normal development, course of a disease, or responses to an intervention.

clinical trial: In experimental medical research, refers to large-scale studies exploring the effectiveness of drugs or vaccines on populations.

closed-ended questions: Questions that can be answered by either *yes* or *no*. This type of question is not considered useful in survey research. The opposite of a closed-ended question is an open-ended question.

coding: A term in qualitative research referring to the systematic categorization of interview responses, focus group conversations, or observed documents with common characteristics (e.g., residents of a community or an occupational group).

cohort: A study sample with some common experience or characteristic.

concurrent validity: A new test's correlation with an established instrument to indicate its accuracy in measuring the variable of interest. For example, a new test for intelligence frequently will be correlated with the Wechsler Intelligence Scales because it has a high reliability and established validity. New tests are developed to update concepts and improve administration, cost, and time considerations.

confidence interval: The area in a sample distribution that most likely contains the population parameter. The width of the confidence interval is affected by the level of statistical confidence desired in the results.

confirmability of qualitative data: Based on the replicability of the methods used by the researcher. The research method should be described in enough detail so that it can be repeated by other researchers.

confounding variable: An extraneous variable affecting research results. For example, test anxiety, fatigue, and lack of sleep may be confounding variables.

construct: A theoretical concept, theme, or idea based on empirical observations. It's a variable that's usually not directly measurable. For example in psychology self-esteem or self-confidence are complex variables that are difficult to measure directly but are described in assessing an individual.

content validity: The most elementary type of validity. It is determined by a logical analysis of test items to see whether the items are consistent and measure what they purport to measure. *See also* face validity.

contingency table: A table of values that includes observed and expected frequencies, such as a chi-square table.

continuous variable: A quantitative measure that can assume an infinite number of values between any two points. Examples of continuous variables are height, weight, and heart rate.

control group: A comparative group included in a study to control for the Hawthorne effect and other extraneous variables. Both the experimental and comparative groups receive equal time or attention.

convenience sample: A sample selected that is readily available. For example, a researcher will select participants who are in a hospital where the researcher is employed.

correlation: A statistical test used to quantify the association between two (usually continuous) variables.

correlation coefficient: A statistical value that indicates the degree of relationship between two variables. It can range from +1.00 through 0 to -1.00.

correlation matrix: A statistical table describing the degree of correlation between pairs of variables, applied to many variables. The correlation matrix indicates the correlation coefficient index for each pair of correlates.

correlational research: Retrospective investigations into the relationship between variables. Variables are not manipulated by the researcher, as they would be in experimental research.

covariate: A suspected or discovered variable important in a study for its effect on the dependent variable.

Cox proportional hazard regression: Statistical test for assessing time to a dichotomous event where the independent variables are nominal or continuous.

credibility of qualitative data: Established through triangulation where the researcher uses multiple methods or tests in measuring a concept or variable. Multiple interviews and sometimes participant journals ensure the validity of the results.

credibility: In qualitative research, the authenticity of the results based on acceptance of the conclusions from the phenomenological evidence. Triangulation (i.e., obtaining data from different perspectives) increases the credibility of the research.

criterion: Standard of performance that is the basis or yardstick for comparisons.

criterion-referenced test: A test based on a standard of performance, competence, or mastery, rather than on a comparison with a normative group. For example, for an individual to pass a test in driver competency, he or she would have to demonstrate mastery of a specific set of criteria. The determination of the criteria is not based on the bell-shaped curve but is based on socially acceptable minimal standards for performance.

critical value: The statistical value displayed in tables that is used to judge whether or not to reject the null hypothesis.

cross-validation: A method to measure test validity by replicating the original testing in other groups.

Cronbach's alpha coefficient: A statistic that is used to measure internal consistency and reliability using continuous data. *See also* Kuder-Richardson coefficient.

culture-free test: A test that is not culturally biased and can be fairly administered across cultures.

D

data: The numerical results of a study. The term is always plural (e.g., data are ...).

decile: A point in a distribution where 10% of the cases fall at or below that point.

deductive reasoning: Inference to particulars from a general principle. For example, proposing a theory and then hypothesizing specific results from an experiment.

degrees of freedom (df): A mathematically derived value that is used in reading statistical tables.

demographic variables: Related to the statistical characteristics of a target population, such as distribution of ages, gender, income, presence of disease (morbidity), death rates (mortality), occupation, accident and injury rates, health status, and nutritional input.

demography: The application of statistical methods to describe human populations regarding factors, such as mortality, morbidity, birth and marriage rates, gender differences, physical and intellectual characteristics, socioeconomic status, and religious beliefs.

dependability of the qualitative data: Confirmed by rigorous research methods being used throughout the research study and any changes in participants and methods for collecting data being described.

dependent variable: Resultant effect of the independent variable. In clinical research, the selection of the dependent variable indicates the desired outcome, such as decrease in anxiety, increase in range of motion, or increase in reading achievement.

descriptive statistics: Statistical tests or procedures to describe a population, sample, or variable. Examples of descriptive statistics are measures of central tendency, measures of variability, frequency distribution, vital statistics, scatter diagram, polygons, and histograms.

developmental test: A measure of a child's performance in age-related areas such as language, perceptual-motor, social, emotional, and ambulation.

dichotomous variable: Variable that only has two possible values.

directional hypothesis: A statement by the researcher predicting that there will be a statistically significant difference between groups in a certain direction. For example, a clinical researcher states, "Aerobic exercise is more effective than anti-depressive medication in reducing anxiety in individuals with clinical depression."

discourse analysis: The study of communication through the forms and mechanisms of verbal interaction.

discrete variable: A variable that is distinct and does not have an infinite number of values between categories. Examples of discrete variables are gender, diagnostic categories, or eye color.

double-blind control: A research design in which neither the researcher nor the participants know whether they are in the experimental or control group.

E

effect modification (interaction): A situation in which two or more independent factors modify the effect of each other with regard to an outcome; thus, the outcome differs depending on whether or not an effect modifier is present.

effect size: A method for determining the relative size of the effect of the independent variable without regard to the degrees of freedom. It is based upon the difference in population means and the size of the population standard deviation and is usually considered to be small, medium, or large (see Cohen, 1988).

empiricism: The philosophy that advocates knowledge based on controlled observation and experiment.

error variance: Variability in measurement due to contaminating factors in the participant, researcher, test instrument, or environment that threaten internal validity. These factors include poor motivation, fatigue, and test anxiety in the participant; researcher bias; unreliability of the test instrument; and a distracting or noisy testing environment.

ethnography: A qualitative research method, where the researcher collects data from naturalistic observations and interviews in order to understand how societies and groups function.

ethnoscience: The study of the characteristics of language as culture in terms of lexical or semantic relations.

evaluation research: The qualitative and systematic evaluation of systems and organizations such as hospitals and educational programs by applying a priori criteria or standards.

evidence-based practice: The use of research studies to inform intervention decisions. The occupational therapist translates the results of study protocols to the current practice setting.

evidence table: A common technique used to extract data to prepare systematic reviews, meta-analyses, and clinical guidelines. An evidence table for a literature review can be less rigorous and detailed than an evidence table used for these other types of publications.

ex post facto design: A retrospective study in which the investigator examines the relationships of variables that have already occurred.

experimental group: The group that is manipulated by the researcher; for example, the experimental group receives an innovative method of teaching.

experimental research: A prospective study in which the investigator seeks to discover cause-and-effect relationships by manipulating the independent variable and observing the effects on the dependent variable.

experimental study: Study that examines groups where an intervention has been allocated.

external validity: The degree to which the results of a study can be generalized to a target population. External validity depends on the representativeness of the sample and the rigor of the experiment. Replication of a study producing consistent results increases the external validity.

extraneous historical factors: Threats to internal validity when unexpected events take place during an experiment that affect the results. These unpredictable events in the participant are extraneous variables.

extraneous variable: A variable other than the independent variable that can potentially affect the results of a study. Extraneous variables can include factors such as gender, intelligence, severity of disability, or socioeconomic status. These variables, if they are uncontrolled, can threaten the internal validity of a study.

F

factor analysis: A statistical method to categorize data into identifiable factors. The procedure is an extension of a correlation matrix where many variables are correlated with each other, and clusters of co-variability are extracted.

factorial design: A research study exploring the interaction between variables, such as a two-factor analysis of variance.

feasible research study: A study in which the investigator has examined in detail and provided solutions for the practical aspects of implementation, such as costs, time, setting, availability of participants, ethics, selection of outcome measures, and procedure for collecting data.

Fisher's exact test: Statistical test used to compare two unpaired (independent) samples where the outcome is dichotomous or nominal and the sample size is small; alternative to the chi-square test.

focus group: A group interview involving a small number of demographically similar people or participants who have other traits/experiences in common depending on the research objective of the study. Their reactions to specific researcher/evaluator-posed questions are studied.

forced choice test items: Items that require participants to make a choice when completing a questionnaire, rating scale, or attitude inventory. Participants select from among items generated by the researcher.

frequency distribution table: A descriptive statistic summarizing data by showing the number of times each score value occurs in a set category or interval.

frequency polygon: A line graph depicting the number of cases that fall into designated categories. It is composed of an X and a Y axis.

Frequency ratio or Fisher ratio (F): Variability among groups divided by variability within groups. A larger F value makes it more likely the null hypothesis can be rejected.

Friedman's test: Statistical test used to compare three or more paired (dependent) samples when the outcome is either ordinal or continuous with a skewed distribution.

functional capacity evaluation (FCE): A comprehensive and systematic approach to measuring a client's overall physical capacity, including muscle strength and endurance.

G

generalizable: The extent to which findings from a study sample can be applied to the entire population.

grounded theory analysis: Referring to qualitative research, the search for regularities by constantly comparing and contrasting similarities and differences in incidents to form categories or themes with distinctive properties and conceptual relationships.

Guttman scale: A cumulative attitude scale that indicates an individual's feelings toward a specific issue. The respondent usually answers *yes* or *no* to a statement.

H

halo effect: A carry-over effect from previous knowledge in an individual, resulting in a bias on the part of a tester or rater. Halo effects typically occur when raters positively prejudge a participant's performance based on the rater's previous experience with him or her. It is a bias in testing.

Hawthorne effect: A confounding variable that creates a positive result that is not caused by the independent variable. The Hawthorne effect is eliminated by introducing a control group or by using the participant as one's own control.

hermeneutics: The study and interpretation of text in which each event is understood by reference to the whole of which it is a part, especially the broader historical context.

heterogeneous: Of different origin or characteristic, such as mixed ages or educational levels.

heuristic research: Investigations that seek to discover relationships between variables through pilot studies and factor analysis. The major purpose is to generate further research.

histogram: A descriptive statistic describing a frequency distribution using attached bars.

historical research: The systematic and objective investigation, through primary sources, into the events and people that shaped history.

homogeneous: Of like origin or characteristic such as age, gender, or occupation.

honeymoon effect: A confounding variable that produces a short-term beneficial effect. It is created by the initial optimism of the researcher desiring to show the positive effects of a specific intervention and the participant wanting the intervention to work. The participant rejects the initial effects of intervention and disregards side effects or negative results. It is controlled by long-term follow-up and reducing researcher bias.

hypothesis: A statement that predicts results and that can be tested. An example of a hypothesis is "Aerobic exercise lowers blood pressure in middle-aged, sedentary men." A hypothesis can be stated in a null (no difference) or in a directional form.

I

idiographic approach: Intensive study of an individual or dynamic case study.

incidence rate: The rate of the initial occurrence or new cases of a disease over a period of time. For example, the incidence of AIDS in the United States for the year 2010 includes all the new cases of AIDS diagnosed during 2010.

independent living evaluation: An assessment tool used to measure a client's ability to perform the activities of daily living. An example is the Barthel Self Care Index.

independent variable: A variable manipulated by the researcher. In clinical research, it represents the intervention, such as sensory integration therapy, or cognitive behavioral therapy.

inductive reasoning: Inferences from particulars or experiments to the general. For example, integrating the results of research studies into a general theory or conclusion.

inferential statistics: Statistical tests for making inferences from samples and populations based on objectively derived data. They include t-tests, analysis of variance, chi-square, correlation coefficients, factor analysis, and multiple regression.

information retrieval systems: Automated system for storing and retrieving information. In the health fields, examples include OT Search, MEDLINE, PubMed, CINAHL, ERIC, or HealthStar.

informed consent form: A voluntary consensual agreement between the investigator and the participant detailing the procedures in the study and the possible psychological and physical risks that could result in harm.

insider perspective: A view of the participant's lived experience in natural settings, sought by the researcher in qualitative studies.

institutional review board (IRB): An interdisciplinary committee established in a university, hospital, or private industry to protect human participants from possible harm that could occur by participating in a research study. It is required at institutions receiving federal funding that all research with human participants be screened with ethical considerations before data are collected or the research is initiated.

internal validity: The degree of rigor in an experiment in controlling for extraneous variables and error variance. Potential threats to internal validity have been identified as extraneous historical factors, maturation, instrumentation, and lack of random sampling. Internal validity is an indication of the trustworthiness of the results. Well-designed studies with good control of variables that could potentially distort the results have high internal validity. The quality of a research study is increased by eliminating the threats to internal validity.

interquartile range (IQR): Measure of spread or dispersion in the data calculated as the difference between the 25th and 75th percentile values.

inter-rater reliability: The degree of agreement and consistency between two independent raters in measuring a variable.

interval scale of measurement: Quantification of a variable in which there are infinite points between each measurement, as well as equal intervals. Examples include the measurement of systolic blood pressure or intelligence scores as measured by the Wechsler scales. An absolute zero is not assumed in measuring a variable, nor are comparative statements assumed, such as X is twice as large as Y.

intra-rater reliability: The degree of consistency over time within a single rater.

Iterative (Interation) means repeating the process of collecting and analyzing data. One has to repeatedly revisit the data or go back and forth repeatedly on the data.

K

Kappa test (k): A statistical procedure to estimate the degree of inter-rater agreement factoring in the probability of chance agreement.

Kendall's coefficient of concordance: Statistical test used to quantify the association between two ordinal variables.

key word: An important word or concept in a study that is identified by the researcher. It is used to electronically retrieve a study when it is part of a database.

knowledge translation: Defined as a dynamic and iterative process that includes synthesis, dissemination, exchange and ethically sound application of knowledge to improve the health of Canadians, provide more effective health services and products and strengthen the health care system. This process takes place within a complex system of interactions between researchers and knowledge users which may vary in intensity, complexity, and level of engagement depending on the nature of the research and the findings as well as the needs of the particular knowledge user.

Kruskal-Wallis test: Nonparametric statistical test used to compare three or more unpaired (independent) samples where the outcome is either ordinal or continuous with a skewed distribution.

Kuder-Richardson coefficient: A statistic that is used to measure internal consistency and reliability using dichotomous data. *See also* Cronbach's alpha coefficient.

L

Likert scale: A measurement scale used in questionnaires to assess a participant's extent of agreement or disagreement with a statement. Likert scales usually include five to seven descriptors (e.g., totally agree, agree, neutral, disagree, totally disagree).

linear regression: Regression analysis used to quantify the association between one independent variable and a continuous dependent variable that is normally distributed.

logical positivism: A philosophical approach of the 1920s and 1930s. Logical positivists asserted that statements about reality must be verified by empirical data.

logistic regression: Regression analysis used to quantify the association between one independent variable and a dichotomous outcome.

M

Mann–Whitney U test: A nonparametric test that is an alternative to the independent *t*-test when testing differences between the means of two independent groups. The normality and equal variances assumptions of the *t*-test need not be satisfied in the Mann–Whitney test.

matched group: A control group selected to use as a comparison to the experimental group. Variables matched typically include age, gender, socioeconomic status, and degree of disability.

maturation: A threat to internal validity that occurs when the researcher does not account for the participant's maturity during an experiment. For example, in testing children, the researcher must consider age in measuring changes from pre- to post-test evaluation. Maturation can also refer to a practice effect and development in the participant during the experiment.

McNemar's test: Statistical test used to compare two paired (dependent) samples when the outcome of interest is dichotomous (or nominal with only two outcomes).

mean: The arithmetic average derived from all scores in a distribution. It is a measure of central tendency.

measurement error: In measuring a variable, errors in test results can occur due to participant anxiety, unreliability of test instrument, noisy setting for testing and tester's inability to follow test protocol accurately.

measures of central tendency: Mean, mode, and median.

measures of variability or dispersion: Range, variance, and standard deviation.

mechanism of change: The underlying causes of change in behavior, attitude, or physiology by an intervention. For example, exercise relieves clinical depression by increasing the neurohormone serotonin that then increases the likelihood of physical activity.

median: The score at the 50th percentile or midpoint where all the cases in a distribution are divided in half. It is a measure of central tendency.

member checking: A validation method to increase the trustworthiness of a qualitative study by providing preliminary results to the participant and receiving feedback.

member checking: A method to increase validity and credibility by sharing the results with the research participants.

meta-analysis: A quantitative analysis of a group of related research studies to determine the overall average effectiveness of an intervention. Meta-analysis is based on the effect size of studies and incorporates consideration of sample sizes and the degree of consistency among studies.

metasynthesis: The systematic review and integration of findings from qualitative studies – an emerging technique in medical research that can use many different methods. Nevertheless, the method must be appropriate to the specific scientific field in which it is used.

methodological research: Objective and systematic investigation for analyzing instruments, tests, procedures, curriculum, software programs, and intervention programs.

mixed method designs: Using qualitative and quantitative research methods in a study. For example, applying interview questions and standardized tests or physiological measures in the same study.

mode: The most frequent score or numerical value in a frequency distribution. A measure of central tendency.

multiple analysis of covariance (MANCOVA): A statistical technique that is based on the analysis of variance where multiple variables are being analyzed and corrected for differences in initial score statistical significance between the groups being compared.

multiple baseline designs: Used in measuring variables for more than one participant, outcome, or setting, before and after intervention.

multiple linear regression: Linear regression used to quantify the association between more than one independent variable and a continuous outcome that is normally distributed.

multiple logistic regression: Logistic regression used to quantify the association between more than one independent variable and a dichotomous outcome.

multiple regression: A statistical method that is used to predict the individual effects of independent variables on a designated dependent variable. Multiple regression has been used in medical research to identify the multiple risk factors in certain diseases, such as cardiovascular disease, stroke, or emphysema. For example, multiple regression is used to predict the effect of designated risk factors (presumed independent variables) on a dependent variable (e.g., heart disease).

multinomial logistic regression: Logistic regression used to quantify the association between one or more independent variables and a nominal outcome having more than 2 levels.

multivariable analysis: Statistical analysis in which there is one dependent variable and more than one independent variable.

N

n: Number of participants in a sub-group

N: Number of participants in the entire study.

narrative analysis: A type of qualitative data analysis that focuses on interpreting the core narratives from a study group's personal stories. Using first-person narrative, data is acquired and organized to allow the researcher to understand how the individuals experienced something.

naturalistic inquiry: Examines the behavior of individuals in their natural settings as they engage in everyday activities.

nominal scale of measurement: Classification of the values of a variable into discrete categories, such as diagnostic groups, professions, or gender. There is no specific order in the categories; no category is more important than any other category. Likewise, each category is mutually exclusive of any other category.

nominal variable: Variable having (descriptive) categorical values.

nomination sampling: The largest values from several independent random samples (nominees) are rank ordered, and an estimate of the population median is formed by interpolating between two of these order statistics.

nomothetic approach: Research leading to general laws in science or universal knowledge.

nonparametric regression: A type of regression used to quantify the association between one or more independent variables and a continuous outcome having a skewed distribution

nonparametric statistical tests: Inferential statistical procedures on samples whose data are not distributed according to the normal curve, or on small samples. These tests include, but are not limited to, the Mann-Whitney U, Kruskall-Wallis, chi-square, Spearman rho correlation, and Wilcoxon tests.

non-response bias: In survey research when those responding to a questionnaire are not representative of non-responders. The non-respondents may have significantly different knowledge, attitudes, practices, or opinions from those who responded to the survey.

normal curve: A bell-shaped curve that describes a mathematical probability distribution of a population where most scores cluster around the mean. Also known as a *Gaussian distribution*.

norm-referenced test: A test used to assess the degree of achievement, aptitude, capacity, interest, or attitude compared to established norms or standard scores based on a population.

null hypothesis (H$_0$): A statement by the researcher that predicts no statistically significant differences between groups or relationships between variables. For example, "There is no statistically significant difference between exercise and splinting in reducing spasticity in children with cerebral palsy."

O

objective psychological test: Standardized test that contains comparative norms for interpreting individual raw scores.

observational study: Descriptive study that examines groups at one or more points in time without allocation of an intervention.

observed statistical value: The value obtained from applying a statistical formula to the data of a study. These values, such as t or F observed, are compared to the critical value that is derived from a statistical table to allow the decision to reject the null hypothesis or not.

one-tailed test of statistical significance: Used when a researcher makes a directional hypothesis that there will be a statistically significant difference between groups or predicts the direction of a correlation.

open-ended questions: Used in survey research. The investigator elicits attitudes, beliefs, and emotions from participants by asking questions that cannot be answered by *yes* or *no*, or by the selection from a limited set of options. The opposite of an open-ended question is a closed-ended question.

operational definition of variable: Specific test, procedure, or set of criteria that defines independent or dependent variables. This definition is crucial for replicating a study or in evaluating a group of studies such as through a meta-analysis.

operationalization: The process by which a non-measurable phenomena is defined by, and its existence denoted by other phenomena. This strategy is more common in psychology, physics, and social and life sciences.

ordinal logistic regression: Logistic regression used to quantify the association between one or more independent variables and an ordinal outcome.

ordinal scale of measurement: Classification of values of a variable into rank order, such as the degree of anxiety, academic achievement, or grade level. The classification defines which group is first, second, third, and so forth; however, it does not define the distance between categories.

ordinal variable: Variable having categories with an implicit ranking.

outcome measure: The specific test or procedure to measure the dependent variable. For example, an outcome measure for pain is the McGill-Melzack Pain Inventory.

outlier: A test result or score outside the normal range of values.

P

paired *t*-test (or correlated *t*-test): Used to compare two paired (dependent) samples where the outcome measure is continuous and normally distributed.

parameter: A descriptive value assigned to a condition in a population. Parameters are set at any given point in time, such as the age characteristics of a specified population.

parametric statistical tests: Inferential statistics that are based on certain assumptions, such as a normal distribution of variable values, equal number of participants in groups, homogeneity of variance, and independence of data.

participatory action research: An approach to action research emphasizing participation and action by members of communities affected by that research. It seeks to understand the world by trying to change it, collaboratively and following reflection.

Pearson product-moment correlation: An inferential test used to determine whether there is a statistically significant linear association between two variables. The derived r coefficient can range from +1.00 (a perfect correlation), to 0.00 (no correlation), to -1.00 (a perfect negative or inverse correlation).

peer checking or debriefing: Consulting colleagues or experts who can objectively review the research methodology to ensure validity of results and lack of bias.

percentage: The number of cases per hundred.

percentile: Value in a distribution below which a given percentage of the cases fall. For example, the 80th percentile is the point where 80% of the cases are at that point or below.

performance test: A test of an individual's skill to enact a task, such as grip strength, range of motion, manual dexterity, or driving skills.

personal equation in measurement: The effect of the presence of the tester on the participant's performance. The tester, as the evaluator, is a variable in the test situation and, if uncontrolled, can distort the test results.

phenomenology: A qualitative research method to understand and analyze a particular experience or event from the participants' perspective.

pilot study: A research study usually with a small number of participants that is innovative but that does not control for all extraneous variables. The primary advantage of a pilot study is that it generates further research.

placebo effect: A confounding variable that occurs when the participant shows signs of improvement or in the reduction of symptoms that is not caused by the intervention under study. It is instead caused by the participant 's belief that an intervention is causing improvement even though the participant is receiving a "dummy" or "sham" intervention. The placebo effect was initially observed in drug studies where an experimental drug was compared to a placebo or nonactive drug. Researchers observed that some of the subjects receiving a placebo improved.

population (N): An entire collection of people (e.g., the entire University of South Dakota student body).

positive correlation: A relationship between two variables where high scores on one variable are associated with high scores on the other, as well as low scores on one with low scores on the other.

post-testing: Testing after the intervention has taken place.

postulate: An unproven, foundational assumption.

power: The ability of a study to detect a difference when one exists; probability of rejecting the null hypothesis when it is false.

predictive validity: The degree to which a test or measuring instrument can predict future performance, functioning, or behavior. For example, a test for performance of ADLs administered during an in-patient stay has good predictive validity in its estimation of ADL performance at home after discharge.

pre-testing: Testing before intervention is applied.

prevalence rate: The number of individuals with a disability or disease divided by the total individuals in a population. For example, the prevalence rate of spinal cord injury in the United States in 2014 is the number of individuals with spinal cord injury living in the United States in 2014 divided by the total population in the United States in 2014.

primary prevention: The prevention of the initial onset of a disease, such as the prevention of polio with a vaccination.

primary source: Published article or conference proceedings that is the original report of data, such as an empirical research study or a theoretical paper.

probability: The mathematical or statistical likelihood that an event will occur.

probability distribution: A description of the probability associated with all possible observed outcomes.

Probability value (p): The probability that the results found were the result of chance and not an actual difference in value. A smaller p-value allows for greater confidence in rejecting the null hypothesis of no difference. For example, $p < .01$ allows more confidence than $p < .05$, and $p < .001$ more than $p < .01$. Also known as *significance*.

problem-oriented research: Applied research initiated by the investigator identifying a significant problem, such as a rapid increase in attention deficit disorders in children or the dramatic rise of individuals who are homeless in urban areas. The research design addresses the problem directly.

Procrustean Bed: Applying an intervention as a panacea for all patients regardless of individual differences and needs. For example, applying a paraffin bath to all patients with arthritis, without regard to the specific needs of individual patients. In this approach, the patient is fitted to the intervention rather than the intervention being selected as the best indicated for this individual.

prolonged engagement: A strategy where researchers place themselves within the actual study to build trust with the participants and to increase the credibility of results.

proportion: Fraction in which the numerator consists of a subset of individuals represented in the denominator.

prospective study: Research that is future oriented and attempts to discover cause-effect relationships between variables. In prospective studies, the investigator manipulates or observes an independent variable that is predicted to affect function or performance and then collects data. Experimental or longitudinal research are examples of prospective designs.

purposive sampling: Selective or nonobjective selection of participants.

p-value: The level of significance, or the risk of making a Type I error when the null hypothesis is rejected. In the social sciences, it is usually established at the .05 or .01 (alpha) level.

Q

qualitative research: Study of people and events in their natural setting. This type of research uses multimodal methods in a naturalistic setting. The researcher using qualitative research methods seeks to explore perceptions and experiences to understand phenomena in terms of the meanings that people ascribe to them. Data sources for this type of research include interviews with open-ended questions, prolonged participant observation, and document analysis.

qualitative variable: Variable that describes attributes (ordinal or nominal).

quantitative research: The application of the scientific method to test hypotheses. The quantitative researcher begins with a testable hypothesis, collects data, and uses statistical analyses to decide whether to accept or reject the hypothesis. Objectivity of the researcher, operational definitions of the variables, and control of extraneous factors are the key points in quantitative research.

quantitative variable: Variable that describes an amount or quantity (continuous or ratio).

quartile: A point in a distribution where 25% of the cases fall at or below that point. Quartiles are values that divide a set of data into four equal parts.

quasi-experimental designs: A term defined by Campbell and Stanley (1963) to identify research studies in which participants are not randomly assigned to equivalent groups. In general, most clinical research studies are within the quasi-experimental model because it is almost impossible to truly select a random sample from a target population or to have truly equivalent experimental and control groups.

quota sampling: Non-random sampling where the researcher tries to maintain proportional groups such as in a population of 60% female vs. 40% male; in this case, the quota sample would reflect this proportion.

R

r: Pearson correlation coefficient.

r^2: A statistic that is associated with a regression model and represents the portion of the observed variance that is accounted for by the regression model. The higher the r^2 value, the better the regression model is at defining the relationship between the independent and dependent variables.

random assignment: Assigning participants to multiple groups with each participant having an equal chance of being selected for any one of the groups.

random errors: The effect of uncontrolled variables in an experiment, such as unexpected events, test procedural errors, and anxiety within the participant. These errors are unpredictable and unsystematic.

random sample: An unbiased portion of a target population that has been selected by chance, such as through random numbers.

randomization: A process that involves selecting a participant or entity for a specific assignment with no predetermined bias, that is, through chance.

randomized controlled trial (RCT): A prospective study where participants are randomly assigned to either an intervention group or a control group, thereby avoiding administrator bias.

range: A measure of variability that is the difference between the highest and lowest values in a distribution of scores.

rank order variables: Examples of ordinal scale measurement in which ranks are assigned in measuring a variable. Most personality tests, such as the Minnesota Multiphasic Personality Inventory, measure rank order variables.

rating scale: An evaluator's appraisal regarding variables such as competence, nonacademic qualities in students, or patient behavior in a psychiatric hospital.

ratio scale of measurement: Quantification of a variable that includes equal intervals and an absolute zero point, such as in measuring heart rate, height, and weight. Comparative statements using "twice as" or "half" are possible with ratio scales.

referral source: A database that lists journal articles and books (e.g., Index Medicus), and information retrieval systems accessed by computer (e.g., OT Search, ERIC, MedLine, email, news lists).

regression analysis: Statistical method used to describe the association between one dependent variable and one or more independent variables; used to adjust for confounding variables.

regression line: A figure that best describes the linear relationship between the X and Y variables. In a high correlation, the researcher is able to predict the unknown value of Y from the known value of X with a certain high level of confidence.

regression to the mean: When an initial very high or very low score usually comes closer to the group mean upon re-measurement.

relative frequency: The ratio of the number of observations having a certain characteristic or value divided by the total number of observations.

reliability: A measure of the consistency of a test instrument. For example, a test has high reliability if it produces consistent results when measuring a variable. Threats to test reliability include ambiguity in the questions and poor implementation of exact test procedures. Reliability is indicated by the correlation coefficient (*r*). An acceptable test reliability is usually an *r* of .7 or above.

repeated measures analysis of variance: Measurements are made repeatedly on each participant (e.g., before, during, and after an intervention). Repeated measures ANOVAs are suited for 2 x 2 (or larger) designs where one or both factors are repeated or where there are repeated factors in a 1 x *n* design.

repeated measures designs: The replication of observations of the effects of interventions over a period of time (e.g., measuring the effects of biofeedback in reducing anxiety after meditation or exercise).

replicate a research design: To carry out a research design for the second time by replicating the research methodology. The purposes are to strengthen generalizability of the findings and to confirm the internal validity of the original study.

representative sample: An unbiased portion of a target population that is representative in terms of demographic characteristics.

research: The systematic and unbiased investigation into a topic by stating a hypothesis, guiding question, or purpose and collecting primary data. It includes quantitative and qualitative designs.

research question (or purpose of the study): The central question that should be answered by the research. A good research article has this labeled clearly, either at the beginning or after reviewing some literature.

response rate: The number and proportion of responses to a researcher's questionnaire or survey. If a researcher sends surveys to 100 people, and 89 respond, then the response rate is 89%.

retrospective study: Research based on causative factors that have already occurred. For example, in a correlational study the researcher may want to examine the relationship between the onset of emphysema and previous smoking behavior. Both variables have already occurred. The researcher tries to reconstruct events and to hypothesize regarding a possible cause-effect relationship. Retrospective research can be used to justify experimental designs to further investigate cause-effect relationships.

rigor: Refers to the systematic control of variables that may affect the results of a study.

risk-benefit ratio: Estimation by the investigator of the possible risks to the research participant and the benefits accrued from the study. The researcher reveals the potential risks and benefits to prospective participants in the study through an informed consent form.

risk of bias assessment (sometimes called "quality assessment" or "critical appraisal"): Helps to establish transparency of evidence synthesis results and findings. A risk of bias assessment is a defining element of systematic reviews and often performed for each included study in the review.

S

sample (n): A subset of a population. For example, a random sample of occupational therapy students from the University of South Dakota.

sampling error: The error that results from estimating a population value from a sample.

scales of measurement: The level at which a test or instrument measures a specific variable such as intelligence, behavior, personality, muscle strength, or academic achievement. Traditionally, scales of measurement are classified into four levels: nominal, ordinal, interval, and ratio.

scattergram, scatter diagram, scatterplot: A figure describing the relationship between the X and Y variables, where pairs of values are plotted as points on a two-dimensional graph.

scientific law: A statement of consistent and uniform occurrences that are predictable (e.g., Mendelian law of genetic determination predicts characteristics of offspring when genetic traits of parents are known).

scientific method: Non-biased, systematic investigation into a subject by stating a hypothesis, collecting empirical data, and considering alternative explanations of the results.

scoping review: A type of knowledge synthesis that uses a systematic and iterative approach to identify and synthesize an existing or emerging body of literature on a given topic.

secondary prevention: The prevention of the recurrence of a disease, such as preventing a second stroke in an individual.

secondary source: A published article or book that reviews primary sources, such as a literature review.

selection bias: Participants selected for a research study are selected in a non-random method and may not be representative of the target population.

self-evaluation method: Participants in a clinical research study assess their own progress. Self-evaluation is an important factor in assessing intervention effectiveness. Other methods used in assessing effectiveness include objective tests, psychophysiological measures, and mechanical procedures.

self-fulfilling prophecy: The expectation by the researcher or rater that a participant will perform at a certain level based on prejudice or bias toward the group to which the participant belongs.

semantic differential: An attitude scale in which the respondent rates concepts such as good-bad, fast-slow, and hard-soft.

semi-structured interview: A qualitative research method that combines a pre-determined set of open questions (questions that prompt discussion) with the opportunity for the interviewer to explore particular themes or responses further.

sensitivity: As applied to test measurement, it is the degree to which a test or assessment measures what it purports to measure. This is also known as *true positive rate*. The reliability and validity of a test instrument would impact its sensitivity to measure a variable. *See also* specificity.

sensitivity check (in meta-analysis): The examination of the extent to which the findings of a meta-analysis are subject to undue influence from a single study.

significance: The probability that the results presented are a result of chance and not an actual difference in values. A smaller significance allows for greater confidence in rejecting the null hypothesis of no difference. Also known as *probability value* or *p-value.*

significance level: In testing a hypothesis, it is the predetermined level of confidence required in order to reject the null hypothesis (alpha level), usually .05 or .01.

simple linear regression: Regression analysis used to quantify the association between one independent variable and a continuous outcome that is normally distributed.

simple logistic regression: Regression analysis used to quantify the association between one independent variable and a dichotomous outcome.

single-case experimental design (SCED): Research design that systematically compares the performance of a participant under experimental and control conditions. It may include more than one participant, but comparisons are made only within each participant's performance. Common designs include ABA and ABAB, where A is the baseline condition and B is the experimental (intervention) condition. Not be confused with a case study.

skewed distribution: A distribution of values that is not symmetric (i.e., not bell-shaped).

- **positively skewed:** Data are distributed such that a greater proportion of the observations have values less than or equal to the mean (i.e., more observations with lower values).

- **negatively skewed:** Data are distributed such that a greater proportion of the observations have values greater than or equal to the mean (i.e., more observations with higher values).

skewness: An indication in a frequency polygon of the asymmetry of a distribution. A distribution can be skewed to the right or left side of the polygon.

slope: The linear direction and angle of a line. It is calculated in the regression line.

snowball or cascading sampling: A recruitment technique in which research participants are asked to assist researchers in identifying other potential subjects

Spearman rank correlation: Nonparametric test used on two ordinal variables to determine the degree of relationship between them. It is an alternative to the Pearson product-moment correlation coefficient (*r*). Also called *Spearman rho.*

specificity: The ability of a test to accurately identify individuals without a specific disease. This is also known as a test's *true negative rate. See also* sensitivity.

split-half reliability: A method to estimate the degree of consistency in a test by correlating one half of the test items, such as even numbered items, with the other half of the test, the odd numbered items.

standard deviation (SD): Statistical measure of the variability of scores from the mean. This is one measure of dispersion or variability. The larger the standard deviation, the more varied the data. Standard deviation equals the square root of the variance.

standard error of measurement (SEM or SE_m): statistical value that indicates the band of error surrounding a test score. For example, a raw score of 90 with an SEM of 4 indicates a true score probably ranging from 86 to 94.

standard score: Calculated by subtracting a raw score from the mean and then dividing the difference by the standard deviation. The sign of the standard score is positive if above the mean or negative if below the mean.

standardized test: A test that has been administered to a target population and for which norms are available.

statistical assumptions: Conditions in research required for a specific statistical test. These assumptions relate to distribution shape of scores, variability of scores, scale of measurement, sample size, and independence of samples.

statistical pie: A descriptive statistic using the circumference of a circle to describe the percentage of cases for each category within a frequency distribution.

statistical sample: A portion of a target population selected to represent the population in an unbiased way.

statistical significance: Probability of the result of a statistical test occurring by chance. For example, a *p* level of 0.01 means that you can be 99% confident that these results did not happen due to chance. Most researchers in occupational therapy accept the .05 level of statistical significance (95% confidence interval).

stem-and-leaf display: Descriptive data analysis that orders and organizes data to display trends and patterns in a distribution. The stem contains the first digit or digits of each observation and the leaf contains the remaining digit or digits of each observation.

survey research: Systematic and objective investigation into the characteristics, attitudes, opinions, and behaviors of target populations through questionnaires or interviews.

systematic review: A comprehensive literature search that tries to answer a focused research question using existing research as evidence. Systematic reviews are a type of literature review of research which require equivalent standards of rigour as primary research. They have a clear, logical rationale that is reported to the reader of the review. They are used in research and policymaking to inform evidence-based decisions and practice.

systematic evidence review: Attempts to find all published and unpublished evidence related to a specific research or policy question, using literature search methodologies designed to be transparent, unbiased, and reproducible.

T

target population: An identified group from which a representative or random sample of participants is selected.

tertiary prevention: The prevention of secondary problems that can result from a disability (e.g., preventing decubiti in individuals with spinal cord injury).

test battery: A group of tests selected to comprehensively measure an individual's capacity (e.g., performance, vocational interests, attitudes, cognition).

test-retest reliability: A method to estimate the degree of consistency of a test. In this method, a test is readministered to the same group of participants after a short period of time. Maturation and changes in the subjects can affect the results and must be considered by the investigator.

theory: A comprehensive model that attempts to explain, for example, how individuals contract and resist disease, learn motoric tasks, or develop cognitive and language functions.

time series research: In experimental research, time series research indicates the measurement of the dependent variable over time intervals (e.g., 2 weeks or 3 months). Its purpose is to evaluate the effect of several interventions or techniques with the same participant or group.

transferability: Refers to whether the results can be generalized to other settings or populations.

transformational research: The use of research as a personal-political activity whereby the research participants become empowered by active engagement in the research process.

treatment effects: In experimental research, the application of the independent variable in producing a desired or predicted outcome (e.g., the use of sensory integration therapy in reducing tactile defensiveness).

treatment protocols: Operational definitions of the methods used by practitioners. The procedure is described in enough detail so that replication is possible. Treatment protocols should be influenced by research findings and are a component of evidence-based practice.

triangulation: The use of multiple approaches in collecting data. For example, in measuring a variable such as functional independence, the investigator would use a standardized ADL scale, make observations in a naturalistic setting, and employ a self-report measure where the patient evaluates his or her performance in self-care activities.

***t*-tests**: Inferential statistics used to determine whether the difference between two means is statistically significant or is too likely to have occurred by chance. They include one-sample *t*-test, independent *t*-test, and correlated or paired-data *t*-test. For testing two independent groups with approximately the same variance, the formula is:

$$t = \frac{mean_1 - mean_2}{\textit{standard error of the difference between the means}}$$

Type I error: The error that results when the null hypothesis is rejected when it is really true; stating there is a difference in outcome when none exists. It is analogous to a false positive in medicine when a physician diagnoses a disease when that disease is not present.

Type II error: The error that results when the null hypothesis is not rejected when it is really false; stating there is no difference in outcome when one actually exists. It is analogous to a false negative in medicine when a physician fails to detect a disease when that disease is present.

U

unobtrusive methodology: A research method in which the investigator collects data from indirect sources, such as patient records, historical documents, letters, and relics.

unpaired (independent) sample: Study design that compares the outcome of two groups where the groups are not matched on any characteristic.

V

validity: As pertaining to measurement, it refers to the degree to which a test or measuring instrument actually measures what it purports to measure. Validity can also refer to the rigor of an experiment in controlling extraneous variables (internal validity) and the generalizability of the results of a study to a target population (external validity).

variability: *See* measures of variability.

variables: Characteristics, factors, or attributes that can be measured qualitatively or quantitatively. Variables can be homogeneous groups, such as physical therapy students, individuals with stroke, or hospital administrators. Variables can also be interventions, such as exercise or biofeedback, or outcomes, such as muscle strength, spasticity, functional capacity, or academic achievement.

variance: The average of each score's deviation from the mean. Variance is an intermediate value that is used in calculating the standard deviation. The variance is the square of the standard deviation. It is a measure of variability or dispersion.

verbatim transcription: A word-for-word literal transcription of a recording or a live event.

vocational interest test: A measure of an individual's preferences toward occupation-related tasks or jobs.

scores from the same participants, such as in before-and-after studies.

within subjects test: The scores of participants in an experimental study that are compared (e.g., pre- and post-intervention or by repeated measures on a test). Each participant is his or her own control.

work samples: Well-defined activities that are similar to an actual job task. Examples include Valpar and Micro-Tower.

W

Wilcoxon signed rank test for correlated samples: Nonparametric test and alternative to the correlated t-test when comparing matched participants or two sets of

Z

z-score: A score based on standard deviation units from the mean (e.g., a z-score of +1 is one standard deviation unit above the mean).

References

Ackerman, E. H. (1982). *A short history of medicine*. The Johns Hopkins University Press.

ACOTE. (2023, February). Draft 1 ACOTE Standards. Accreditation Council for Occupational Therapy Education Education Statards Rview Committee. https://acoteonline.org/accreditation-explained/standards/

Ad Hoc Document Development Committee. (2022). Occupational therapy doctoral capstone: Purpose and value. *American Journal of Occupational Therapy, 76*. doi.org/10.5014/ajot.2022.76S3004

Adamit, T., Shames, J., & Rand, D. (2021). Effectiveness of the functional and cognitive occupational therapy (FaC$_O$T) intervention for improving daily functioning and participation of individuals with mild stroke: A randomized controlled trial. *International Journal of Environmental Research and Public Health, 18*(15), 7988. doi.org/10.3390/ijerph18157988

Adler, P. A., & Adler, P. (1994). Observational techniques. In N. K. Denzin & Y. S. Lincoln (Eds.), *Handbook of qualitative research* (pp. 377–392). Sage Publications.

AERA, APA, & NCME. (2014). *Standards for educational and psychological testing*. American Educational Research Association.

AJOT. (2007). Accreditation standards for a doctoral-degree-level educational program for the occupational therapist. *American Journal of Occupational Therapy, 61*(6), 641–651. https://doi.org/10.5014/ajot.61.6.641

AJOT. (2018). 2018 Accreditation Council for Occupational Therapy Education (ACOTE®) standards and interpretive guide (effective July 31, 2020). *American Journal of Occupational Therapy, 72*(Supplement_2), 7212410005p1–7212410005p83. https://doi.org/10.5014/ajot.2018.72S217

Alve, Y. A., Islam, A., Hatlestad, B., & Mirza, M. P. (2023). Participation in everyday occupations among Rohingya refugees in Bangladeshi refugee camps. *The American Journal of Occupational Therapy, 77*(3), 7703205060. https://doi.org/10.5014/ajot.2023.050006

AMA Manual of Style Committee. (2020). *AMA manual of style: A guide for authors and editors*. Oxford University Press. https://doi.org/10.1093/jama/9780190246556.001.0001

American Occupational Therapy Association. (2014). Occupational therapy practice framework: Domain and process. *The American Journal of Occupational Therapy, 68*(Supplement_1), S1–S48. https://doi.org/10.5014/ajot.2014.682006

American Occupational Therapy Association. (2020). Occupational therapy practice framework: Domain and process (4th ed.). *American Journal of Occupational Therapy, 74*(Supplement_2). https://doi.org/10.5014/ajot.2020.74S2001

American Psychological Association. (1974). *Standards for educational & psychological tests*. APA.

American Psychological Association. (2020). *Publication manual of the American Psychological Association* (7th ed.). APA. http://doi.org/10.1027/0000165-000

Anderson, M. H., Bechtol, C. O., & Sollars, R. E. (1959). *Clinical prosthetics for physicians and therapists: A handbook of clinical practices related to artificial limbs*. Charles C. Thomas.

Anastasi, A., & Urbina, S. (1997). *Psychological testing* (7th ed.). Prentice Hall.

Angell, A. M., Goodman, L., Walker, H. R., McDonald, K. E., Kraus, L. E., Elms, E. H., Frieden, L., Sheth, A. J., & Hammel, J. (2020). "Starting to live a life": Understanding full participation for people with disabilities after institutionalization. *The American Journal of Occupational Therapy, 74*(4), 7404205030p1–7404205030p11. https://doi.org/10.5014/ajot.2020.040097

Anonymous. (2022). BestMedicalDegrees.com. www.bestmedical-degrees.com/30-of-the-oldest-medical-schools-in-the-world/

Anonymous. (2023a). How to order. www.pearsonassessments.com/professional-assessments/ordering/how-to-order/qualifications/qualifications-policy.html

Anonymous. (2023b). Student guide for Voice Thread. www.csuohio.edu/sites/default/files/Student_Guide_for_Voice_Thread.pdf

AOTA. (2006). TriAlliances addresses clinicians on cap exceptions process. *American Occupational Therapy Association*. www.aota.org/~/media/Corporate/Files/Advocacy/Reimb/News/Archives/Archived-Letters/Lymphedema%20letter%20to%20MedCAC.pdf

AOTA. (2023). *Representative Assembly definition of occupational therapy practice*. American Occupational Therapy Association. www.aota.org/community/volunteer-groups/representative-assembly-ra

Armstrong, M. J., & Okun, M. S. (2020). Diagnosis and treatment of Parkinson disease: A review. *JAMA, 323*(6), 548–560. https://doi.org/10.1001/jama.2019.22360

Aromataris, E., & Munn, Z. (Eds.). (2020). *Joanna Briggs Institute manual for evidence synthesis*. JBI. https://doi.org/10.46658/JBIMES-20-01

Atwater, E. C. (1973). The medical profession in a new society, Rochester, New York (1811–1860). *Bulletin of the History of Medicine, 47*(3), 221–235.

Ayres, A. J. (1972). *Sensory integration and praxis tests (SIPT)*. Western Psychological Services.

Ayres, A. J. (1973). *Sensory integration and learning disorders*. Western Psychological Services.

Babik, I., Cunha, A. B., & Lobo, M. A. (2021). Assistive and rehabilitative effects of the Playskin Lift™ exoskeletal garment on reaching and object exploration in children with arthrogryposis. *The American Journal of Occupational Therapy, 75*(1), 7501205110p1–7501205110p10. https://doi.org/10.5014/ajot.2020.040972

Bagatell, N., Lamarche, E., & Klinger, L. (2023). Roles of caregivers of autistic adults: A qualitative study. *The American Journal of Occupational Therapy, 77*(2), 7702205030. https://doi.org/10.5014/ajot.2023.050117

Bailliard, A. L. (2015). Habits of the sensory system and mental health: Understanding sensory dissonance. *The American Journal of Occupational Therapy, 69*(4), 6904250020p1–6904250020p8. doi.org/10.5014/ajot.2015.014977

Baker, N. A., & Tickle-Degnen, L. (2001). The effectiveness of physical, psychological, and functional interventions in treating clients with multiple sclerosis: A meta-analysis. *The American Journal of Occupational Therapy, 55*(3), 324–331. doi.org/10.5014/ajot.55.3.324

Bamm, E. L., Rosenbaum, P., Wilkins, S., Stratford, P., & Mahlberg, N. (2015). Exploring client-centered care experiences in in-patient rehabilitation settings. *Global Qualitative Nursing Research, 2,* 2333393015582030. doi.org/10.1177/2333393615000030

Bartnik, L. M., & Rice, M. S. (2013). Comparison of caregiver forces required for sliding a patient up in bed using an array of slide sheets. *Workplace Health & Safety, 61*(9), 393–400. doi.org/10.1177/216507991306100904

Barzun, J. (1974). *Clio and the doctors: Psycho-history, quanto-history, & history.* University of Chicago Press.

Bayley, N. (2006). *Bayley scales of infant and toddler development* (3rd ed.). Harcourt Assessment, Psych Corp.

Beall's List of Predatory Journals and Publishers. (2023). *Beallslist. net.* beallslist.weebly.com

Beard, J. D. (2008). Which is the best revascularization for critical limb ischemia: Endovascular or open surgery? *Journal of Vascular Surgery, 48*(6), 11S–16S. doi.org/10.1016/j.jvs.2008.08.036

Benham, S., Enam, N., & Ivaturi, S. (2022). A mindfulness program addressing sleep quality and stress: Transition to a telehealth format for higher education students during COVID-19. *International Journal of Telerehabilitation, 14*(1). doi:10.5195/ijt.2022.6439

Benison, S. (1972). The history of polio research in the United States: Appraisal and lessons. In G. Holton (Ed.), *The twentieth-century sciences: Studies in the biography of ideas* (pp. 308–343). W.W. Norton.

Bennett, A. E., Power, T. J., Eiraldi, R. B., Leff, S. S., & Blum, N. J. (2009). Identifying learning problems in children evaluated for ADHD: The academic performance questionnaire. *Pediatrics, 124*(4), e633–e639. doi:10.5195/ijt.2022.6439

Bennett, S., Laver, K., Voigt-Radloff, S., Letts, L., Clemson, L., Graff, M., Wiseman, J., & Gitlin, L. (2019). Occupational therapy for people with dementia and their family carers provided at home: A systematic review and meta-analysis. *BMJ Open, 9*(11), e026308. doi.org/10.1136/bmjopen-2018-026308

Bergström, A., Vik, K., Haak, M., Metzelthin, S., Graff, L., & Hjelle, K. M. (2023). The jigsaw puzzle of activities for mastering daily life; service recipients and professionals' perceptions of gains and changes attributed to reablement—A qualitative meta-synthesis. *Scandinavian Journal of Occupational Therapy, 30*(5), 604–615. doi.org/10.1080/11038128.2022.2081603

Bernard, C. (1957). *An introduction to the study of experimental medicine* (H. C. Greene, Trans.). Dover. (Original work published 1865)

Berndt, A., Hutchinson, C., Tepper, D., & George, S. (2022). Professional reasoning of occupational therapy driver rehabilitation interventions. *Australian Occupational Therapy Journal, 69*(4), 436–446. doi.org/10.1111/1440-1630.12804

Best, J. W. (1977). *Research in education* (3rd ed.). Prentice-Hall.

Best, J. W., & Kahn, J. V. (2016). *Research in education.* Pearson Education India.

Bettelheim, B. (1967). *The empty fortress: Infantile autism and the birth of the self.* The Free Press.

Bhandari, P. (2023, June 22). External validity: Definition, types, threats & examples. *Scribbr.* www.scribbr.com/methodology/external-validity/

Bockoven, J. S. (1971). Occupational therapy—A historical perspective: Legacy of moral treatment—1800s to 1910. *The American Journal of Occupational Therapy, 25*(5), 223–225.

Bono, G. L., Achermann, P., Rückriem, B., Lieber, J., & van Hedel, H. J. (2022). Goal-directed personalized upper limb intensive therapy (PULIT) for children with hemiparesis: A retrospective analysis. *The American Journal of Occupational Therapy, 76*(6). doi.org/10.5014/ajot.2022.049008

Bootes, K., & Chapparo, C. J. (2002). Cognitive and behavioural assessment of people with traumatic brain injury in the workplace: Occupational therapists' perceptions. *Work, 19*(3), 255–268.

Borgetto, B., Born, S., Bünemann-Geißler, D., Düchting, M., Kahrs, A., Kasper, N., Menzel, M., Netzband, A., Reichel, K., & Reßler, W. (2007). Die Forschungspyramide-Diskussionsbeitrag zur Evidenz-basierten Praxis in der Ergotherapie. *Ergoscience, 2*(2), 56–63. doi:10.1055/s-2007-963004

Boshoff, K., Bowen-Salter, H., Gibbs, D., Phillips, R. L., Porter, L., & Wiles, L. (2021). A meta-synthesis of how parents of children with autism describe their experience of accessing and using routine healthcare services for their children. *Health & Social Care in the Community, 29*(6), 1668–1682. doi.org/10.1111/hsc.13369

Bouteloup, Z., & Beltran, R. (2007). Application of the occupational adaptation framework in child and adolescent occupational therapy practice. A case study. *Australian Occupational Therapy Journal, 54*(3), 228–238. doi.org/10.1111/j.1440-1630.2007.00620.x

Brin, D. (n.d.). David Brin Quotes. BrainyQuote.com. www.brainyquote.com/authors/david-brin-quotes

Brown, C. L., & Finlayson, M. L. (2013). Performance measures rather than self-report measures of functional status predict home care use in community-dwelling older adults: Utiliser des mesures du rendement plutôt que des instruments d'autoévaluation des capacités fonctionnelles pour prédire l'utilisation des soins à domicile chez des aînés vivant dans la collectivité. *Canadian Journal of Occupational Therapy, 80*(5), 284–294. doi.org/10.1177/0008417413501467

Brown, C., Geiszler, L. C., Lewis, K. J., & Arbesman, M. (2018). Effectiveness of interventions for weight loss for people with serious mental illness: A systematic review and meta-analysis. *The American Journal of Occupational Therapy, 72*(5), 7205190030p1–7205190030p9. doi.org/10.5014/ajot.2018.033415

Bureau of Labor Statistics, US Department of Labor. (2022). *Occupational outlook handbook.* www.bls.gov/ooh/Burgess, J., Wenborn, J., Di Bona, L., Orrell, M., & Poland, F. (2021). Taking part in the community occupational therapy in dementia UK intervention from the perspective of people with dementia, family carers and occupational therapists: A qualitative study. *Dementia, 20*(6), 2057–2076. doi: 10.1177/1471301220981240

Burke, H. (2022, April 14). Top 10 new medical technologies 2022. *Proclinical.* www.proclinical.com/blogs/2022-4/top-10-new-medical-technologies-2022

Cannon, W. B. (1932). *The wisdom of the body.* W.W. Norton & Company.

Carrera, P., Boshoff, K., Wiles, L., Phillips, R., Gibbs, D., & Porter, L. (2023). Understanding parents' experiences with mainstream schooling for their children with autism spectrum disorder: A meta-analysis. *The American Journal of Occupational Therapy, 77*(4). doi: 10.5014/ajot.2023.050025

Carter, N., Bryant-Lukosius, D., DiCenso, A., Blythe, J., & Neville, A. J. (2014). The use of triangulation in qualitative research. *Oncol Nurs Forum, 41*(5), 545–547. doi: 10.1188/14.ONF.545-547

Case-Smith, J. (1995). The relationships among sensorimotor components, fine motor skill, and functional performance in preschool children. *The American Journal of Occupational Therapy, 49*(7), 645–652. doi: 10.5014/ajot.49.7.645

Case-Smith, J., O'Brien, J. C., & Miller-Kuhaneck, H. (2020). *Case-Smith's occupational therapy for children and adolescents* (8th ed.). Elsevier.

Cavalera, C., Rovaris, M., Mendozzi, L., Pugnetti, L., Garegnani, M., Castelnuovo, G., Molinari, E., & Pagnini, F. (2018). Online meditation training for people with multiple sclerosis: A randomized controlled trial. *Multiple Sclerosis Journal, 25*, 610–617. doi.org/10.1177/1352458518761187

CDC. (2023). *Center for Disease Control and Prevention.* www.cdc.gov/

Chang, L. H., Chen, P. Y., Wang, J., Shih, B. H., & Tseng, Y. H., Mao, H. F. (2021). High-ecological cognitive intervention to improve cognitive skills and cognitive-functional performance for older adults with mild cognitive impairment. *The American Journal of Occupational Therapy, 75*(5), 7505205050. doi: 10.5014/ajot.2021.041996

Chang, P., Tsai, K., Richard, C., Davidson, H. A., & Hersch, G. (2023). Rest and sleep patterns and activities of residents in long-term care facilities: A descriptive study. *The Open Journal of Occupational Therapy, 11*(1), 1–7. doi.org/10.15453/2168-6408.2000

Chen, X., Liu, F., Lin, S., Yu, L., & Lin, R. (2022). Effects of virtual reality rehabilitation training on cognitive function and activities of daily living of patients with poststroke cognitive impairment: A systematic review and meta-analysis. *Archives of Physical Medicine and Rehabilitation, 103*(7), 1422–1435. doi: 10.1016/j.apmr.2022.03.012

Chilton, R. L., Weaver, J. A., Doerrer, S., & Ideishi, R. (2022). Addressing OT practitioners' knowledge and attitudes about older adult sexual health and sexual activity through continuing education. *The American Journal of Occupational Therapy, 76*(Supplement_1), 7610505107p1. doi.org/10.5014/ajot.2022.76S1-PO107

Christensen, C. B. (2008). *Self and world: From analytic philosophy to phenomenology.* Walter de Gruyter.

Christiansen, C. H., Clark, F., Kielhofner, G., & Rogers, J. (1995). Position paper: Occupation. American occupational therapy association. *The American Journal of Occupational Therapy: Official Publication of the American Occupational Therapy Association, 49*(10), 1015–1018.

Clark, F. (1993). Occupation embedded in a real life: Interweaving occupational science and occupational therapy. *The American Journal of Occupational Therapy, 47*(12), 1067–1078. doi: 10.5014/ajot.47.12.1067

Clarke, G. N., Rohde, P., Lewinsohn, P. M., Hops, H., & Seeley, J. R. (1999). Cognitive-behavioral treatment of adolescent depression: Efficacy of acute group treatment and booster sessions. *Journal of the American Academy of Child & Adolescent Psychiatry, 38*(3), 272–279. doi: 10.1097/00004583-199903000-00014

Coburn, K. L., Kurtz, M. R., Rivera, D., & Kana, R. K. (2022). Behavioral and neurobiological evidence for the effects of reading interventions on autistic children: A systematic review. *Neuroscience and Biobehavior Review, 139*, 104748. doi: 10.1016/j.neubiorev.2022.104748

Cohen, J. (1988). *Statistical power analysis for the behavioral sciences* (2nd ed.). Erlbaum.

Creswell, J. W., & Creswell, J. D. (2023). *Research design: Qualitative, quantitative, and mixed methods approaches* (6th ed.). Sage Publications.

Crocker, M. D., MacKay-Lyons, M., & McDonnell, E. (1997). Forced use of the upper extremity in cerebral palsy: A single-case design. *The American Journal of Occupational Therapy, 51*(10), 824–833. doi: 10.5014/ajot.51.10.824

Crowther, J. G., Whiddington, R., & Sutton, R. M. (1949). Science at war. *Physics Today, 2*(2), 29–37.

Dallas, M. E. (2021, September 10). The 10 most common surgeries in the US. *Healthgrades.* www.healthgrades.com/right-care/tests-and-procedures/the-10-most-common-surgeries-in-the-u-s

Daniels, L. (1956). *Muscle testing: Techniques of manual examination* (2nd ed.). Saunders.

DARPA. (2023). Revolutionizing prosthetics. *Defence Advanced Research Project Agency.* www.darpa.mil/program/revolutionizing-prosthetics

Davidson, M., Kapara, O., Goldberg, S., Yoffe, R., Noy, S., & Weiser, M. (2015). A nation-wide study on the percentage of schizophrenia and bipolar disorder patients who earn minimum wage or above. *Schizophrenia Bulletin, 42*(2), 443–447.

Deno, S. L. (1985). Curriculum-based measurement: The emerging alternative. *Exceptional Children, 52*(3), 219–232. doi: 10.1177/001440298505200303

Denzin, N. K. (1994). Introduction: Entering the field of qualitative research. *Handbook of Qualitative Research.* Sage.

Dépelteau, A., Lagueux, É., Pagé, R., & Hudon, C. (2021). Occupational adaptation of people living with fibromyalgia: A systematic review and thematic synthesis. *The American Journal of Occupational Therapy, 75*(4), 7504190040. doi: 10.5014/ajot.2021.047134

DePoy, E., & Gitlin, L. N. (2019). *Introduction to research e-book: Understanding and applying multiple strategies.* Elsevier Health Sciences.

Dial, J. G. (1986). The McCarron-Dial system—an approach to clinical, vocational, and educational evaluation. http://eric.ed.gov/ERICWebPortal/detail?accno=ED171739

Dickerson, A. E., & Brown, L. E. (2007). Pediatric constraint-induced movement therapy in a young child with minimal active arm movement. *The American Journal of Occupational Therapy, 61*(5), 563–573. doi: 10.5014/ajot.61.5.563

Dickinson, D., Tenhula, W., Morris, S., Brown, C., Peer, J., Spencer, K., Li, L., Gold, J. M., & Bellack, A. S. (2010). A randomized, controlled trial of computer-assisted cognitive remediation for schizophrenia. *American Journal of Psychiatry, 167*(2), 170–180. doi: 10.1176/appi.ajp.2009.09020264

Ding, R., & Logemann, J. A. (2000). Pneumonia in stroke patients: A retrospective study. *Dysphagia, 15*, 51–57. doi.org/10.1007/s004550010001

Division of HIV/AIDS Prevention. (2014). HIV surveillance report. *Centers for Disease Control and Prevention.* www.cdc.gov/hiv/library/reports/surveillance/

Doarn, C. R., McVeigh, F., & Poropatich, R. (2010). Innovative new technologies to identify and treat traumatic brain injuries: Crossover technologies and approaches between military and civilian applications. *Telemedicine Journal and E-Health: The Official Journal of the American Telemedicine Association, 16*(3), 373–381. doi: 10.1089/tmj.2010.0009

Doig, E., Fleming, J., Cornwell, P. L., & Kuipers, P. (2009). Qualitative exploration of a client-centered, goal-directed approach to community-based occupational therapy for adults with traumatic brain injury. *The American Journal of Occupational Therapy: Official Publication of the American Occupational Therapy Association, 63*(5), 559–568. doi: 10.5014/ajot.63.5.559

Dole, J. E., Baker, N., & Roll, S. C. (2021). Carpal tunnel treatment options: Developing consolidated guidelines for best practice—a meta-synthesis. *The American Journal of Occupational Therapy, 75*(S2), 7512510275–7512510275p1. doi: 10.5014/ajot.2021.75S2-RP275

Downer, A. H. (1988). *Physical therapy procedures* (4th ed.). Thomas.

Dubos, R. (1959). *Mirage of health: Utopias, progress, and biological change.* Rutgers University Press.

Dunn, L. M. (1968). Special education for the mildly retarded—Is much of it justifiable? *Exceptional Children, 35*(1), 5–22.

Eaton, S. E. (2023, March 4). Artificial intelligence and academic integrity, post-plagiarism. *University World News.* www.universityworldnews.com/post.php?story=20230228133041549

Ellis, H., & Abdalla, S. (2019). *A history of surgery* (3rd ed.). CRC Press. https://doi.org/10.1201/9780429461743

Epps, S., & Tindal, G. (1987). The effectiveness of differential programming in serving students with mild handicaps: Placement options and instructional programming. *Handbook of Special Education: Research and Practice, 1*, 213–248.

Escalona-Noguero, C., López-Valls, M., & Sot, B. (2021). CRISPR/CAS technology as a promising weapon to combat viral infections. *Bioessays, 43*(4), 2000315.

Espín-Tello, S. M., Dickinson, H. O., Bueno-Lozano, M., Jiménez-Bernadó, M. T., & Caballero-Navarro, A. L. (2018). Functional capacity and self-esteem of people with cerebral palsy. *The American Journal of Occupational Therapy, 72*(3), 7203205120p1–7203205120p8. doi: 10.5014/ajot.2018.025940

FDA. (2019, October). Regulated products and facilities. *FDA at a Glance.* www.fda.gov/media/131874/download

Ferguson, P. M., Ferguson, D., & Taylor, S. J. (1992). *Interpreting disability: A qualitative reader*. Teachers College Press.

Ferguson, G. A., & Takane, Y. (1989). *Statistical analysis in psychology and education* (6th ed.). McGraw-Hill.

Finlayson, K. W., & Dixon, A. (2008). Qualitative meta-synthesis: A guide for the novice. *Nurse Researcher, 15*(2), 59–71. https://doi.org/10.7748/nr2008.01.15.2.59.c6330

Fleming, M. H. (1991). The therapist with the three-track mind. *The American Journal of Occupational Therapy, 45*(11), 1007–1014. doi: 10.5014/ajot.45.11.1007

Flick, U., & Metzler, K. (2014). *The Sage handbook of qualitative data analysis* (1st ed.). Sage Publications. https://doi.org/10.4135/9781446282243

Fogel, Y., Rosenblum, S., & Barnett, A. L. (2022). Handwriting legibility across different writing tasks in school-aged children. *Hong Kong Journal of Occupational Therapy, 35*(1), 44–51. https://doi.org/10.1177/15691861221075709

Ford, A. R., Smith, D. L., & Banister, G. E. (2021). Recruitment and retention of occupational therapy practitioners and students of color: A qualitative study. *The American Journal of Occupational Therapy, 75*(1), 7501205150p1–7501205150p8.

Forness, S. R., & Kavale, K. A. (1984). Education of the mentally retarded: A note on policy. *Education and Training of the Mentally Retarded, 19*(4), 239–245. www.jstor.org/stable/23877265

Fox, V., & Bailliard, A. L. (2021). Liminal space of first-episode psychosis: Health management and its effect on social participation. *The American Journal of Occupational Therapy, 75*(6), 7506205090. https://doi.org/10.5014/ajot.2021.046953

Fraenkel, J. R., Wallen, N. E., & Hyun, H. H. (2012). *How to design and evaluate research in education*. McGraw-Hill.

Frank, G. (1992). Opening feminist histories of occupational therapy. *The American Journal of Occupational Therapy, 46*(11), 989–999. doi: 10.5014/ajot.46.11.989

Frank, G., Bernardo, C. S., Tropper, S., Noguchi, F., Lipman, C., Maulhardt, B., & Weitze, L. (1997). Jewish spirituality through actions in time: Daily occupations of young Orthodox Jewish couples in Los Angeles. *The American Journal of Occupational Therapy, 51*(3), 199–206. doi: 10.5014/ajot.51.3.199

Frankenburg, W. K., Dodds, J., Archer, P., Bresnick, B., Maschka, P., Edelman, N., & Shapiro, H. (1990). *Denver Developmental Screening Test II*. Denver Developmental Materials.

Frankenburg, W. K., Dodds, J., Archer, P., Shapiro, H., & Bresnick, B. (1992). The Denver II: A major revision and restandardization of the Denver Developmental Screening Test. *Pediatrics, 89*(1), 91–97. doi: 10.1542/peds.89.1.91

Freeman, D. (1983). *Margaret Mead and Samoa: The making and unmaking of an anthropological myth*. Australian National University Press.

French, S. (Ed.). (1994). *On equal terms: Working with disabled people*. Oxford: Butterworth/Heinemann.

Frey, J. H., & Fontana, A. (1991). The group interview in social research. *The Social Science Journal, 28*(2), 175–187. doi: 10.1016/0362-3319(91)90003-M

Friedland, J., & Silva, J. (2008). Evolving identities: Thomas Bessell Kidner and occupational therapy in the United States. *The American Journal of Occupational Therapy, 62*(3), 349–360. doi: 10.5014/ajot.62.3.349

Fuchs, D., Fuchs, L. S., & Fernstrom, P. (1993). A conservative approach to special education reform: Mainstreaming through transenvironmental programming and curriculum-based measurement. *American Educational Research Journal, 30*(1), 149–177. https://doi.org/10.3102/0002831203000114

Gagnier, J. J., Kienle, G., Altman, D. G., Moher, D., Sox, H., & Riley, D. (2013). The CARE guidelines: consensus-based clinical case reporting guideline development. *Global Advances in Health and Medicine, 2*(5), 38–43. https://doi.org/10.1136/bcr-2013-201554

García-Pérez, P., Rodríguez-Martínez, M. d. C., Lara, J. P., & Cruz-Cosme, C. d. l. (2021). Early occupational therapy intervention in the hospital discharge after stroke. *International Journal of Environmental Research and Public Health, 18*(24), 12877. https://doi.org/10.3390/ijerph182412877

Geertz, C. (1973). *The interpretation of cultures* (Vol. 5019). Basic Books.

Gesell, A. (1928a). The control of developmental observation. In *Infancy and human growth* (pp. 23–55). MacMillan Co. https://doi.org/10.1037/14664-002

Gesell, A. (1928b). *Infancy and human growth*. Macmillan.

Gesell, A., Thompson, H., & Amatruda, C. S. (1934). *Infant behavior: Its genesis and growth*. McGraw-Hill Book Company. https://doi.org/10.1037/11333-000

Getz, C. J. (1987). *The effects of altruism on activity productivity in elderly women in skilled-care nursing facilities*. Western Michigan University.

Gewurtz, R., Stergiou-Kita, M., Shaw, L., Kirsh, B., & Rappolt, S. (2008). Qualitative meta-synthesis: Reflections on the utility and challenges in occupational therapy. *Canadian Journal of Occupational Therapy, 75*(5), 301–308. https://doi.org/10.1177/000841740807500513

Glaser, B. G., & Strauss, A. L. (1967). *The discovery of grounded theory: Strategies for qualitative research*. Aldine Publishing.

Glaser, R. (1963). Instructional technology and the measurement of learning outcomes: Some questions. *American Psychologist, 18*(8), 519. https://doi.org/10.1037/h0049294

Glass, G. V. (1976). Primary, secondary, and meta-analysis of research. *Educational Researcher, 5*(10), 3–8. https://doi.org/10.3102/0013189X005010003

Goldberg, R. T. (1974). Rehabilitation research—New directions. *Journal of Rehabilitation, 40*(3), 12–14.

Good, B. J. (1993). *Medicine, rationality and experience: An anthropological perspective*. Cambridge University Press.

Gordon, E. E. (1968). A view of the target population. In A. J. Tannenbaum (Ed.), *Special education programs for disadvantaged children and youth* (pp. 5–18). The Council for Exceptional Children.

Gravetter, F. J., & Wallnau, L. R. (2016). *Statistics for the behavioral sciences* (10th ed.). Cengage.

Guba, E. G. (1981). Criteria for assessing the trustworthiness of naturalistic inquiries. *ECTJ, 29*(2), 75–91.

Guba, E. G. (1990). Carrying on the dialog. In E.G. Guba (Ed.), *The paradigm dialog* (pp. 368–378). Sage.Gustafsson, L., Patterson, E., Marshall, K., Bennett, S., & Bower, K. (2016). Efficacy of compression gloves in maintaining edema reductions after application of compression bandaging to the stroke-affected upper limb. *The American Journal of Occupational Therapy, 70*(2), 7002290030p1–7002290030p9. https://doi.org/10.5014/ajot.2016.017939

Gutman, S. A. (1995). Influence of the US military and occupational therapy reconstruction aides in World War I on the development of occupational therapy. *The American Journal of Occupational Therapy, 49*(3), 256–262. https://doi.org/10.5014/ajot.49.3.256

Gutman, S. A., Raphael-Greenfield, E. I., & Rao, A. K. (2012). Effect of a motor-based role-play intervention on the social behaviors of adolescents with high-functioning autism: Multiple-baseline single-subject design. *The American Journal of Occupational Therapy, 66*(5), 529–537. https://doi.org/10.5014/ajot.2012.003756

Gutwinski, S., Schreiter, S., Deutscher, K., & Fazel, S. (2021). The prevalence of mental disorders among homeless people in high-income countries: An updated systematic review and meta-regression analysis. *PLoS Medicine, 18*(8), e1003750. https://doi.org/10.1371/journal.pmed.1003750

Hæger, K., & Edlund, Y. (1988). *The illustrated history of surgery*. Bell Pub. Co.

Hallahan, D. P., & Kauffman, J. M. (Eds.). (1981). *Handbook of special education*. Prentice-Hall.

Hallahan, D. P., & Kauffman, J. M. (1993). *Exceptional children: Introduction to special education* (6th ed.). Allyn and Bacon.

Hamera, E., & Brown, C. E. (2000). Developing a context-based performance measure for persons with schizophrenia: The test of grocery shopping skills. *The American Journal of Occupational Therapy, 54*(1), 20–25. https://doi.org/10.5014/ajot.54.1.20

Hamlin, R. B. (1992). Embracing our past, informing our future: A feminist re-vision of health care. *The American Journal of Occupational Therapy, 46*(11), 1028–1035. https://doi.org/10.5014/ajot.46.11.1028

Hansen, C., Steinmetz, H., & Block, J. (2022). How to conduct a meta-analysis in eight steps: A practical guide. *Management Review Quarterly*, 1–19. https://doi.org/10.1007/s11301-021-00247-4

Harper, K. J., Mast, E., Carter, G., Katnich, T., Oldham, V., & Morrisby, C. (2023). Prioritising patients for hospital occupational therapy to reduce inpatient falls: A retrospective case-control study to identify predictive patient falls risk factors. *British Journal of Occupational Therapy, 86*(11), 747–754. https://doi.org/10.1177/03080226231181019

Harvey, W. (1938). On the motion of the heart and blood in animals (R. Willis, Trans.). In C. W. Elliot (Ed.), *The Harvard classics scientific papers* (pp. 273–274). P. E. Collier and Sons.

Hasselkus, B. R., & Dickie, V. A. (1994). Doing occupational therapy: Dimensions of satisfaction and dissatisfaction. *The American Journal of Occupational Therapy, 48*(2), 145–154. https://doi.org/10.5014/ajot.48.2.145

Hatter, J. K., & Nelson, D. L. (1987). Altruism and task participation in the elderly. *The American Journal of Occupational Therapy, 41*(6), 379–381. https://doi.org/10.5014/ajot.41.6.379

Haynes, M. C., & Jenkins, J. R. (1986). Reading instruction in special education resource rooms. *American Educational Research Journal, 23*(2), 161–190. https://doi.org/10.3102/00028312023002161

Haynes, R. B., Devereaux, P. J., & Guyatt, G. H. (2002). Physicians' and patients' choices in evidence based practice: Evidence does not make decisions, people do. *BMJ, 324*(7350), 1350. https://doi.org/10.1136/bmj.324.7350.1350

He, K., Jiang, J., Chen, M., Wang, T., Huang, X., Zhu, R., Zhang, Z., Chen, J., & Zhao, L. (2023). Effects of occupational therapy on quality of life in breast cancer patients: A systematic review and meta-analysis. *Medicine, 102*(31), e34484. https://doi.org/10.1097/MD.0000000000034484

The Health Foundation. (2015). Evaluation: What to consider. www.health.org.uk/publications/evaluation-what-to-consider

Hernandez, A. V., Marti, K. M., & Roman, Y. M. (2020). Meta-analysis. *Chest, 158*(1), S97–S102. https://doi.org/10.1016/j.chest.2020.03.003

Hersch, G., Hutchinson, S., Davidson, H., Wilson, C., Maharaj, T., & Watson, K. B. (2012). Effect of an occupation-based cultural heritage intervention in long-term geriatric care: A two-group control study. *The American Journal of Occupational Therapy, 66*(2), 224–232. https://doi.org/10.5014/ajot.2012.002394

Higgs, J. (1997). *Qualitative research: Discourse on methodologies*. Hampden Press.Hinkle, D. E., Wiersma, W., & Jurs, S. G. (2003). *Applied statistics for the behavioral sciences*. Houghton Mifflin.

Hinojosa, J., & Kramer, P. (2014). *Evaluation in occupational therapy: Obtaining and interpreting data*. American Occupational Therapy Association.

Hinshelwood, J. (1917). *Congenital word-blindness*. HK Lewis & Company.

Hoffmann, M., Gustafsson, L., & Di Tommaso, A. (2022). Exploring stroke survivors' experiences and understandings of occupational therapy. *Scandinavian Journal of Occupational Therapy, 29*(2), 165–174. https://doi.org/10.1080/11038128.2020.1831060

Holstein, J. A., & Gubrium, J. F. (1995). *Qualitative research methods series: The active interview* (Vol. 37). Sage Publications.

Horghagen, S., Josephsson, S., & Alsaker, S. (2007). The use of craft activities as an occupational therapy treatment modality in Norway during 1952–1960. *Occupational Therapy International, 14*(1), 42–56. https://doi.org/10.1002/oti.222

Hoogerwerf, A. E. W., Bol, Y., Lobbestael, J., Huppers, R., & Van Heugten, C. M. (2017). Mindfulness-based cognitive therapy for severely fatigued multiple sclerosis patients: A waiting list controlled study. *Journal of Rehabilitation Medicine, 49*, 497–504. https://doi.org/10.2340/16501977-2237

HPI. (2019, October). *Prescription drugs*. Health Policy Institute, McCourt School of Public Health, Georgetown University. https://hpi.georgetown.edu/rxdrugs/

Huebsch, J. A., Kottke, T. E., McGinnis, P., Nichols, J., Parker, E. D., Tillema, J. O., & Hanson, A. M. (2015). A qualitative study of processes used to implement evidence-based care in a primary care practice. *Family Practice, 32*(5), 578–583. https://doi.org/10.1093/fampra/cmv045

Hughes, S. O. (2002). *Altruism and occupational performance in the elderly*. Unpublished manuscript.

Hunt, N., & Marshall, K. (2012). *Exceptional children and youth*. Wadsworth, Cengage Learning.

Husserl, E. (1913). *Ideas: General introduction to pure phenomenology* (W. R. Boyce Gibson, Trans.). Routledge.

Hutchins, R. M. (1952). *Hippocratic writings* (F. Adams, Trans.; Vol. 10). W. Benton.

Ikiugu, M. N., Nissen, R. M., Bellar, C., Maassen, A., & Van Peursem, K. (2017). Clinical effectiveness of occupational therapy in mental health: A meta-analysis. *The American Journal of Occupational Therapy, 71*(5), 7105100020p1–7105100020p10. https://doi.org/10.5014/ajot.2017.024588

Illingworth, W. H. (1910). *History of the education of the blind*. S. Low, Marston.

Izadi-Najafabadi, S., Gunton, C., Dureno, Z., & Zwicker, J. G. (2022). Effectiveness of cognitive orientation to occupational performance intervention in improving motor skills of children with developmental coordination disorder: A randomized waitlist-control trial. *Clinical Rehabilitation, 36*(6), 776–788. https://doi.org/10.1177/0269215521086188

Jackson, J., Carlson, M., Mandel, D., Zemke, R., & Clark, F. (1998). Occupation in lifestyle redesign: The well elderly study occupational therapy program. *The American Journal of Occupational Therapy, 52*(5), 326–336. https://doi.org/10.5014/ajot.52.5.326

Jacob, T., & Shapira, A. (2010). Quality of life and health conditions reported from two post-polio clinics in Israel. *Journal of Rehabilitation Medicine, 42*(4), 377–379. https://doi.org/10.2340/16501977-0515

Jacobson, N. S., Dobson, K. S., Truax, P. A., Addis, M. E., Koerner, K., Gollan, J. K., Gortner, E., & Prince, S. E. (1996). A component analysis of cognitive-behavioral treatment for depression. *Journal of Consulting and Clinical Psychology, 64*(2), 295–304. https://doi.org/10.1037//0022-006x.64.2.295

Jensen, L. A., & Allen, M. N. (1996). Meta-synthesis of qualitative findings. *Qualitative Health Research, 6*(4), 553–560. https://doi.org/10.1177/104973239600600407

Johns Hopkins University Library. (2023). Core QDAS functions. https://guides.library.jhu.edu/QDAS

Juckett, L. A., Robinson, M. L., Malloy, J., & Oliver, H. V. (2021). Translating knowledge to optimize value-based occupational therapy: Strategies for educators, practitioners, and researchers. *The American Journal of Occupational Therapy, 75*(6). https://doi.org/10.5014/ajot.2021.756003

Kehoe, R., & Rice, M. (2016). Reality, virtual reality, and imagery: Quality of movement in novice dart players. *British Journal of Occupational Therapy, 79*(4), 244–251. https://doi.org/10.1177/0308022615616820

Keith, R. A. (1984). Functional assessment measures in medical rehabilitation: Current status. *Archives of Physical Medicine and Rehabilitation*, 65(2), 74–78.

Kendall, H. O., Kendall, F. P., & Wadsworth, G. E. (1971). *Muscles, testing and function* (2nd ed.). Williams and Wilkins.

Kendi, I. X. (2023). *How to be an antiracist*. One World.

Kensky, J. (2016, April 20–23). 2016 Welcome Ceremony Keynote: A story of recovery and resilience. 2016 American Occupational Therapy Association Annual Conference & Expo, Chicago, IL.

Kerlinger, F. N. (1986). *Foundations of behavioral research* (3rd ed.). Holt, Rinehart and Winston.

Kibele, A. (1989). Occupational therapy's role in improving the quality of life for persons with cerebral palsy. *The American Journal of Occupational Therapy*, 43(6), 371–377. https://doi.org/10.5014/ajot.43.6.371

Kielhofner, G. (1982). Qualitative research: Part One, paradigmatic grounds and issues of reliability and validity. *The Occupational Therapy Journal of Research*, 2(2), 67–79. https://doi.org/10.1177/153944928200200201

Kim, D. (2020). The effects of a recollection-based occupational therapy program of Alzheimer's disease: A randomized controlled trial. *Occupational Therapy International*, 6305727. https://doi.org/10.1155/2020/6305727

Kipfer, B. A. (2010). *Roget's international thesaurus* (7th ed.). Collins Reference.

Kirk, S. A. (1963). Behavioral diagnosis and remediation of learning disabilities. In *Proceedings of the annual meeting: Conference on exploration into the problems of the perceptually handicapped child* (Vol. 1, pp. 1–7). Evanston, IL.

Kirk, S. A., Gallagher, J. J., & Coleman, M. R. (2022). *Educating exceptional children* (15th ed.). Wadsworth.

Kliebsch, U., Stürmer, T., Siebert, H., & Brenner, H. (1998). Risk factors of institutionalization in an elderly disabled population. *The European Journal of Public Health*, 8(2), 106–112. https://doi.org/10.1093/eurpub/8.2.106

Klinkman, M. S. (2009). Assessing functional outcomes in clinical practice. *American Journal of Managed Care*, 15(11), S335–S342.

Kokorelias, K. M., Lu, F. K., Santos, J. R., Xu, Y., Leung, R., & Cameron, J. I. (2020). "Caregiving is a full-time job" impacting stroke caregivers' health and well-being: A qualitative meta-synthesis. *Health & Social Care in the Community*, 28(2), 325–340. https://doi.org/10.1111/hsc.12869

Koller, K., Woods, L., Engel, L., Bottari, C., Dawson, D. R., & Nalder, E. (2016). Loss of financial management independence after brain injury: Survivors' experiences. *The American Journal of Occupational Therapy*, 70(3), 7003180070p1–7003180070p8. https://doi.org/10.5014/ajot.2016.020198

Krefting, L. (1991). Rigor in qualitative research: The assessment of trustworthiness. *The American Journal of Occupational Therapy*, 45(3), 214–222. https://doi.org/10.5014/ajot.45.3.214

Kwon, I. (2022). The value of medical humanities in medical education: Focusing on the history of medicine. *Korean Journal of Medical History*, 31(3), 495–517. https://doi.org/10.13081/kjmh.2022.31.495

Landsberger, H. A. (1958). *Hawthorne revisited: Management and the worker, its critics, and developments in human relations in industry*. Cornell University Press.

Lane, H. (1976). *The wild boy of Aveyron*. Harvard University Press.

Lane, J. D., Ledford, J. R., & Gast, D. L. (2017). Single-case experimental design: Current standards and applications in occupational therapy. *The American Journal of Occupational Therapy*, 71(2), 7102300010p1–7102300010p9. https://doi.org/10.5014/ajot.2017.022210

Larson, R. E., Murtagh, E. M., & Rice, M. S. (2018). Forces involved when sliding a patient up in bed. *Work*, 59(3), 439–448. https://doi.org/10.3233/WOR-182688

Lau, S. C. L., Judycki, S., Mix, M., DePaul, O., Tomazin, R., Hardi, A., Wong, A. W. K., & Baum, C. (2022). Theory-based self-management interventions for community-dwelling stroke survivors: A systematic review and meta-analysis. *The American Journal of Occupational Therapy*, 76(4), 7604205010. https://doi.org/10.5014/ajot.2022.049117

Laverdure, P., & Beisbier, S. (2021). Occupation- and activity-based interventions to improve performance of activities of daily living, play, and leisure for children and youth ages 5 to 21: A systematic review. *The American Journal of Occupational Therapy*, 75(1), 7501205050p1–7501205050p24. https://doi.org/10.5014/ajot.2021.039560

Lawson, L. M., & Foster, L. (2016). Sensory patterns, obesity, and physical activity participation of children with autism spectrum disorder. *The American Journal of Occupational Therapy*, 70(5), 7005180070p1–7005180070p8. https://doi.org/10.5014/ajot.2016.021535

Lawton, E. B. (1956). *Activities of daily living: Testing, training and equipment*. NYU-Bellevue Medical Center.

Lehr, R. (1992). Sixteen S-squared over D-squared: A relation for crude sample size estimates. *Statistics in Medicine*, 11(8), 1099–1102. https://doi.org/10.1002/sim.4780110811

Leibold, M. L., Holm, M. B., Raina, K. D., Reynolds III, C. F., & Rogers, J. C. (2014). Activities and adaptation in late-life depression: A qualitative study. *The American Journal of Occupational Therapy*, 68(5), 570–577. https://doi.org/10.5014/ajot.2014.011130

Levi, M. K., Schreuer, N., Granovsky, Y., Bar-Shalita, T., Fogel, I. W., Hoffman, T., & Gal, E. (2023). "Feeling unwanted, when nobody wants you around": Perceptions of social pain among people with autism. *The American Journal of Occupational Therapy*, 77(2), 7702185050. https://doi.org/10.5014/ajot.2023.050061

Levitt, O., Gilbert-Hunt, S., Murray, C., Baker, A., & Boshoff, K. (2021). International allied health student placements: A meta-synthesis. *Scandinavian Journal of Occupational Therapy*, 28(4), 251–263. https://doi.org/10.1080/11038128.2020.1809703

Lezak, M. D., Howieson, D. B., Bigler, E. D., & Tranel, D. (2012). *Neuropsychological assessment* (5th ed.). Oxford University Press.

Liberati, A., Altman, D. G., Tetzlaff, J., Mulrow, C., Gøtzsche, P. C., Ioannidis, J. P., Clarke, M., Devereaux, P. J., Kleijnen, J., & Moher, D. (2009). The PRISMA statement for reporting systematic reviews and meta-analyses of studies that evaluate health care interventions: Explanation and elaboration. *PLoS Medicine*, 6(7), e1000100. https://doi.org/10.1371/journal.pmed.1000100

Lin, C. L., Lin, C. K., & Yu, J. J. (2018). The effectiveness of parent participation in occupational therapy for children with developmental delay. *Neuropsychiatric Disease and Treatment*, 14, 623–630. https://doi.org/10.2147/NDT.S158688

Lin, K., Wu, Y., Chen, I., Tsai, P., Wu, C., & Chen, C. (2015). Dual-task performance involving hand dexterity and cognitive tasks and daily functioning in people with schizophrenia: A pilot study. *The American Journal of Occupational Therapy*, 69(3), 6903250020p1–6903250020p7. https://doi.org/10.5014/ajot.2014.014738

Lindsay, S., Ahmed, H., Tomas, V., & Vijayakumar, A. (2023). Exploring the lived experiences of ethnic minority youth with disabilities: A systematic review and meta synthesis of qualitative data. *Disability and Rehabilitation*, 45(4), 588–601. https://doi.org/10.1080/09638288.2022.2040614

Lindström, M. (2023). The Covid-19 pandemic and the Swedish strategy: Central aspects of the strategy in relation to evidence and evidence-based medicine criteria. In *Sweden's pandemic experiment* (pp. 90–105). Routledge.

Linkov, I., Loney, D., Cormier, S., Satterstrom, F. K., & Bridges, T. (2009). Weight-of-evidence evaluation in environmental assessment: Review of qualitative and quantitative approaches. *Science of the Total Environment*, 407(19), 5199–5205. https://doi.org/10.1016/j.scitotenv.2009.05.004

Llewellyn, G. (1995). Qualitative research with people with intellectual disability. *Occupational Therapy International*, 2(2), 108–127. https://doi.org/10.1002/oti.6150020206

Lockwood, K. J., & Porter, J. (2022). Effectiveness of hospital-based interventions by occupational therapy practitioners on reducing readmissions: A systematic review with meta-analyses. *The American Journal of Occupational Therapy*, 76(1). https://doi.org/10.5014/ajot.2022.048959

Lofquist, L. H. (1957). *Vocational counseling with the physically handicapped*. Appleton-Century-Crofts.

López-López, J. A., Davies, S. R., Caldwell, D. M., Churchill, R., Peters, T. J., Tallon, D., Dawson, S., Wu, Q., Li, J., & Taylor, A. (2019). The process and delivery of CBT for depression in adults: A systematic review and network meta-analysis. *Psychological Medicine*, 49(12), 1937–1947. https://doi.org/10.1017/S003329171900120X

Luborsky, M. R., & Lysack, C. (2017). Design considerations in qualitative research. In *Kielhofner's research in occupational therapy: Methods of inquiry for enhancing practice* (pp. 180–195). F.A. Davis Company.

Luria, A. R. (1961). *The role of speech in the regulation of normal and abnormal behavior*. Pergamon.

Lynch, H., Moore, A., O'Connor, D., & Boyle, B. (2023). Evidence for implementing tiered approaches in school-based occupational therapy in elementary schools: A scoping review. *The American Journal of Occupational Therapy*, 77(1), 7701205110. https://doi.org/10.5014/ajot.2023.050027

Madhoun, H. Y., Tan, B., Feng, Y., Zhou, Y., Zhou, C., & Yu, L. (2020). Task-based mirror therapy enhances the upper limb motor function in subacute stroke patients: A randomized control trial. *European Journal of Physical and Rehabilitation Medicine*, 56(3), 265–271. https://doi.org/10.23736/S1973-9087.20.06070-0

Magnusson, L., Håkansson, C., Brandt, S., Öberg, M., & Orban, K. (2021). Occupational balance and sleep among women. *Scandinavian Journal of Occupational Therapy*, 28(8), 643–651. https://doi.org/10.1080/11038128.2020.1721558

Mannion, N., & Sullivan, N. (2021). Occupational therapy for functional impairments resulting from COVID-19 infection: A case report. *The American Journal of Occupational Therapy*, 75(Supplement_1). https://doi.org/10.5014/ajot.2021.049215

Marini, R. P. (2003). Approaches to analyzing experiments with factorial arrangements of treatments plus other treatments. *Horticultural Science*, 38(1), 117–120. https://doi.org/10.21273/HORTSCI.38.1.117

Marston, D. (1987–1988). The effectiveness of special education: A time series analysis of reading performance in regular and special education settings. *The Journal of Special Education*, 27, 466–480.

Martí-Ibáñez, F. (1962). *The epic of medicine*. Bramhall House.

Martin, R. P., Hooper, S., & Snow, J. (1986). Behavioral rating scale approaches to personality assessment in children and adolescents. In H. M. Knoff (Ed.), *The assessment of child and adolescent personality* (pp. 309–351). Guilford.

Mashimo, I., Yotsumoto, K., Fujimoto, H., & Hashimoto, T. (2020). Effects of home-visit occupational therapy using a management tool for daily life performance on severe mental illness: A multicenter randomized controlled trial. *Kobe Journal of Medical Sciences*, 66(4), E119.

Masri, A. F., Rice, M. S., Miller, B. K., & Foster, R. N. (2019). Influence of altruism on engagement with craft activity among women in long-term care and assisted living facilities. *Annals of International Occupational Therapy*, 2(1), 16–22. https://doi.org/10.3928/24761222-20180723-02

Mathiowetz, V. (2019). Effects of meditative movements for persons with chronic health conditions. *The American Journal of Occupational Therapy*, 73(4_Supplement_1), 7311515355p1. https://doi.org/10.5014/ajot.2019.73S1-PO5023

Mathiowetz, V., Wiemer, D. M., & Federman, S. M. (1986). Grip and pinch strength: Norms for 6- to 19-year-olds. *The American Journal of Occupational Therapy*, 40(10), 705–711. https://doi.org/10.5014/ajot.40.10.705

Mattox, J. G. (1995). *Altruistic engagement in a retirement community*. Unpublished manuscript.

McAlonan, S. (1996). Improving sexual rehabilitation services: The patient's perspective. *The American Journal of Occupational Therapy*, 50(10), 826–834. https://doi.org/10.5014/ajot.50.10.826

McBride, M. R., & Lewis, R. D. (2004). African American and Asian American elders: An ethnogeriatric perspective. *Annual Review of Nursing Research*, 22(1), 161–214.

McCartney, W. M. (2007). Radiation dose during barium enema. *Radiologic Technology*, 79(1), 91–93.

McCuaig, M., & Frank, G. (1991). The able self: Adaptive patterns and choices in independent living for a person with cerebral palsy. *The American Journal of Occupational Therapy*, 45(3), 224–234. https://doi.org/10.5014/ajot.45.3.224

McDermott, D. E. (1994). Jean Itard: The first child and youth counselor. *Journal of Child and Youth Care*, 9, 59–71.

McGowan, J. F. (1967). *An introduction to the vocational rehabilitation process*. US Department of Health, Education, and Welfare, Vocational Rehabilitation.

McGrath, M., Lever, S., McCluskey, A., & Power, E. (2019). How is sexuality after stroke experienced by stroke survivors and partners of stroke survivors? A systematic review of qualitative studies. *Clinical Rehabilitation*, 33(2), 293–303. https://doi.org/10.1177/0269215518793483

McGruder, J. (1999). *OT634 Course Syllabus*. University of Puget Sound, Tacoma WA. Unpublished Document.

McGruder, J., Cors, D., Tiernan, A. M., & Tomlin, G. (2003). Weighted wrist cuffs for tremor reduction during eating in adults with static brain lesions. *The American Journal of Occupational Therapy*, 57(5), 507–516. https://doi.org/10.5014/ajot.57.5.507

McIntosh, V., Carter, F. A., Bulik, C. M., Frampton, C., & Joyce, P. R. (2011). Five-year outcome of cognitive behavioral therapy and exposure with response prevention for bulimia nervosa. *Psychological Medicine*, 41(5), 1061–1071. https://doi.org/10.1017/S0033291710001583

McCarthy, A., Galvin, R., Dockery, F., McLoughlin, K., O'Connor, M., Corey, G., Whiston, A., Carey, L., Steed, F., Tierney, A., & Robinson, K. (2023). Multidisciplinary inpatient rehabilitation for older adults with COVID-19: A systematic review and meta-analysis of clinical and process outcomes. *BMC Geriatrics*, 23(1), 391. https://doi.org/10.1186/s12877-023-04098-4

McMichael, A. J. (2015). Extreme weather events and infectious disease outbreaks. *Virulence*, 6(6), 543–547. https://doi.org/10.4161/21505594.2014.975022

Mead, M. (1928). *Coming of age in Samoa*. Blue Ribbon Books.

Meckler, L., & Hitt, G. (2010, March 24). Obama signs landmark health bill. *Wall Street Journal*, p. A4.

Mercer, C. D. (1983). *Students with learning disabilities* (2nd ed.). Merrill.

Mercer, C. D., Mercer, A. R., & Pullen, P. C. (2014). *Teaching students with learning problems* (8th ed.). Pearson.

Merriam-Webster, I. (1998). *Merriam-Webster's collegiate dictionary*. Merriam-Webster.

Meyen, E. L., & Skrtic, T. M. (1988). *Exceptional children and youth* (3rd ed.). Love.

Miles, M. B., & Huberman, A. M. (1994). *Qualitative data analysis: An expanded sourcebook*. (2nd ed.). Sage Publications.

Miles, M. B., Huberman, A. M., & Saldaña, J. (2014). *Qualitative data analysis: A methods sourcebook* (3rd ed.). Sage.

Miller, L. J. (1988). *Miller assessment for preschoolers*. Person/PsyCorp.

Minichiello, V., Aroni, R., & Hays, T. N. (2008). *In-depth interviewing: Principles, techniques, analysis*. Pearson Education Australia.

Mitchell, P. (2009). Mental health care roles of non-medical primary health and social care services. *Health & Social Care in the Community, 17*(1), 71–82. https://doi.org/10.1111/j.1365-2524.2008.00800.x

Modern Language Association of America (MLA). (2016). *MLA handbook* (8th ed.). MLA.

Moen, E., McLean, A., Boyd, L. A., Schmidt, J., & Zwicker, J. G. (2022). Experiences of children and youth with concussion: A qualitative study. *The American Journal of Occupational Therapy, 76*(4), 7604205040. https://doi.org/10.5014/ajot.2022.047597

Montessori, M. (1912). *The Montessori method* (A. E. George, Trans.). Frederick A. Stokes.

Morse, J. M. (1994). *Critical issues in qualitative research methods.* Sage.

Mulcahey, M. J., Smith, B. T., Betz, R. R., & Weiss, A. A. (1995). Outcomes of tendon transfer surgery and occupational therapy in a child with tetraplegia secondary to spinal cord injury. *The American Journal of Occupational Therapy, 49*(7), 607–617. https://doi.org/10.5014/ajot.49.7.607

Mullen, E. M. (1995). *Mullen scales of early learning.* American Guidance Service.

Mulligan, S. (2003). *Occupational therapy evaluation for children: A pocket guide.* Lippincott Williams & Wilkins.

Muluk, N. B., Bayoğlu, B., & Anlar, B. (2016). A study of language development and affecting factors in children aged 5 to 27 months. *Ear, Nose & Throat Journal, 95*(1), 23–29. https://doi.org/10.1177/014556131609500107

Munn, Z., Peters, M. D., Stern, C., Tufanaru, C., McArthur, A., & Aromataris, E. (2018). Systematic review or scoping review? Guidance for authors when choosing between a systematic or scoping review approach. *BMC Medical Research Methodology, 18*, 1–7. doi: 10.1186/s12874-018-0611-x

Muñoz, J. P., Moreton, E. M., & Sitterly, A. M. (2016). The scope of practice of occupational therapy in US criminal justice settings. *Occupational Therapy International, 23*(3), 241–254. doi: 10.1002/oti.1427

Murphy, S., & Tickle-Degnen, L. (2001). The effectiveness of occupational therapy-related treatments for persons with Parkinson's disease: A meta-analytic review. *The American Journal of Occupational Therapy, 55*(4), 385–392. doi: 10.5014/ajot.55.4.385

Nadolsky, J. M. (1974). The work sample in vocational evaluation: A consistent rationale. *Vocational Evaluation and Work Adjustment Bulletin, 7*(2), 2–5.

Nas, K., Yazmalar, L., Şah, V., Aydin, A., & Öneş, K. (2015). Rehabilitation of spinal cord injuries. *World Journal of Orthopedics, 6*(1), 8.NCES. (2022). *Students with disabilities: Condition of education.* National Center for Education Statistics, US Department of Education, Institute of Education Sciences. https://nces.ed.gov/programs/coe/indicator/cgg/students-with-disabilities

Nelson, D. L., & Jepson-Thomas, J. (2003). Occupational form, occupational performance, and a conceptual framework for therapeutic occupation. In *Perspectives in human occupation: Participation in life* (pp. 87–155). Lippincott Williams & Wilkins.

Newton, I. (1675). Newton letter to Hooke. https://digitallibrary.hsp.org/index.php/Detail/objects/9792

Njelesani, J., Teachman, G., & Bangura, I. R. (2021). "The strength to leave": Women with disabilities navigating violent relationships and occupational identities. *The American Journal of Occupational Therapy, 75*(4). doi: 10.5014/ajot.2021.045542

Noblit, G. W., & Hare, R. D. (1988). *Meta-ethnography* (1st ed.). Sage Publications.

Nygård, L., Ryd, C., Astell, A., Nedlund, A., Boger, J., Mäki Petäjä Leinonen, A., Issakainen, M., & Larsson Lund, M. (2022). Self-initiated management approaches in everyday occupations used by people with acquired cognitive impairment. *Scandinavian Journal of Occupational Therapy, 29*(2), 139–151. doi: 10.1080/11038128.2021.1925740

Ogden, C. L., Fryar, C. D., Martin, C. B., Freedman, D. S., Carroll, M. D., Gu, Q., Hales, C. M. (2020). Trends in obesity prevalence by race and Hispanic origin—1999-2000 to 2017-2018. *JAMA, 324*(12), 1208–1210. doi:10.1001/jama.2020.14590.

Olds, G. (1938). Distribution of the sum of squares of rank differences for small numbers of individuals. *Annals of Mathematical Statistics, 9*, 133–148.

Olds, G. (1949). The 5 percent significance levels of sums of squares of rank differences and a correction. *Annals of Mathematical Statistics, 20*, 117–118.

Oliver, M. (1991). *Social work: Disabled people and disabling environments.* Jessica Kingsley.

Österholm, J., Nedlund, A., & Ranada, Å L. (2022). Collaboration and coordination of health and care services for older people with dementia by multidisciplinary health and care providers: A scoping review protocol. *BMJ Open, 12*(12), e066578. doi: 10.1136/bmjopen-2022-066578

Ottenbacher, K. J. (1986a). *Evaluating clinical change: Strategies for occupational and physical therapists.* Williams & Wilkins.

Ottenbacher, K. J. (1986b). Reliability and accuracy of visually analyzing graphed data from single-subject designs. *The American Journal of Occupational Therapy, 40*(7), 464–469. doi: 10.5014/ajot.40.7.464

Ownsworth, T., Fleming, J., Tate, R., Beadle, E., Griffin, J., Kendall, M., Schmidt, J., Lane-Brown, A., Chevignard, M., & Shum, D. H. (2017). Do people with severe traumatic brain injury benefit from making errors? A randomized controlled trial of error-based and errorless learning. *Neurorehabilitation and Neural Repair, 31*(12), 1072–1082. doi: 10.1177/1545968317740635

Oxford Grice, K., Vogel, K. A., Le, V., Mitchell, A., Muniz, S., & Vollmer, M. A. (2003). Adult norms for a commercially available Nine Hole Peg Test for finger dexterity. *The American Journal of Occupational Therapy, 57*(5), 570–573. doi: 10.5014/ajot.57.5.570

Pajević, A., Pajević, I., Jakovljević, M., Hasanović, M., Kravić, N., & Žigić, N. (2021). Ibn Sina (Avicenna) as a psychiatrist: A view from today's perspective. *Psychiatria Danubina, 33*(suppl 4), 1218–1226.

Paracheck, J. F. (1986). *Paracheck geriatric rating scale.* Center for Neurodevelopmental Studies.

Parsons, T. (1964). *The theory of social and economic organization* (First Free Press paperback ed.). The Free Press.

Patterson, C. H. (1958). *Counseling the emotionally disturbed.* Harper and Brothers.

Patton, M. Q. (1990). *Qualitative evaluation and research methods.* Sage Publications.

Pedersen, J. P., Ehrlich-Jones, L. S., Heinemann, A. W., & LaVela, S. L. (2023). Informal caregivers' perceptions of facilitators of successful weight management for people with spinal cord injury. *The American Journal of Occupational Therapy, 77*(3), 7703205110. doi: 10.5014/ajot.2023.050093

Peloquin, S. M. (1991). Occupational therapy service: Individual and collective understandings of the founders, Part 2. *The American Journal of Occupational Therapy, 45*(8), 733–744. doi: 10.5014/ajot.45.8.733

Pérez-Corrales, J., Huertas-Hoyas, E., García-Bravo, C., Güeita-Rodríguez, J., & Palacios-Ceña, D. (2022). Volunteering as a meaningful occupation in the process of recovery from serious mental illness: A qualitative study. *The American Journal of Occupational Therapy, 76*(2). doi: 10.5014/ajot.2022.045104

Peters, H. T., Pisegna, J., Faieta, J., & Page, S. J. (2017). Functional brain stimulation in a chronic stroke survivor with moderate impairment. *The American Journal of Occupational Therapy, 71*(3), 7103190080p1–7103190080p6. doi: 10.5014/ajot.2017.025247

Pettigrew, J., Robinson, K., & Moloney, S. (2017a). The bluebirds: World War I soldiers' experiences of occupational therapy. *The American Journal of Occupational Therapy, 71*(1), 7101100010p1–7101100010p9. doi: 10.5014/ajot.2017.023812

Piaget, J. (2010). *Thea language and thought of the child* (3rd. ed., repr. ed.). Routledge Classics.

Pinninti, N. R., Rissmiller, D. J., & Steer, R. A. (2010). Cognitive-behavioral therapy as an adjunct to second-generation antipsychotics in the treatment of schizophrenia. *Psychiatric Services, 61*(9), 940–943. doi: 10.1176/ps.2010.61.9.940

Plantinga, L. C., Johansen, K. L., Schillinger, D., & Powe, N. R. (2012). Lower socioeconomic status and disability among US adults with chronic kidney disease, 1999–2008. *Preventing Chronic Disease, 9*, E12.

Pollock, N. (1993). Client-centered assessment. *The American Journal of Occupational Therapy, 47*(4), 298–301. doi: 10.5014/ajot.47.4.298

Portney, L. G., & Watkins, M. P. (2009). *Foundations of clinical research: Applications to practice.* Pearson/Prentice Hall.

Preissner, K. (2010). Use of the occupational therapy task-oriented approach to optimize the motor performance of a client with cognitive limitations. *The American Journal of Occupational Therapy, 64*(5), 727–734. doi: 10.5014/ajot.2010.08026

Progeria Research Foundation. (2023). *Progeria quick facts.* Progeria Research Foundation. www.progeriaresearch.org/quick-facts/

Purdue University. (2023). *Purdue OWL.* https://owl.english.purdue.edu

Rapolienė, J., Endzelytė, E., Jasevičienė, I., & Savickas, R. (2018). Stroke patients' motivation influence on the effectiveness of occupational therapy. *Rehabilitation research And Practice, 2018*, 9367942. https://doi.org/10.1155/2018/9367942

Rashid, M., Harish, S. P., Mathew, J., Kalidas, A., & Raja, K. (2022). Comprehensive rehabilitation outcome measurement scale (CROMS): Development and preliminary validation of an interdisciplinary measure for rehabilitation outcomes. *Health and Quality of Life Outcomes, 20*(1), 1–17. doi: 10.1186/s12955-022-02048-z

Reason, P. (1988). *Human inquiry in action: Developments in new paradigm research.* Sage.

Reid, W. M., Seavor, C., & Taylor, R. G. (1991). Application of a computer-based zero-one methodology to the assignment of nurses to a clinical rotation schedule. *Computers in Nursing, 9*(6), 219–223.

Reitz, S. M. (1992). A historical review of occupational therapy's role in preventive health and wellness. *The American Journal of Occupational Therapy, 46*(1), 50–55. doi: 10.5014/ajot.46.1.50

Reynolds, C. R. (2008). RTI, neuroscience, and sense: Chaos in the diagnosis and treatment of learning disabilities. In E. Fletcher-Janzen & C. R. Reyanolds (Eds.), *Neurophsychological perspectives on learning disabilities in the era of REI* (pp. 14–53). Wiley.

Ribeiro, J., Mira, E., Lourenço, I., Santos, M., & Braúna, M. (2019). The intervention of occupational therapy in drug addiction: A case study in the Comunidade Terapêutica Clínica do Outeiro—Portugal. Intervenção da Terapia Ocupacional na toxicodependência: estudo de caso na Comunidade Terapêutica Clínica do Outeiro—Portugal. *Ciencia & saude coletiva, 24*(5), 1585–1596. https://doi.org/10.1590/1413-81232018245.04452019

Rice, M. S., Dusseau, J. M., & Miller, B. K. (2011). A questionnaire of musculoskeletal injuries associated with manual patient lifting in occupational therapy practitioners in the state of Ohio. *Occupational Therapy in Health Care, 25*(2–3), 95–107. https://10.3109/07380577.2011.566308

Rich, T., Hicks, B., Dahl, A., Sullivan, E., Barrett, B., & Bedore, B. (2022). Preliminary experiences in acute occupational therapy for in-patients with coronavirus-19 (COVID-19): Leveraging assistive technology in three case studies of male veterans. *Disability and Rehabilitation: Assistive Technology, 17*(3), 283–289. doi: 10.1080/17483107.2020.1852326

Riley, D. S., Barber, M. S., Kienle, G. S., Aronson, J. K., von Schoen-Angerer, T., Tugwell, P., Kiene, H., Helfand, M., Altman, D. G., & Sox, H. (2017). CARE guidelines for case reports: Explanation and elaboration document. *Journal of Clinical Epidemiology, 89*, 218–235. doi: 10.1016/j.jclinepi.2017.04.026

Rivett, P., & Ackoff, R. L. (1963). *A manager's guide to operational research.* Wiley.

Rocamora-Montenegro, M., Compañ-Gabucio, L., & Garcia de la Hera, M. (2021). Occupational therapy interventions for adults with severe mental illness: A scoping review. *BMJ Open, 11*(10), e047467. doi: 10.1136/bmjopen-2020-047467

Rodakowski, J., Skidmore, E. R., Reynolds III, C. F., Dew, M. A., Butters, M. A., Holm, M. B., Lopez, O. L., & Rogers, J. C. (2014). Can performance on daily activities discriminate between older adults with normal cognitive function and those with mild cognitive impairment? *Journal of the American Geriatrics Society, 62*(7), 1347–1352. doi: 10.1111/jgs.12878

Rogers, J. C., & Holm, M. B. (2016). Functional assessment in mental health: Lessons from occupational therapy. *Dialogues in Clinical Neuroscience, 18*(2), 145–154. https://doi.org/10.31887/DCNS.2016.18.2/jrogers

Ross F. L. (1992). The use of computers in occupational therapy for visual-scanning training. *The American Journal of Occupational Therapy: Official Publication of the American Occupational Therapy Association, 46*(4), 314–322. https://doi.org/10.5014/ajot.46.4.314

Rousseau, J. J. (1883). *Emile: Or, concerning education* (E. J. Steeg & T. E. Worthington, Eds.). DC Health & Co. (Original work published 1762)

Rubin, S. E., Chan, F., & Thomas, D. L. (2003). Assessing changes in life skills and quality of life resulting from rehabilitation services. *Journal of Rehabilitation, 69*(3), 4–9.

Runyon, R. P., & Haber, A. (1967). *Fundamentals of behavioral statistics.* Addison-Wesley.

Rushmer, R. F. (1972). *Medical engineering: Projections for health care delivery.* Academic Press.

Rusk, H. A. (1971). *Rehabilitation medicine.* Mosby.

Sackett, D. L., Rosenberg, W. M., Gray, J. M., Haynes, R. B., & Richardson, W. S. (1996). Evidence based medicine: What it is and what it isn't. *BMJ, 312*(7023), 71–72. doi: 10.1136/bmj.312.7023.71

Sailor, W. (1991). Special education in the restructured school. *Remedial and Special Education, 12*(6), 8–22. doi. org/10.1177/074192591012006

Sand, R. (1952). *The advance to social medicine.* Staples Press.

Sandelowski, M., & Barroso, J. (2006). *Handbook for synthesizing qualitative research.* Springer Publishing.

Sattler, J. M. (1992). *Assessment of children* (3rd ed., Rev.). Author.

Sattler, J. M. (2020). *Assessment of children: Cognitive foundations and applications* (6th ed.). Author.

Schmid, H. (1981). Qualitative research and occupational therapy. *The American Journal of Occupational Therapy, 35*(2), 105–106. doi.org/10.5014/ajot.35.2.105

Schmidt, P., Reiss, A., Dürichen, R., & Van Laerhoven, K. (2019). Wearable-based affect recognition—A review. *Sensors, 19*(19), 4079. doi: 10.3390/s19194079

Schoen, S., & Miller, L. (1985). Miller Assessment for Preschoolers (MAP). In *Encyclopedia of Autism Spectrum Disorders* (pp. 1861–1863). Springer. https://10.1007/978-1-4419-1698-3_625

Schwartz, C., Meisenhelder, J. B., Ma, Y., & Reed, G. (2003). Altruistic social interest behaviors are associated with better mental health. *Psychosomatic Medicine, 65*(5), 778–785. doi: 10.1097/01.psy.0000079378.39062.d4

Scull, A. (2015). *Madness in civilization: A cultural history of insanity, from the Bible to Freud, from the madhouse to modern medicine.* Princeton University Press.

Selye, H. (1956). *The stress of life.* McGraw-Hill.

Shankman, P. (2010). The trashing of Margaret Mead: How Derek Freeman fooled us all. *Skeptic, 15*(3), 24–28.

Sharpe, P. A., & Ottenbacher, K. J. (1990). Use of an elbow restraint to improve finger-feeding skills in a child with Rett Syndrome. *The American Journal of Occupational Therapy*, 44(4), 328–332. https://10.5014/ajot.44.4.328

Shea, T. M., & Bauer, A. M. (1994). *Learners with disabilities: A social systems perspective of special education.* Brown & Benchmark.

Siengsukon, C. F., Aldughmi, M., Kahya, M., Bruce, J., Lynch, S., Norouzinia, A. N. Glusman, M., & Billinger, S. (2016). Randomized controlled trial of exercise interventions to improve sleep quality and daytime sleepiness in individuals with multiple sclerosis: A pilot study. *Multiple Sclerosis Journal—Experimental, Translational and Clinical, 2*, 1–9. doi: 10.1177/2055217316680639

Sibley, L., & Armbruster, D. (1997). Obstetric first aid in the community—Partners in safe motherhood a strategy for reducing maternal mortality. *Journal of Nurse-Midwifery, 42*(2), 117–121. doi: 10.1016/s0091-2182(97)00022-0

Sigmon, S. B. (1987). *Radical analysis of special education: Focus on historical development and learning disabilities.* Falmer Press.

Skrtic, T. (1991). The special education paradox: Equity as the way to excellence. *Harvard Educational Review, 61*(2), 148–207. doi. org/10.17763/haer.61.2.0q70275158oh0617

Sledziewski, L., Schaaf, R. C., & Mount, J. (2012). Use of robotics in spinal cord injury: A case report. *The American Journal of Occupational Therapy, 66*(1), 51–58. doi: 10.5014/ajot.2012.000943

Smith, D. D., & Tyler N. C. (2010). *Introduction to special education: Making a difference* (7th ed.). Merrill/Pearson.

Smith, J., Halliwell, N., Laurent, A., Tsotsoros, J., Harris, K., & DeGrace, B. (2023). Social participation experiences of families raising a young child with autism spectrum disorder: Implications for mental health and well-being. *The American Journal of Occupational Therapy, 77*(2), 7702185090. doi: 10.5014/ajot.2023.050156

Song, B.-N. (2015). A meta-analysis on the effects of occupational therapy program intervention for dementia in the community. *Korean Journal of Occupational Therapy, 23*(1), 53–72.

Spradley, J. (1980). *Participant observation.* Holt, Rineart and Winston.

Stainback, W., & Stainback, S. (1992). *Controversial issues confronting special education: Divergent perspectives.* ERIC.

Stanford Encyclopedia of Philosophy. (2022). Edmund Husserl. https://plato.stanford.edu/entries/husserl

Stein, F. (1976). *Anatomy of research in allied health.* Schenkman Publishing Company.

Stein, F. (1988). Research analysis of OT assessments used in mental health. In B. J. Hemphill-Pearson (Ed.), *The mental health assessment in occupational therapy: An integrative approach to the evaluative process* (pp. 225–247). Slack.

Stein, F. (2020). The impact of clinical research and evidence-based practice in occupational therapy. *Cadernos Brasileiros de Terapia Ocupacional.* https://doi.org/10.4322/2526-8910.ctoED2801

Stevens, P. A. (Ed.). (2022). *Qualitative data analysis: Key approaches.* Sage Publications.

Strauss, A. A., & Kephart, N. C. (1940). Behavior differences in mentally retarded children measured by a new behavior rating scale. *American Journal of Psychiatry, 96*(5), 1117–1124. doi. org/10.1176/ajp. 96.5.1117

Strauss, A. A., & Lehtinen, L. E. (1947). *Psychopathology and education of the brain-injured child.* Grune & Stratton.

Strauss, A. A., & Werner, H. (1941). The mental organization of the brain-injured mentally defective child. *American Journal of Psychiatry, 97*(5), 1194–1203. doi: 10.1016/j.nicl.2021.102621

Strauss, A., & Corbin, J. (1998). *Basis of qualitative research techniques: Techniques and procedures for developing grounded theory.* Sage Publications.

Strunk Jr, W., & White, E. B. (1979). *The elements of style* (3rd ed.). Macmillan.

Strunk Jr, W., & White, E. B. (1999). *The elements of style* (4th ed.). Macmillan.

Swinth, Y., Tomlin, G., & Luthman, M. (2015). Content analysis of qualitative research on children and youth with autism, 1993–2011: Considerations for occupational therapy services. *The American Journal of Occupational Therapy, 69*(5), 6905185030p1–6905185030p9. doi: 10.5014/ajot.2015.017970

Tanta, K. J., Deitz, J. C., White, O., & Billingsley, F. (2005). The effects of peer-play level on initiations and responses of preschool children with delayed play skills. *The American Journal of Occupational Therapy, 59*(4), 437–443. doi: 10.5014/ajot.59.4.437

Tate, R. L., Perdices, M., Rosenkoetter, U., Shadish, W., Vohra, S., Barlow, D. H., Horner, R., Kazdin, A., Kratochwill, T., & McDonald, S. (2016). The single-case reporting guideline in behavioural interventions (SCRIBE) 2016 statement. *Physical Therapy, 96*(7), e1–e10. doi: 10.5014/ajot.2016.704002

Taylor, L. P. S., & McGruder, J. E. (1996). The meaning of sea kayaking for persons with spinal cord injuries. *The American Journal of Occupational Therapy, 50*(1), 39–46. doi: 10.5014/ajot.50.1.39

Taylor, M. L., & Marks, M. (1955). *Aphasic rehabilitation: Manual and workbook.* NYU—Bellevue Medical Center.

Taylor, R. R., Braveman, B., & Hammel, J. (2004). Developing and evaluating community-based services through participatory action research: Two case examples. *The American Journal of Occupational Therapy, 58*(1), 73–82. doi: 10.5014/ajot.58.1.73

Tesch, R. (1990). *Qualitative research: Analysis types and software tools.* Falmer.

Thomas, J., & Harden, A. (2008). Methods for the thematic synthesis of qualitative research in systematic reviews. *BMC Medical Research Methodology, 8*(1), 1–10. doi: 10.1186/1471-2288-8-45

Thorwald, J. (1963). *Science and secrets of early medicine.* Harcourt, Brace and World.

Tofani, M., Ranieri, A., Fabbrini, G., Berardi, A., Pelosin, E., Valente, D., Fabbrini, A., Costanzo, M., & Galeoto, G. (2020). Efficacy of occupational therapy interventions on quality of life in patients with Parkinson's disease: A systematic review and meta-analysis. *Movement Disorders Clinical Practice, 7*(8), 891–901. doi: 10.1002/mdc3.13089

Tomlin, G. S., & Borgetto, B. (2011). Research pyramid: A new evidence-based practice model for occupational therapy. *The American Journal of Occupational Therapy, 65*(2), 189–196. doi: 10.5014/ajot.2011.000828

Tomlin, G. S., & Swinth, Y. (2015). Contribution of qualitative research to evidence in practice for people with autism spectrum disorder. *The American Journal of Occupational Therapy, 69*(5), 6905360010p1–6905360010p4. doi: 10.5014/ajot.2015.017988

Tong, A., Flemming, K., McInnes, E., Oliver, S., & Craig, J. (2012). Enhancing transparency in reporting the synthesis of qualitative research: ENTREQ. *BMC Medical Research Methodology, 12*(1), 181. https://10.1186/1471-2288-12-181

Tryon, W. W. (1982). A simplified time-series analysis for evaluating treatment interventions. *Journal of Applied Behavior Analysis, 15*(3), 423–429. doi: 10.1901/jaba.1982.15-423

Tukey, J. W. (1977). *Exploratory data analysis.* Addison-Wesley.

Turabian, K. L. (2018). *A manual for writers of research papers, theses, and dissertations: Chicago style for students and researchers.* University of Chicago Press.

Turnbull III, H. R., & Turnbull, A. P. (1998). *Free appropriate public education: The law and children with disabilities.* ERIC.

Twisk, F. N., & Maes, M. (2009). A review on cognitive behavorial therapy (CBT) and graded exercise therapy (GET) in myalgic encephalomyelitis (ME)/chronic fatigue syndrome (CFS): CBT/GET is not only ineffective and not evidence-based, but also potentially harmful for many patients with ME/CFS. *Neuro Endocrinology Letters, 30*(3), 284–299.

Uhlig, T., Fongen, C., Steen, E., Christie, A., & Ødegård, S. (2010). Exploring Tai Chi in rheumatoid arthritis: A quantitative and qualitative study. *BMC Musculoskeletal Disorders, 11*(1), 1–7. doi: 10.1186/1471-2474-11-43

Umeda, C., & Deitz, J. (2011). Effects of therapy cushions on classroom behaviors of children with autism spectrum disorder. *The American Journal of Occupational Therapy, 65*(2), 152–159. https://10.5014/ajot.2011.000760

Uomoto, J. M., & Williams, R. M. (2009). Post-acute polytrauma rehabilitation and integrated care of returning veterans: Toward a holistic approach. *Rehabilitation Psychology, 54*(3), 259. doi: 10.1037/a0016907

US Congress. (2004). *Individuals with disabilities education improvement act of 2004.* Paper presented at Washington, DC, US Congress.

US Department of Education. (2000). *To assure the free appropriate public education of all children with disabilities.* Paper presented at the Twenty-First Annual Report to Congress on the Implementation of the Individuals with Disabilities Education Act (IDEA). US Government Printing Office.

US Department of Education, Office of Special Education and Rehabilitative Services, Office of Special Education Programs. (2009) *2007 annual report to Congress on the Individuals with Disabilities Education Act, Part D.* Author.

Van Heest, K. N. L., Mogush, A. R., & Mathiowetz, V. G. (2017). Effects of a one-to-one fatigue management course for people with chronic conditions and fatigue. *The American Journal of Occupational Therapy, 71*(4), 7104100020p1–7104100020p9. https://10.5014/ajot.2017.023440

VanderKaay, S., Letts, L., Jung, B., & Moll, S. E. (2019). Online ethics education for occupational therapy clinician–educators: A single-group pre-/post-test study. *Disability and Rehabilitation, 41*(23), 2841–2853. doi: 10.1080/09638288.2018.1473510

Varni, J. W., & Limbers, C. A. (2009). The pediatric quality of life inventory: Measuring pediatric health-related quality of life from the perspective of children and their parents. *Pediatric Clinics of North America, 56*(4), 843–863. doi: 10.1016/j.pcl.2009.05.016

Venes, D. (2017). *Taber's cyclopedic medical dictionary.* FA Davis.

Vergason, G. A., & Anderegg, M. L. (1992). Preserving the least restrictive environment. In *Controversial issues confronting special education: Divergent perspectives* (pp. 45–54). Allyn & Bacon.

Virues-Ortega, J., Julio, F. M., & Pastor-Barriuso, R. (2013). The TEACCH program for children and adults with autism: A meta-analysis of intervention studies. *Clinical Psychology Review, 33*(8), 940–953. doi: 10.1016/j.cpr.2013.07.005

Vroman, K., & Stewart, L. (2013). *Occupational therapy evaluation for adults: A pocket guide.* Lippincott Williams & Wilkins.

Vygotsky, L. S. (1934). *Thought and language.* Wiley.

Waldman-Levi, A., Cope, A., & Olson, L. (2022). Understanding father-child joint play experience using a convergent mixed-methods design. *The American Journal of Occupational Therapy: Official Publication of the American Occupational Therapy Association, 76*(5), 7605205070. https://doi.org/10.5014/ajot.2022.046573

Wallis, W. A., Roberts, H. V., & Shultz, G. P. (2014). *The nature of statistics.* Dover Publications.

Warner, G., Baird, L. G., McCormack, B., Urquhart, R., Lawson, B., Tschupruk, C., Christian, E., Weeks, L., Kumanan, K., & Sampalli, T. (2021). Engaging family caregivers and health system partners in exploring how multi-level contexts in primary care practices affect case management functions and outcomes of patients and family caregivers at end of life: A realist synthesis. *BMC Palliative Care, 20*, 1–30. doi: 10.1186/s12904-021-00781-8

Watling, R. L., & Dietz, J. (2007). Immediate effect of Ayres's sensory integration-based occupational therapy intervention on children with autism spectrum disorders. *The American Journal of Occupational Therapy, 61*(5), 574–583. doi: 10.5014/ajot.61.5.574

Westby, M. D., & Backman, C. L. (2010). Patient and health professional views on rehabilitation practices and outcomes following total hip and knee arthroplasty for osteoarthritis: A focus group study. *BMC Health Services Research, 10*(1), 1–15. doi: 10.1186/1472-6963-10-119

Wiener, N. (1948). *Cybernetics or control and communication in the animal and the machine.* Wiley and Sons.

Wilcox, J., Peterson, K. S., Lewis, C. M., & Margetis, J. L. (2021). Occupational therapy during COVID-19-related critical illness: A case report. *The American Journal of Occupational Therapy, 75*(Supplement_1). doi: 10.5014/ajot.2021.049196

Will, M. C. (1986). Educating children with learning problems: A shared responsibility. *Exceptional Children, 52*(5), 411–415. doi: 10.1177/001440298605200502

Willard, H. S., & Spackman, C. S. (1971). *Occupational therapy* (4th ed.). J. B. Lippincott.

Winkler, A. C., & McCuen, J. R. (1979). *Writing the research paper: A handbook.* Harcourt.

Winkler, A. C., & McCuen, J. (1998). *From idea to essay: A rhetoric, reader, and handbook.* Allyn & Bacon.

Winnie, A. J. (1912). *History and handbook of day schools for the deaf and blind: A bulletin of information concerning the origin, maintenance, advantages and standing of the day schools for the deaf and blind in Wisconsin.* Democratic Printing, State Printer.

Wolfensberger, W. P., Nirje, B., Olshansky, S., Perske, R., & Roos, P. (1972). *The principle of normalization in human services.* National Institute on Mental Retardation.

Woods, K., Karrison, T., Koshy, M., Patel, A., Friedmann, P., & Cassel, C. (1997). Hospital utilization patterns and costs for adult sickle cell patients in Illinois. *Public Health Reports, 112*(1), 44.

Woodside, H. H. (1971). The development of occupational therapy 1910–1929. *The American Journal of Occupational Therapy: Official Publication of the American Occupational Therapy Association, 25*(5), 226–230.

World Health Organization (WHO). (1996). *WHOQOL-BREF: Introduction, administration, scoring and generic version of the assessment: Field trial version, December 1996.* WHO.

World Health Organization (WHO). (2021). *Key facts (World Health Organization).* www.who.int/news-room/fact-sheets/detail/rehabilitation,

World Health Organization (WHO). (2023). World Health Organization. www.who.int/

Xakellis Jr, G. C., Frantz, R. A., Lewis, A., & Harvey, P. (1998). Cost-effectiveness of an intensive pressure ulcer prevention protocol in long-term care. *Advances in Wound Care: The Journal for Prevention and Healing, 11*(1), 22–29.

Yanlin, C., Jianhua, G., Jiangwei, G., Fang, Y., Jianyun, L. I., Libing, Z., Junjie, Y., Zhipeng, X., & Dongmei, C. (2018). Comprehensive rehabilitation intervention with medical treatment and education among autism children aged 3–6 years old. *School of Health in China, 39*(3), 343–345, 349.

Yerxa, E. J., & Locker, S. B. (1990). Quality of time use by adults with spinal cord injuries. *The American Journal of Occupational Therapy, 44*(4), 318–326. doi: 10.5014/ajot.44.4.318

Yu, X., Wu, R., Ji, Y., & Feng, Z. (2023). Assisted living technology with artificial intelligence in occupational therapy. *Frontiers in Public Health.* www.frontiersin.org/research-topics/46422/assisted-living-technology-with-artificial-intelligence-in-occupational-therapy

Yuen, H. K. (2002). Impact of an altruistic activity on life satisfaction in institutionalized elders: A pilot study. *Physical & Occupational Therapy in Geriatrics, 20*(3–4), 125–135. doi.org/10.1080/J148v20n03_08

Zinsser, W. (1990). *On writing well: An informal guide to writing nonfiction* (4th ed.). Harper Collins.

INDEX

Note: **Bold** page numbers refer to tables and *italic* page numbers refer to figures.

Printed in the United States
by Baker & Taylor Publisher Services